AF869697

Children's Well-Being: Indicators and Research

Volume 26

Series Editor

Asher Ben-Arieh, Paul Baerwald School of Social Work & Social Welfare, The Hebrew University of Jerusalem, Jerusalem, Israel

Editorial Board Members

J. Lawrence Aber, New York University, New York, USA
Johnathan Bradshaw, University of York, York, UK
Ferran Casas, University of Girona, Girona, Spain
Ick-Joong Chung, Duksung Women's University, Seoul, Korea (Republic of)
Howard Dubowitz, University of Maryland, Baltimore, USA
Ivar Frønes, University of Oslo, Oslo, Norway
Frank Furstenberg, University of Pennsylvania, Philadelphia, USA
Robbie Gilligan, Trinity College Dublin, Dublin, Ireland
Robert M. George, University of Chicago, Chicago, USA
Ian Gough, University of Bath, Bath, UK
An-Magritt Jensen, Norwegian University of Science and Technology, Trondheim, Norway
Sheila B. Kamerman, Columbia University, New York, USA
Jill. E Korbin, Case Western Reserve University, Cleaveland, USA
Dagmar Kutsar, University of Tartu, Tartu, Estonia
Kenneth C. Land, Duke University, Durham, USA
Bong Joo Lee, Seoul National University, Seoul, Korea (Republic of)
Jan Mason, University of Western Sydney, Sydney, Australia
Kristin A. Moore, Child Trends, Maryland, USA
Bernhard Nauck, Chemnitz University of Technology, Chemnitz, Germany
Usha S. Nayar, Tata Institute of Social Sciences, Mumbai, India
Shelley Phipps, Dalhousie University, Halifax, NS, Canada
Jackie Sanders, Massey University, Palmerston North, New Zealand
Giovanni Sgritta, University of Rome, Rome, Italy
Thomas S. Weisner, University of California, Los Angeles, USA
Helmut Wintersberger, University of Vienna, Vienna, Austria

This series focuses on the subject of measurements and indicators of children's well being and their usage, within multiple domains and in diverse cultures. More specifically, the series seeks to present measures and data resources, analysis of data, exploration of theoretical issues, and information about the status of children, as well as the implementation of this information in policy and practice. By doing so it aims to explore how child indicators can be used to improve the development and the well being of children.

With an international perspective the series will provide a unique applied perspective, by bringing in a variety of analytical models, varied perspectives, and a variety of social policy regimes.

Children's Well-Being: Indicators and Research will be unique and exclusive in the field of measures and indicators of children's lives and will be a source of high quality, policy impact and rigorous scientific papers.

Naomi Anne Shmuel

Children's Wellbeing in Immigrant Families

Ethiopian Jews in Israel

Springer

Naomi Anne Shmuel
Hebrew University of Jerusalem
Jerusalem, Israel

ISSN 1879-5196 ISSN 1879-520X (electronic)
Children's Well-Being: Indicators and Research
ISBN 978-3-031-31916-7 ISBN 978-3-031-31917-4 (eBook)
https://doi.org/10.1007/978-3-031-31917-4

0th edition: © Author 2020

© The Editor(s) (if applicable) and The Author(s), under exclusive license to Springer Nature Switzerland AG 2023
This work is subject to copyright. All rights are solely and exclusively licensed by the Publisher, whether the whole or part of the material is concerned, specifically the rights of reprinting, reuse of illustrations, recitation, broadcasting, reproduction on microfilms or in any other physical way, and transmission or information storage and retrieval, electronic adaptation, computer software, or by similar or dissimilar methodology now known or hereafter developed.
The use of general descriptive names, registered names, trademarks, service marks, etc. in this publication does not imply, even in the absence of a specific statement, that such names are exempt from the relevant protective laws and regulations and therefore free for general use.
The publisher, the authors, and the editors are safe to assume that the advice and information in this book are believed to be true and accurate at the date of publication. Neither the publisher nor the authors or the editors give a warranty, expressed or implied, with respect to the material contained herein or for any errors or omissions that may have been made. The publisher remains neutral with regard to jurisdictional claims in published maps and institutional affiliations.

This Springer imprint is published by the registered company Springer Nature Switzerland AG
The registered company address is: Gewerbestrasse 11, 6330 Cham, Switzerland

To my sister Stella, because once we were immigrant children together

Preface

Childhood Between Cultures

As a child I always wanted a Star of David. It seems like an easy request to gratify, but in our home, it caused havoc: before I was born my parents agreed there would be no religious symbols and the children would not be labelled. My father was an atheist from a Christian family and my mother a Jew who had come to England as a 15-year-old child refugee fleeing Nazi Germany on the Kindertransport in 1938. About 10,000 children ranging in age from three to 17 entered England in this way before the Second World War broke out, they came from Austria, Germany, Czechoslovakia, and Poland. My mother never saw her parents again, they were killed in the Holocaust with many of her extended family. When my parents met, they were both adverse to categorizing people, they saw this as the source of all evil causing the utmost human suffering. But reality did not have mercy on them: society always likes to label people, to demand allegiance to a specific group. My mother (Gershon, 1990)[1] wrote:

When we went out of Germany
carrying six million lives
that was Jewish history
but each child was one refugee
we unlike the Egyptian slaves
were exiled individually
and each in desolation has
created his own wilderness.

She avoided talking about her past until I, her fourth child, was born. A year after my birth she made her first visit back to her hometown, Bielefeld, and began writing poems that have become the voice of her generation. On that journey familiar streets aroused childhood memories of her grandfather, Adolf Schönfeld, who was the head

[1] She was born Kaethe Loewenthal and wrote under the name Karen Gershon, which was her father's Jewish name.

of the Jewish community in Bielefeld and the first victim of the Nazis after they came to power in 1933. The emotions aroused by this visit in 1963 awoke her Jewish roots and produced a flood of poetry, some of which was published in several books (Gershon, 1966, 1972, 1975) and in Zionist magazines that reached the then president of Israel Zalman Shazar. He invited her to join a delegation of British authors for a visit to Israel in 1966. Overcome by the fulfilment of her childhood dream to reach the Promised Land, Gershon sent my father a letter to say she was not coming back. My father reminded her she had left four children in England, and two years later, in 1968, the family emigrated to Israel. I was six, my sister 13 and both my brothers over 18. It was a transition destined to fail, despite my mother's relentless efforts to settle us in our new country. As a pacifist with an aversion to religious ceremonies and rituals, my father found it almost impossible to reconcile himself to Israeli reality. My mother, who had already changed languages once, could not bring herself to write in Hebrew. Five years after we arrived, we went back to England. I was eleven and still did not have a Star of David.

Every child is born into a story which shapes who they will become and what they will do with their life. The home I grew up in was festival-free, I think my parent's will to celebrate had been eroded by tragic life experiences. And yet I remember a Christmas tree with the desired Star of David on top, well out of my reach. There were many political arguments at home, which usually reduced my mother to tears and ended in long heavy silences. As a child the unsurmountable barriers between my parents led me to speak of living in the sea so as not to have to choose between them. As a teenager making cultural adjustments for the second time, the question of my own identity was unresolved.

The country I had been born in and returned to did not receive me with open arms as I had felt Jerusalem did. My mother became morose and withdrawn. In Israel she had been full of vitality, singing aloud the Zionist songs she had learnt as a child in the Maccabi youth group, at ease with strangers, initiating conversations as if we were all one big family. Infected by her enthusiasm at being in Jerusalem I flourished, soon fluent in Hebrew and always surrounded by friends. I learnt how to swim at the YMCA,[2] to draw at the Israel Museum, to act at the Jerusalem Theatre, and I was an enthusiastic young Israeli scout. Coming back to England after the Yom Kippur war (1973) shattered my world. I could speak English, but could not read or write very well, so was placed in a group of low achievers. I had to wear a uniform for the first time, including a skirt and tie, and was expected to use the respectful *sir* and *miss* when addressing my teachers. To them I was a stranger, no one took an interest in the world I had come from. After I moved to high school in a London suburb, I was no longer the only stranger; amongst my peers were immigrants from Kenya, Ghana, Pakistan, and India. Naturally I found my place amongst them, we were *the others* together.

---

[2]The Jerusalem international YMCA is an educational, cultural, and sports center for all the residents of Jerusalem.

Under the grey skies of England I tried, like my mother years before, to connect to the universal human experience that did not require labels. I read anthropology books about people in different places in the world and was fascinated by the multitude of ways humanity chose to live. All the while a gaping void opened within me, the absence of connection to a viable identity of my own to give meaning to my life. I felt this emptiness as hopelessness. My parents attributed the change in me to my age, believing I had simply become a grumpy teenager.

Only after I completed a degree in anthropology at London University did I go back to Israel, ten years after I had left, and began to face the big questions of *who am I and where do I belong?* On my return I was overwhelmed by a sense of homecoming. Before long it became clear to me that I had a long way to go before I was entitled to feel at home: my childish Hebrew and Scandinavian looks made people answer me automatically in English and ask me bluntly if I was Jewish. Once again, I was *the other* in the eyes of my surroundings. And yet in a surreal, uncanny way Jerusalem never failed me—every street and flower, every breath-taking view and honey-coloured stone welcomed me back. The sound of Hebrew all around me was like music to my ears, every cell of my body told me: *this is where you belong.* It was a powerful feeling which sent me to meet my parents' friends, people who had been surrogate families to us as new immigrants, almost the grandparents I never had. They were all welcoming and encouraging, offering me hospitality and a haven, which I politely rejected, sensing that this journey I needed to take alone. They echoed this sense of homecoming to me but being *the other* had already been embedded into the fabric of who was, it was the only identity I had.

I never knew much about my father's childhood, except that his father grew up in an orphanage from which he escaped at the age of 16 to join the British army. My father was the middle one of three children, I don't think they had much of a family life. My mother's childhood stories were happier, three sisters raised by a successful architect, with family holidays on the coast of the Baltic Sea. Their lives were good until Hitler came to power when my mother was ten years old. I collected the rest of the story like pieces of a puzzle throughout my adult life, the whole picture was just too horrific to tell a child (documented in her books: Gershon, 1993, 2009).[3]

My mother used to read me bedtime stories till long after I could already read to myself. Often the protagonists were orphans struggling to survive without parents. I have little or no memory of the stories themselves, it is my mother's tears and trembling voice I remember. Being almost a lone survivor of her family was something she carried her whole life as a responsibility to justify her own existence. She expected us, her children, to do the same. I always felt her story was mine, that the grandparents I had not known expected me to be a continuation, it was through them that I belonged here, in Israel.

My meeting with the Ethiopian community in Israel was a turning point in my life: here were new immigrants who looked so different from their surroundings, yet had no doubt whatsoever about their identity or their right to belong here. They

[3] Forthcoming in her biography which I am currently writing.

became an inspiration to me. Many of them had walked for months across a formidable desert, crossing thc border between Ethiopia and Sudan to reach the Promised Land. Their stories fascinated me; their culture of open hospitality made me a frequent house guest. The rest is history: amongst them I found Emmanuel, who gave me the desired Star of David and four children (we were married for 35 years and to date have four grandchildren).

During our venture into joint parenthood, I began to understand that we had different expectations about family life and parenting based on different basic cultural concepts. Looking for the glue that binds families together and fills that inner void I had felt within me for years, I found the power of Jewish traditions, folklore, and cultural heritage. These are passed between the generations naturally, through everyday acts of living which bind parents and children, define identity and belonging to one's cultural, religious, social, or community group. And yet this transferal can be interrupted or blocked—customs and traditions disappear, languages are forgotten, relationships unravel, children grow up with an inner void. It was realizing this and witnessing the breakdown in communication and connection between the generations in the Ethiopian immigrant community that sent me to study this subject. As my children grew older, I began to wonder if they too sometimes felt alienated from their surroundings either through their own experiences as dark-skinned teenagers in Israeli society or as direct inter-generational transferal from us, their immigrant parents. Was the unsurmountable barrier based on identity and cultural background I had witnessed between my parents repeating itself through a mysterious inter-generational transferal threatening us too—as we struggled with different perspectives on reality, different attitudes towards parenting and education—were my own children also growing up on a painful cultural divide? These thoughts bothered me, but seeing some of the inter-generational clashes in our home mirrored in other immigrant families made me realize that these were the result of parenting in transition, of children growing up with immigrant parents. Every family develops in context, embedded in and influenced by history, the surrounding environment and culture. Transition rocks the boat—family members react to it differently, adjust at different paces, cling to the familiar regardless of its utility, or adjust to the local scene and change to varying degrees.

The two transitions I experienced as a child were formative experiences in my life, my own narrative about them has changed over the years. As is the case for many immigrant children, my parents were busy with their own struggles during these periods of time and were often unaware of the challenges faced by us children as new immigrants. Issues of wellbeing were never paramount considerations as my parents struggled to survive financially and socially, life inevitably always seemed to contain a certain element of suffering. Compared to what had happened to the previous generation this must have seemed trivial to them; it took many years for me to turn my attention to the issue of my own wellbeing as a legitimate concern.

Before my marriage to Emmanuel I travelled to Ethiopia on a daring and somewhat reckless journey to look for his family. Amongst the discoveries on this trip was the fact that Shy, a frequent visitor to our home who had been introduced to me by Emmanuel as his brother, was in fact a cousin. On my return I shared this revelation with Shy, who laughed at me saying, 'don't worry Naomi, all our childhood I thought we were brothers!' Shy and Emmanuel grew up in a small village in the province of Gondar. When Emmanuel was very young his father died, and the father's brother—Shy's father—took responsibility for him together with his own elder brothers. There is no contradiction here—the whole village raised the children together. In Western societies we tend to think of families as *nuclear* or *extended* as if it is just a matter of numbers. But in Ethiopia the concept of *beta-saab* refers to people who live under the same roof, which can also mean people who are not blood relations. The term *zamad* refers to relatives in a wider sense. What defines family is mutual responsibility and connection, therefore children who grew up together referred to each other as brothers. In Ethiopia social belonging and status are a derivative of genealogy, therefore the ability to name relatives seven or eight generations back was crucial.

In contrast, I grew up bereft of relatives, with only my parents as the pillars of my childhood. I learnt the meaning of community when my son Michael, then eight years old, went missing on one cold dark winter evening in Jerusalem. At some point the police officer accompanying me suggested taking me home to check phone messages (there were no mobile phones back then). As we neared the house, I was amazed to see about 15 Ethiopian neighbours sitting on the wall outside our building, waiting for me. Some of them I did not even know. Apparently, the rumour of the missing boy brought everybody out to look for him. Seeing them there was very moving to me, it made me feel that I was not alone in this world. The child was found safe and sound, the details are irrelevant, the point is that I learnt what it means to be part of a community.

My family of origin was not close, based on Western values of self-expression and self-fulfilment, in which privacy was more important that connection. I was fascinated and impressed by the cohesiveness and mutual responsibility I saw in Emmanuel's extended family, his stories from the village where children looked after each other and shared food from the same plate, where siblings and cousins cared for one another. I made a conscious decision that these were values I wanted to instil in my children, and so it was: they received snacks in one dish to teach them to share, all toys and games in the house belonged to everyone, when we moved into a bigger apartment, they all shared a bedroom, and the spare room became their playroom. As they grew older, in their teenage years when they wore the same size clothes, these also became common property, even if they bought them themselves. When my eldest son left home, he said to me: 'Mum, I don't know what clothes to take, everybody wears them!' Until today they keep close connection and share whatever they have.

Parental expectations of children are dependent on their world view, therefore the clash between Emmanuel and me on educational issues was inevitable. Emmanuel grew up in a hierarchical society where age and gender determined everything. As a father, he expected his children to be obedient and respectful to their elders, while I expected *mutual* respect and attentiveness. He expected modesty, humility, and emotional restraint, while I expected them to verbalize their emotions, to practice open discussion which reflected their feelings and thoughts. He expected me to back him up as a father, to help him preserve the respectful distance customary between adults and children in Ethiopia. But I did not grow up with a *respectful distance* and wanted my children to be able to speak freely, listen honestly, and share their feelings and experiences without reservations. I did not believe in punishing children; in my parent's home, no child was ever hit.

During his most rebellious teenage years, when he was sixteen, our son Michael took upon himself the task of writing the first children's book in Hebrew on the journey from Ethiopia to Sudan on foot, through the eyes of a child (Shmuel, 2006). He set out with a recording device to interview immigrants who had made this journey as children. This was a time when the communication between Michael and us, his parents, was difficult and challenging. Emmanuel was absent from the long list of people interviewed for his book, as he was from the event marking its publication at the Hebrew University. When Michael stood at the podium to address the crowd, he called the journey *our journey*. Later I asked him why, his answer was, *I feel this is my story too*.

Writing the story and identifying with the journey which he never heard about from his own father was a turning point in Michael's turbulent life, but it took a while to mend the rift and improve communication with us, his parents. This illustrates how hard it is for immigrant parents to provide a stable protective base for the next generation, to offer them an anchor as they grow, based on connection, a meaningful supportive relationship, roots, and a strong cultural identity. The research on which this book is based deals precisely with this issue, and the tensions created between the generations in immigrant families. Inevitably such families contain opposing processes of change and continuance—how do these affect family life and personal development? How do the second generation, growing up on the cultural divide, experience the different cultures? Sometimes the connection between family members may become frayed or fragile, or in the parent's effort to hold on, unyielding and restrictive. How can parents find the right balance between holding on too tightly or letting go completely, as the next generation seem to be slipping further and further away from them? It takes wisdom and determination to keep reconnecting despite all the hardships, and yet there are families who manage to do so. These issues are relevant to all immigrant families, my hope is that the insights in this book will help in understanding the world of immigrants and the second generation.

For many years I could see only difficulties in my hybrid identity and believed that my life would have been easier if I had grown up in one place and not been forced to choose my own identity, language, and country. My university studies and my research have helped me see the advantages of growing up on the cultural divide and having a complex identity. Seeing the world as complicated and people as impossible to divide according to set categories, a clearer vision of reality becomes apparent, enabling empathy and understanding for all humanity. It took me a long time to come to terms with all the elements of my identity, perhaps this only really happened when I found a place to belong and watched my own children growing up rooted in country and community. I believe that accepting ourselves is the first step to accepting others, and realizing that in different contexts, we are all *others* of sorts.

Jerusalem, Israel
June 2022

Naomi Anne Shmuel

References

Gershon, K. (1966). *Selected poems*. Gollancz.
Gershon, K. (1972). *Legacies and encounters*. Gollancz.
Gershon, K. (1975). *My daughters, my sisters*. Gollancz.
Gershon, K. (1990). The children's exodus. In K. Gershon. *Collected poems* (p. 22). Papermac, Macmillan. (Originally published by Gollancz 1966).
Gershon, K. (1993). *A lesser child*. Peter Owen.
Gershon, K. (2009). *A tempered wind*. Northwestern University Press.
Shmuel, M. (2006). *Coming out of Ethiopia*. Hippy Program (Etgar), The Institute for Advancement of Education, Hebrew University Jerusalem.

Acknowledgements

Firstly, I wish to thank each one of the people from the Ethiopian Jewish community in Israel who agreed to be interviewed, thus enabling the research on which this book is based. With appreciation and gratitude for their friendly hospitality and the open conversations which provided insights into their experiences and perceptions of cultural transition.

A deep thank you to my friend Bossana who translated the interviews in Amharic and added important interpretations and perceptions of her own which form a vital contribution to the research.

I thank my university supervisor Professor Hagar Salamon of the Department of Folklore at the Hebrew University in Jerusalem for her guidance during my research, her constant availability, patience, and valuable instruction in the art of conducting interviews and analysing them.

I am grateful also to Dr. Rita Sever and Dr. Gadi-Ben Ezer for their participation in the accompanying committee for my doctoral research and to Dr. Rafi Youngman and Professor Steve Kaplan for their amicable judging of my PhD dissertation.

The research was supported by several grants and academic prizes, which I am very grateful for:

- A grant from the Israeli Organization for Women Academics
- The Folklore Department at the Hebrew University of Jerusalem for two prizes: the Tamar and Dov Noy prize for a research proposal, and the Raphael Patai award of excellence for PhD dissertation
- The Memorial Foundation for Jewish Culture doctoral scholarship

My appreciation also to Professor Dorit Roer-Strier, Professor Yochai Nadan, and the NEVET team—an international and multidisciplinary research and training venue at the Hebrew University's School of Social Work that serves as a greenhouse for capacity building of young scholars and practitioners.

A special thank you to Professor Jill Korbin for connecting me to Springer and to Professor Asher Ben-Arieh for endorsing my manuscript, both enabling the publication of this book.

Lastly, but of course most importantly, with deep appreciation and gratitude to my family, especially my former husband Emmanuel Shmuel, who taught me more than anyone else about Ethiopian culture and traditions.

Contents

About the Author

Dr. Naomi Anne Shmuel is a British Israeli author, illustrator, anthropologist, and parent group counsellor. She did her research via the Folklore Department at the Hebrew University in Jerusalem, concentrating on the process of continuance and change across the generations amongst Ethiopian immigrant families in Israel. Her connection to this community is both professional and personal; her husband for 35 years, Emmanuel, made the long and difficult journey on foot from Ethiopia to Sudan to reach Israel, they have four sons and four grandchildren. Naomi began writing books for her children following their encounter with prejudice, these were the first children's books in Hebrew to include brown-skinned characters. In all she has published eight books for children, four for youth and three books for adults. These have won her many prizes, including the prestigious Prime Minister's Prize for literature, and are used by educators to foster inter-cultural understanding and appreciation for diversity in Israeli schools and pre-schools. Naomi teaches at various academic institutions in Israel and runs workshops training professionals for working in culturally diverse environments. She is an active member of NEVET, an international, multidisciplinary research and training venue at the Hebrew University's School of Social Work, which produces context-informed practice and policy research for professionals working with families and children in multicultural contexts.

To contact the author: www.naomis-books.com; naomi.shmuel@mail.huji.ac.il

Abbreviations

G1	The *first generation* refers to people who emigrated as adults over the age of 21.
G1.5	The *one and a half generation* are people who emigrated between the ages of eight and 20 and were thus educated both in Ethiopia and in Israel.
G2	The *second generation* refers to participants who were either born in Israel or Sudan (emigrating as babies) or emigrated up until the age of seven.

Chapter 1
Introduction

1.1 Voices from Two Studies

Up three flights of stairs in what looked like a nice neighbourhood I knocked on the door and was invited in to see a surprising number of people waiting for me. I had been apprehensive on the long journey to get there, now a tingling excitement ran through my body in anticipation: they had all gathered for my sake! Aside from two lovely students I had interviewed, I did not seem to be getting very far with my grand idea of three generation interviews. Most people I asked said they would check with their families and then either never got back to me or said that some family members did not want to be interviewed. I had shared my frustration with Genet, a social worker I met in connection with her work, and she had invited me to her mother's home for what turned out to be my first successful day of multiple interviews. I had instantly been impressed by Genet when I met her, she was self-assured, eloquent, and cheerful, and turned out to be an asset to my research and later also a good friend. You will hear a lot more about Genet and her family in this book, but on this initial meeting I wondered what motivated her so much to help me, a relative stranger. The answer was twofold; on the one hand, her familiarity with my books, which she regularly read to her children. On the other hand, it was the reason she gave to her grandfather to convince him to talk to me: "the next generation will ask us who we are, we need to be able to give them answers".

In the following chapters, you will hear the voices of participants in two qualitative studies conducted in Israel amongst the Ethiopian Amhara Jewish immigrant community:[1] the first between 2008–2010 included seven parents (two fathers and five mothers) with the aim of understanding parenting methods and educational traditions in Ethiopia and how these are changing with the transition to Israel

[1] Mostly from Gondar region, one interviewee from Addis Ababa and one from the Tigray region.

© The Author(s), under exclusive license to Springer Nature Switzerland AG 2023

N. A. Shmuel, *Children's Wellbeing in Immigrant Families*, Children's Well-Being: Indicators and Research 26,
https://doi.org/10.1007/978-3-031-31917-4_1

(Shmuel, 2010). The second between 2014–2017 included fifty participants (31 women and 19 men), thirty-four who emigrated to Israel from Ethiopia (28 via the perilous journey on foot to Sudan) and sixteen who were born in Israel or arrived as infants (Shmuel, 2018). Participants in this second study ranged in age between 13 and 90, with varied educational backgrounds, from no schooling at all (14) to academic degrees (11 with undergraduate degrees, 3 with master's degrees, all first-generation academics to their families). In each family I interviewed anybody who was willing to talk to me, thus in some families three generations, in others a mix of siblings, cousins, aunts, and uncles. I wanted to hear about their experiences, both within the family and in Israeli society, in their own words. Their narratives form the basis of this book, which connects folklore studies and the study of families in transition. The aim is to enhance an understanding of the processes and challenges faced by parents and children in their endeavour to belong, the place of cultural heritage in inter-generational relations, and what are the factors fostering or hindering resilience and adaptation. And to hear answers to the question posed by Genet—what should we tell the next generation?

1.2 Ethiopian Jews in Israel

Today there are 155,300 members of the Ethiopian Jewish community in Israel, of these 67,800 were born in Israel (CBS[2]). The community is diverse, coming from different parts of Ethiopia (Tigray, Gondar, and Simien Mountains), speak various languages (Amharic, Tigrinya), emigrated at different times (via Sudan or Addis Ababa) and from different family, educational, economic, and other backgrounds (Trevisan Semi & Weil, 2011). Most of the immigrants came from rural areas, the transition involved many sudden changes in their way of life, these will be discussed in more detail in the following chapters.

The first Ethiopian Jews to arrive in Israel were a group of youngsters brought to the Kfar Batya children's village in 1955, after completing their schooling they were sent back to Ethiopia as educators and community leaders.

The majority of the Jews from Ethiopia came to Israel in three distinct waves of immigration, the first of which began at the end of the 1970s and culminated in Operation Moses (1984–1985). At this time the young adults of the community (including many teenagers) were the first to make the perilous journey on foot from Ethiopia to Sudan, where they stayed in refugee camps under difficult conditions, experiencing trauma, separation from and loss of family members. 8000 Jews arrived in this immigration wave, an additional 4000 lost their lives on the journey. The second wave, known as Operation Solomon, which took place in 1991, 14,000 people were covertly airlifted from temporary transition camps near the Israeli Embassy in Addis Ababa within 34 h. The third wave has continued since then until

[2] The Central Bureau of Statistics in Israel November 11, 2020 report.

today, bringing 22,000 members of the Falashmura community to Israel. The Falashmura are Jews who converted to Christianity because of proselytization during the nineteenth and twentieth centuries.

Before discussing the consequences of immigration to Israel, it is important to recognize the historical perspective on the connection between *Beta Yisrael* [Ethiopian jews] and world Jewry. From Mediaeval times, the Jews of Ethiopia had many things in common with their Christian neighbours: their clothing, traditional meals, and family structure. They were distinguished primarily through craftsmanship: the Jews of Ethiopia were the potters, weavers, and metalworkers. Both communities prayed in Geez and were led by spiritual leaders who called their flock the 'children of Israel' (Kaplan & Rosen, 1998).

The first non-Ethiopian Jew to visit the Jewish villages in Ethiopia was Yosef Halevi in 1867 (Kaplan, 2007). He described many thousand members of the community living in small autonomous independent villages, each led by a *Kes* (Rabbi and spiritual leader). It was not until the middle of the nineteenth century that a persistent connection was formed with the Beta Yisrael, beginning with the visit of Faitlovich, an orientalist researcher, in 1904. The following century led to serious transformation for the Beta Yisrael community, as local hierarchy and religious traditions were matched to the acceptable format of world Jewry.

There were also many historical events which influenced the Beta Yisrael community: the meeting with Protestant missionaries in 1860, revolutions and new governments in 1974 and 1987, the war with Somalia from 1977 to 1978, and with Eritrea from 1961 to 1991. All these events are reflected in the interviews with the participants of my study: those conscripted (Mahari), those taken to the town to study in mission schools (Shy), those who participated in national projects to improve education and literacy in peripheral areas (Yafit).

Ethiopia is a multi-ethnic society, where over eighty languages are spoken (Nigusie, 2018).

It is important to recognize that the changes undergone by the *Beta Yisrael* community began long before they came to Israel. Perhaps it is in Israel that the final transformation to becoming *Ethiopian Jewry* occurred, but the changes began in the nineteenth century and continue until today. This is not necessarily the tragic loss of traditions, but more akin to an inevitable historical process following transition and new inter-cultural relations (Kaplan & Rosen, 1998; Rosen, 1985; Freedman & Freedman, 1987).

1.3 Culture and Context

Culture is a socially interactive process occurring within and between generations creating shared activity and shared meaning (Greenfield et al., 2003). Societies tend to lean towards one of two specific pathways to human development and knowledge acquisition, that stressing independence (predominant in individualistic societies) or that stressing interdependence (predominant in collectivistic societies). Parental ethnotheories of child development and concepts of the *ideal child* guiding parental priorities and methods of childcare are derived out of these paradigms (Greenfield et al.).

Folklore, culture, and traditions are interwoven into people's lives in such a way that they are not obviously recognizable. Daily activities create and unravel cultural constructs, bind or divide connections, form the basis for joint family strategies for coping with change or sew familial or personal disruption and instability. Coping mechanisms and an on-going family dialogue with cultural change and adjustment after transition are influenced by many factors: family processes and functioning before emigration, the experiences of the journey, arrival and initial absorption, the availability of family support networks, who arrived when, separations and losses, communication patterns, quality of family relationships, economic status as well as personal and cultural flexibility. Immigrant families from collectivistic societies entering individualistic societies are also influenced by the tensions and confusion caused by clashing conceptual paradigms guiding towards opposing cultural pathways—interdependence or dependence (Greenfield et al., 2003). Children of the second generation are born into this often fragile and unstable reality while the family is still in various stages of adjustment and change. Often their first experiences involve repeated moves until the family finds a permanent or semi-permanent home. This is frequently a time when the adults around them are busy settling in, overcoming their own emotions about the transition, perhaps also coping with painful loss and separation, while struggling to support their families financially. All these factors often lead to situations where the younger generation's needs, problems, and challenges are not perceived or deemed significant as the adults are preoccupied with other more pressing issues of survival and adjustment.

The conceptual framework for organizing ideas on culture, traditions, and knowledge influences our approach to research and interpretation of results. In the context of understanding family life in transition and the resultant balance between often conflicting cultures after immigration, it is useful to use the paradigm proposed by Swidler (1986) which defines culture as a toolkit of symbols, stories, rituals, and worldview enabling people to navigate their lives. The specifics of the toolkit are formed, recreated, and renewed constantly in time and place, and include diverse and inconsistent elements belonging to the same culture—this is part of the complexity of human culture which makes it both fascinating and difficult to study. The distinction which Swidler makes between settled and unsettled lives, the latter referring to people in transition, such as migrants and refugees, forms a clarifying basis from which to start. People in settled lives experience culture as a natural continuity between the generations, providing an often invisible or unperceived organizing conceptual framework comprised of values and patterns of action. These are not static, but change is integrated into the flow of life, in the sense that culture and circumstances reinforce each other. While people in transition, in the flux of social transformation, are experiencing their home culture in contrast to other cultures, where its role is emphasized to sustain previous life strategies or aid in constructing new ones. In this case, principles, symbols, and rituals are harnessed to shape action while learning and adjusting to new, often challenging, surroundings. The distinction between settled and unsettled lives is not a dichotomy, people may be more or less settled, cultural transmission between the generations more or less harmonious, life strategies more or less enduring. But specifically, transition heightens awareness of previously taken-for-granted assumptions about life, coupled with the fact that in face of uncertainty people tend to cling to the familiar for a sense of security (Janoff-Bulman, 2010).

I come from a very interdisciplinary professional and academic background combining perspectives from anthropology, folklore, education and social work. I find that approaching the complexity of the human experience from the combined theoretical basis of various academic disciplines is profoundly enlightening, enabling an all-encompassing holistic perspective. Often when asked to give lectures explaining complex ideas in a short period of time, to professional audiences who are eager to hear the bottom line for practical everyday practice, I am concerned by *limitational distortion*. Meaning that the necessity of limitation can lead to oversimplistic binary descriptions distorting the intricacies of human experience. In fact, it is precisely this reductionist tendency which leads to misunderstandings and stereotypical thinking, enhancing hierarchical perspectives which denote preference for one way of doing or being over another. Especially when discussing the multifaceted reality of inter-cultural relations, a much more edifying approach is provided by Boer's (2006) focus on the grey area between all categories—defining boundaries as a *space-between* rather than a divisive definitive line. For it is precisely the categorization of people according to spatial, ethnic, religious, and gender boxes that creates the proverbial other, thereby obscuring from view diversity within cultures, what people in different groups have in common, and the ambiguous blurry edges of all pre-defined groups. This is of utmost significance when discussing the experiences of immigrants after transition for the following reasons. Firstly, immigrants are in effect living in the grey area, the children in immigrant families are growing up on that fine illusive divide between cultures. Therefore, our interpretation of that divide—as a boundary or as a space for negotiation—influences the way we interpret their experiences. In the former case—the divide as a definitive boundary—this opens the way for the justification of exclusion (both within the family and outside it, as shall be illustrated). While the latter—the divide as a space for negotiation—opens countless opportunities for constructive dialogue between cultures and the potential for healthy hybridity. Secondly, the common tendency of attributing this divide to an inherent difference of cultures blurs or negates entirely the social structures that have created such a boundary. These social structures include historical, geopolitical factors that define the legitimacy of crossing boundaries, meaning both the official acceptance as immigrants and the social conceptual acceptance as fellow citizens. These social structures also carry the very concepts giving meaning to crossing boundaries, including inherent assumptions on the hierarchy of cultures and appropriate or inappropriate ways of living. The common rhetoric in Israel on the *gaps* immigrants must overcome, is often a reflection of such binary views (Shmuel, 2015). The concept of gaps between cultures leads to perceptions of cultural deficit that must be corrected by educating the immigrants in local ways, rather than basing their integration on immigrants' strength, resilience, and inherent human adaptability. Thirdly, considering the cultural divide as a space in which change and conservation are negotiated, both individually and within families, reflects its potential potency as an area of growth, not empty and meaningless but essential and significant in the process of transition. It is this understanding of the *necessity of process* which is crucial as a basis for understanding and helping immigrant families.

Assumptions and concepts about children and childhood are social constructs which shape parental and social expectations of children (James & Prout, 1997). This includes the premise that children are significant as future adults or the perception of childhood as a period of life worthy of consideration, not just in view of its later consequences. This last perspective has encouraged attention to the wellbeing of children as entitlement, focusing on children as active agents in the creation of their own realities (McAuley & Rose, 2010). Children grow up in diverse contexts which influence their lives in many ways, determine life circumstances and opportunities, and are subject to change (Roer-Strier & Nadan, 2020). Transition, especially to new geographical and cultural settings, as is resultant from emigration, has both immediate and long-term far-reaching consequences for both children and their families. As reflected in the content of this book, understanding the significance of context in people's lives, especially the changing effects of using the cultural toolkit in different contexts, is of paramount significance in understanding families in transition.

1.4 Three Generations of Immigrants

While conducting the interviews it became apparent that the age of emigration is crucial and seemed to influence both the level of people's cultural competency in each culture as well as perspectives about identity and belonging. Thus, the participants have been categorized as belonging to one of three groups: the *first generation* (G1) refers to people who emigrated as adults over the age of 21. The *second generation* (G2) refers to participants who were either born in Israel or Sudan (emigrating as babies) or emigrated up until the age of seven. This group was educated primarily in Israel, and thus is different from the other two groups, and would be expected to be more *Israeli*.

Fitting to the previous discussion on the nature of boundaries, there are various definitions in the academic literature for the intermediate, one and a half generation (G1.5). For example, Amit (2018) defines them as having arrived in the destination country under the age of 12, while Remennick and Prashizky (2019) define them as having arrived between the ages of nine and 18, Sharaby (2021) also defines them as having arrived over the age of eight. In my study G1.5 are people who emigrated between the ages of eight and 20 and were thus educated both in Ethiopia and in Israel. They emigrated at various stages of puberty; their experiences with cultural transition are more complex. I chose these cut-off ages following what seemed appropriate for the people I interviewed, the exact numerical definitions seem less critical than the overall concept that arriving in a new country at different stages of maturity influences people's subjective experience of the transition and capacity to cope with the period of ambiguity which follows, which may last a lifetime. This is precisely the significance of transcending boundaries and living unsettled lives, henceforth negotiated both within the family and as individuals. While certain patterns of behaviour are evident in same-generation participants, this is not unequivocal, for example Naama and Habtam belong to the second generation (G2), but in many ways their behaviour fits the pattern of the intermediate generation (G1.5), especially regarding the responsibility they take for their younger siblings. Similarly, there are big differences between members of the G1 group, for example Shy, Dany, Abigail, Yafit, and Abraham are all more or less fluent in Hebrew, they work and are involved in Israeli society, in contrast to the rest of this group who mostly do not speak or read Hebrew and live relatively isolated from Israeli society in what might be considered ethnic enclaves.[3]

The participants of the studies were located through *snowballing*, some of them were familiar to me from family or work encounters, others I was referred to by these. Most participants chose to remain anonymous and appear in this book under pseudonyms, which adhere to the language of the name (those who introduced themselves with their Amharic names have an Amharic pseudonym).[4]

The interviews were semi-structured, initially I asked people to describe their parents or children and their daily routines. I had a list of topics I was interested in, such as what language was spoken at home or who they sought out for advice in times of need, but the interview was primarily an open conversation in which I listened to their narratives and occasionally prompted them with relevant questions. There were participants whose narrative was detailed and uninterrupted, and others who required more prompting.

Narrative ethnographic studies are possibly the only way of understanding the full complexity of family transition in context (Tardiff-Williams & Fisher, 2009). Narrative studies are especially useful for understanding the complexities involved in the lives of second-generation immigrants, as Portes et al. (2005) have pointed out, quantitative data alone cannot do this.

An in-depth analysis of people's own words provides unique insights into their perspectives and has been found most beneficial by other researchers on families (such as Lam, 2005; Uttal & Han, 2011). Ungar (2003) also found qualitative methods invaluable in contributing to the understanding of resilience by revealing detailed descriptions of specific contexts, eliciting minority voices accounting for local outcomes, promoting attentive tolerance for these localized constructions, and encouraging researchers to face their own bias.

[3] A full list of participants according to generations appears in the appendix.

[4] To make the reading easier for English readers some of the pseudonyms were changed for this publication.

The narratives of the participants in my study open a window onto their experiences, feelings, and perspectives. This view may be momentary and limited, but at the same time contains an element of both personal and collective experiences. Listening to different members of the same family provides an array of viewpoints on what is happening in the family, comparing different families reveals patterns that repeat themselves and can be recognized as phenomena connected to the process of transition itself. All of these reflect both challenges and coping mechanisms. Thus, the fragile intertwining of cultures can almost be observed, and the breaking points mapped on the inter-generational interface where efforts to change or conserve cultural practices become palpable and often conflictual. As cultures merge, old assumptions become questioned, cultural symbols and traditions gain new meanings in different contexts or become redundant. All this complicates relationships, fosters misunderstandings, arouses in some family members a sense of progress and in others a sense of loss. One can only understand this complexity within families by listening to people, hearing them talk about relationships and their daily dilemmas and concerns.

For most people daily family life involves automatic responses and habits which do not easily translate into a verbal narrative about values, beliefs, and world views. Parental ethnotheories are assumed as common knowledge, often acted upon without explicit awareness. Yet at the meeting point between cultures these may surface as beliefs which clash with the new culture (Harkness & Super, 2006). At the same time, declared changes in perceptions do not necessarily involve a change in behaviour, for example someone might declare an attitude of gender equality and yet their parental behaviour does not support this in practice. Most people's parenting is instinctive, actions precede ideas, routines formulate perspectives. Parental expectations of children are based on perceptions of *normal* and *appropriate* behaviour (Rubin & Chung, 2006). It is easier to ask people *what* they do than *why* they do it, listening to their instinctive descriptions of their daily experiences and interactions with family members can be the best way of learning about their lives and perceptions (Goodnow, 2006).

Culture is not a static phenomenon that can be observed or examined, but an intricate combination of events and experiences that are constantly evolving and changing (Schmidt-Lauber, 2012). Accordingly, the research material was collected and analysed in an on-going process throughout the study. The topics which arose and were noted while transcribing and listening to the interviews became the central themes of the study, comparable in intensity and expression between the different families. This process involved careful attention to the narratives of the participants, including their pauses and contradictions, intonation, and expressions, revealing hidden meanings which become apparent only after repeated listening. The words of participants who spoke in Amharic were simultaneously translated by relatives present during the interview, often this involved additional conversations between them. These interviews were further translated and analysed together with my very patient and extremely helpful Ethiopian Israeli friend Bossana, who was also interviewed in the first study. Bossana contributed valuable insights as she translated recordings, noted as distinct from the translation itself. These on-going conversations between us during the analysis proved to be very useful for understanding the complexity reflected by the dialogue of the interviews. Certain themes repeated themselves in different families, especially when discussing relationships between the generations, changing communication patterns, and the challenges faced by parents raising children in Israel. Because of the complexity of the issues involved and the importance of deriving meaning from the interviews, the analysis was based on a combination of repetitive listening to recorded interviews and rereading transcribed narratives, often together with Bossana. I did not use any software to analyse the interviews.

Narrative analysis is based on the premise that knowledge and understanding is grounded in field work, in an interactive on-going process throughout the study between researcher and participants (Backman & Kyngäs, 1999; Heath & Cowley, 2004). The aim in such a study is to reflect simultaneously both particular and shared phenomenon, forming a holistic view of reality in its full complexity, from which one might be able to reach relevant conclusions. Grounded theory embedded in field work rests on identifying recurrent themes in the interviews, that can be subcategorized and compared between the narratives collected. The initial themes in the current study were language, communication, gender, cultural authority, identity, and representation. As the interviews were collected sub-categories arose, for example within communication: listening, consulting, conflicts, support, description, etc. The categories themselves are an abstraction since they represent all the data and not a specific case. Sometimes categories overlap, for example in the intersection between communication and gender, reflecting the inter-relatedness of phenomenon that form the complexity of reality. The theory is grounded since it is created as a hypothesis inspired by field work, then to be examined in further interviews and becomes theory during the process of data analysis (Glasner & Strauss, 1967).

In linguist terminology, ethnographic research searches for the *emic* description—explaining culture through the eyes of the interviewed narrator rather than the *etic* description, through the eyes of the researcher (Lieblich et al., 1998). Inevitably, as is demonstrated by this study, this leads to multiple perceptions of reality, ultimately combined with the perceptions and analysis of the researcher.

1.5 Challenges and Limitations of the Interviews

I began with the intention of interviewing three generations in each family, but this proved impossible in some families since not everybody was willing to participate. Therefore, I decided to interview anybody who was willing in each family, and in this way came to have a different combination of relatives interviewed each time. In some families I managed to conduct each interview separately, in others they insisted on all sitting together in the living room, which probably influenced the content of the interviews. I have detailed below in the description of the families how and where the interviews took place.

I admit that I was unable to document sufficiently facial expressions and body language during the interviews, since sensitivity and respect for the participants required my undivided attention to listen to them while they were talking. There was one instance when Bossana, translating an interview in Amharic, stopped to say,

> I need to read his face, there could be many intentions, I cannot understand just from the words, I need to see his face to know what he meant, if he was smiling or cross, I cannot tell just from the words.

Parents often describe their children in relation to a cultural ideal of the child (Harkness and Super, 2006, p. 63) but they may also be in denial or defensive or trying to impress. When adults talk about their own childhood their memory is selective, tending to conform to a positive or negative attitude they have developed about it over the years, and therefore is not necessarily accurate. Immigrant parents tend to be nostalgic about their childhood in Ethiopia, to see the past through the prism of present struggles in the new society. Doleve-Gandelman (1990) called this 'a lost imaginary cultural space'.

While open questions which require a detailed response are better than questions which can be answered by a yes or no answer (Schmidt-Lauber, 2012), the depth and detail gained in the interview is comprised of a delicate balance between the ability of the researcher to wait in silence for more explanations and the willingness of the interviewee to divulge information. Prior knowledge of culture and customs can have a great impact on this, for example I discovered that older people were much harder to interview, since they tended to adhere to a narrative unconnected to my questions, generally about their lives in Ethiopia or about the journey to Israel. I came to realize that asking them initially to describe their children could even be considered rude, that it was more respectful to first show an interest in them as people irrespective of their role as parents or grandparents.

Even if I did not know the interviewees in advance, most of them knew who I was as an author who published the first children's books in Hebrew to include dark-skinned characters and as the wife (at this time) of an Ethiopian man. I feel that this contributed to people's openness and willingness to talk to me, but it also made me feel obligated to abide by the customary codes of respect and politeness, which sometimes made it hard to ask difficult questions or pursue sensitive topics in the interview. It is also possible that some people wishing to impress me may have filtered their narrative or omitted discussing personal family difficulties. It is important to recognize the context in which the interviews took place as *social fields*, Bourdieu's (1988) terminology, indicating that interviews are never detached from reality but form a process of creating meaning through interaction (Briggs, 2007). As such the narratives are time and place specific; another time or place may have produced different answers and therefore different conclusions.

Perhaps it is pertinent to note that as a parent counsellor who has run numerous parenting workshops within the Ethiopian community, the voices of other parent were present in my mind while conducting my research, although none of the interviewees were from any of my parent groups.

A difference of cultures between interviewer and interviewee can have a significant influence on the outcome of the interview (Sands et al., 2007). If language is considered shared codes for effective communication (Dittmann, 1962), then the inter-cultural interview contains many potential challenges which may interfere with full mutual understanding: interpretation of words or phrases, a sense of obligation, power relations, trust issues, differing cultural assumptions, interpretations of body language and facial expressions. While this may be openly discussed, nevertheless in some cases assumed understanding may miss the point entirely. Therefore, double checking meanings using someone from the interviewees culture and language was a suitable precaution, as suggested by Kopperberg (2010), although without any guarantee of accuracy. An active awareness of my own cultural assumptions and interpretations was also important, I considered empathy and responsiveness as more appropriate than objectivity, as discussed in Duranti (1997). In some instances, the interview was followed by a request for parent counselling, such private conversations were not recorded or included in the study.

The voices in this book are not representative of the Ethiopian Israeli Jewish community in Israel, they are a random sample from a particular section of a diverse community who happened to be interviewed by me. As such further studies on families from other segments of this community, by other researchers in a different time and place, could well serve to illuminate further the issues addressed here.

1.6 Introducing the Immigrant Families[5]

The Demse Family

I met Dana as a student in her final year of undergraduate study in a course I taught, she volunteered to be interviewed and later introduced me to her mother Yael and uncle Dany. All the interviews took place after the end of the course. Dana's parents live in a poor area of a big city, the uncle in a nearby city, her younger brother was in the army at this time. The other three brothers are resident in psychiatric hospitals. This last fact I only realized towards the end of the interview with Dana, who described them as 'unsuccessful', before the interview I had no idea that her family situation was so difficult. The interviews with Dana's mother and uncle took place rather awkwardly in the living room of her parent's home, although we had scheduled this in advance when I arrived it did not seem like a suitable time. The very distressful situation of this family as a result of the mental illness of three members, was a central theme to the interviews. The family arrived in Israel on the difficult journey on foot via Sudan with three healthy little boys (aged one, three, and five). Dana and her younger brother were born in Israel. The way Dana and her mother talked about the situation reflected their obvious distress about it, their personal explanations and fears, as well as sense of guilt and shared responsibility. When Yael spoke about the journey to Israel she said, 'maybe their illness started there',

[5] All information relates to the time of the interview.

to which Dana interrupted her and stated emphatically 'it's not because of Sudan'. There was a lot of tension between mother and daughter, especially on this issue. Yael was much more reserved about it, but her obvious distress was heart breaking.

The Abebe Family

Ester, a student, was introduced to me by a mutual acquaintance. After I interviewed her, she invited me to the family home in another city, where her mother Modesh and sister Leah agreed to be interviewed. The father and two brothers did not.

Ester described her parents as not having integrated into Israeli society 'perhaps because we live in a place where there are only Ethiopians, maybe if we had lived somewhere else it would have been different'. She said that her father 'mixes more' because of his work, her mother is a housewife. Leah described their neighbourhood as 'not very good'. Despite living in what can only be described as a slum, the apartment itself was renovated and beautifully decorated with traditional Ethiopian art, pictures, ornaments, and colourful woven baskets. The parents left Ethiopia on foot to Sudan as a young couple with two small children aged three and four, both of whom died on the journey. 'When they stopped on the way, their children died', said Ester sadly. The bereaved young couple arrived in Israel to begin a new life, where four more children were born. Ester was obviously very moved by her parents' story, saying, 'Sometimes I think about my parents, how they coped with what they went through'. The father has always been sole provider for the family while Modesh looked after the children. There is a strong sense of plenty in this home which seems unconnected to their financial situation. Despite refusing to be interviewed, the father and brothers were friendly and hospitable, and impressed me by their apparent caring cohesiveness.

The Desta Family

I have already introduced Genet, whose family I met and interviewed in her mother's apartment: her mother Almaz, her grandfather Berihun (Almaz's father), her uncle Mamu (Berihun's brother), her sister's son Avi and her cousin Addis. I met them all in the large family living room and interviewed them one by one in the dining area, which was not partitioned from the living room but set apart from it. There was a low buzz of conversations going on in the background during the interviews, at one point Genet shushed her mother gently but assertively saying 'be quiet, we are working here'.

The second generation comprised Avi, a recently discharged soldier born in Israel, and Addis, who arrived at the age of five and was serving in the army. The family appeared very supportive of one another; in the pre-interview introductions they explained how over the years they had deliberately bought apartments in close proximity to one another. Almaz spoke of the language difficulties when they first arrived in Israel, and the longing for members of her family who had arrived but remained geographically far away from her. Genet explains:

> She was in the *ulpan* [Hebrew class] thinking about her parents, it was the first time she was ever separated from them.

Genet effectively grew up in a single-parent family, Almaz was her father's second wife (while he was still married to the first). He did not take part in raising her, she referred to her grandfather as a 'father figure'. Avi was also raised only by his mother (Genet's sister) and the extended family, explaining that his father did not live with them and died when he was thirteen. His mother, for whom he has great admiration, was his source of security:

> I grew up without a father, I had a mother who gave me everything I needed. She took care of the house and two boys. She was only 25 when she arrived in Israel, but she managed on her own.

Addis grew up with two parents but described their home as including 'tough discipline'.

The entire family made the difficult journey via Sudan to Israel, Genet was 12 when she arrived. Nine years ago, one of her brothers was killed in a car accident, the loss was a devastating event in the family as Addis described:

> It's unpleasant when someone is lost, when everybody is crying. It's the moment that you never want to happen, and then it does.

Almaz was a midwife in Ethiopia, she administered the birth of Genet's first child in the family home ('right where you are sitting' she laughs). Genet describes this as a reconciliation between them after her conflictual teenage years following their immigration. Today they run workshops for mothers and daughters within the community, encouraging inter-generational connection.

The Fikre Family

I have known Naama and her mother Yafit since they arrived in Israel over thirty years ago, when I was working in an Absorption Centre. I first interviewed Naama in her rented apartment, and later Yafit in the family home. I also interviewed Naama's brother Yisrael (who was serving in the army with my son), and the father Mahari (with his wife and son present). Later I interviewed Naama's cousin Shani and her husband Teruneh, each separately in their family home. On a separate occasion I interviewed Yafit and Shani's parents, grandfather Gebre, Grandmother Fasika, and their son (Yafit and Shani's brother) Abraham, all of them together in the grandparents' home.

All family members arrived separately via Sudan except for Teruneh and Mahari, who arrived via Addis Ababa. The first person to arrive in Israel was young Yafit with her friends, two years later her parents arrived with her daughter Naama (then seven) and sister Shani (then five). Mahari had been conscripted in Ethiopia and all contact with him lost for many years, miraculously he arrived about 10 years later. Yafit told me the whole story in great detail in her interview, but later asked me not to use this information. Yisrael was the first of three children born in Israel after their reunion.

Aside from Naama they all live in a small settlement within walking distance of each other. The prolonged separations in this family had far-reaching consequences which were discussed in the interviews. Shani described the journey via Sudan as

> a dramatic event that influenced my life. You think you are going to die, and then the plot changes, to your advantage.

Yafit, was a single parent for many years until her husband Mahari arrived, she describes their financial hardships in Israel in contrast to their self-sufficiency in Ethiopia:

> In Ethiopia we were a lot of children, but our father [Gebre] had enough money to raise us. We were raised like corn. Nobody was neglected because there were a lot of children, everybody was treated the same, clothed and fed the same, firstly the children. Ethiopian custom is first the adults, but my father always put the children first.

The Shmuel Family

Shy is Emmanuel's (my former husband) cousin, who offered to come to our family home for the interview. Afterwards I visited his in-laws Emebet and Tareke, and then his home to interview his wife Liora and their daughter Shira. I was not able to interview their two sons, one of whom was in the army and the other a discharged soldier who was working.

Liora and Shy have worked within the Ethiopian community in different capacities for many years, they often give guidance and support to members of their extended family and others. Liora's father, Tareke, is the nephew of Yona Bogale (1908–1987) who was the manager of the chain of Ort schools created for the Beta Yisrael community in Ethiopia, known educator and social activist (Weil, 1987; Bogale, 1985). Tareke spoke extensively of his uncle who had a great influence upon him. Yona Bogale met with Doctor Yaacov Feitlovich and Professor Tammeret Emmanuel in 1921 and was sent as a young man to study in Israel, France, and Germany. Tareke himself took an active part in helping Jews leave Ethiopia and has been recognized by the Israeli authorities as a *prisoner of Zion*. This extensive extended family has made great efforts to maintain their cohesiveness in Israel, a subject which came up in the interviews with all of them.

Tareke and Emebet have five children, all living in close proximity and in constant contact with their parents. The grandparents take an active role in raising the next generation from babyhood, their home is a centre for frequent family gatherings. During the interview the living room was full of children of various ages, Liora made sure there was a quiet room in which I could interview her parents (separately) undisturbed, she also translated for us.

Shy also has an extended family nearby (about an hour away by car). For several years, Shy and Liora fostered two orphaned children from Ethiopia, one of who accompanied them on their visit there some years previously. I was impressed by the fact that Shy and Liora went to sit in the garden while I interviewed Shira (13) in their home, to give us privacy. Without them listening Shira could say anything but showed nothing but respect and admiration for her parents.

The Gedamu Family

In this family I interviewed Worknesh, her daughters Noa and Lee, her son Matan and Noa's husband Miki. Noa and Miki have been living in America for several years. Worknesh, who divorced a few years ago, gave birth to ten children: four of them were unavailable to be interviewed, two died in Ethiopia, and one retarded daughter with chronic health problems was present in the living room during the interviews. Worknesh spoke in Amharic and her daughters translated, later I went over the recording with Bossana.

The whole family survived the difficult journey to Sudan on foot. The first to arrive, separately, were the eldest girls, teenagers at the time, they were sent to boarding schools. One year later the whole family was reunited. Worknesh repeatedly gave praise to God for enabling all her family to arrive safely, and described how ill they had been in Sudan, and that she had not expected them all to survive.

The family live in a large city, in a neighbourhood where there are few Ethiopian immigrants. They are obviously a very cohesive and supportive family, demonstrated by the fact that although they do not all live in the same city, the adult children take turns helping their mother care for the handicapped daughter who cannot be left alone in the house.

The Solomon Family

Lemlem was the only one interviewed from this family. She is an academic who works in education, gives lectures, and is generally widely respected and appreciated both within the Ethiopian community and outside. She arrived in Israel at the age of fifteen with her parents via Addis Ababa, they came from the Tigray region. She is the only daughter in a family with many sons. Lemlem and her husband have three children and live in a town in a neighbourhood with few Ethiopians.

The Aharon Family

Mulu is her mother's daughter from a previous marriage, Noam and Yaniv are her brothers from her mother's current marriage. Mulu was 12 when she arrived in Israel after the difficult journey via Sudan, a few months later she was sent to a boarding school. She described this with anger as something that was arranged by the authorities and was very traumatic for both herself and her parents. Noam was only two years old when he arrived, Yaniv was born in Israel. A few years ago, their eldest brother was killed in a car accident. Two other children died in Ethiopia and the mother's brother died on the journey to Israel in Sudan. There are other half-brothers in this family, but I was able to interview only these three, Mulu in her home and each brother separately in a private room in the parents' home.

As the eldest sister and a very resourceful social worker, Mulu has a crucial role in this family, her brothers repeatedly mentioned her as the one person they could rely on to listen to them and help them. Both parents have worked in menial jobs since their arrival in Israel and have recently managed to move out of a poor area of the city to more amenable accommodation in a nicer neighbourhood.

The Metiku Family

I interviewed three sisters, whose mother had nine children from two different marriages. Aberash and Rachel were children from the first marriage, Tsehai the second. The mother was widowed when Aberash was a baby, Aberash and Tsehai came to Israel with their mother in Operation Solomon in 1991. Aberash was then 12 and Tsehai nine. Rachel, the eldest sister, made the journey to Israel via Sudan with her uncle seven years before them, when she was only eight. Her mother sent her away because she did not get along with her stepfather. Rachel recollects these years with tears in her eyes as lonely and full of difficulties as she was moved between an orphanage, foster homes, and her grandmother.

All three sisters are married and have formed new families in Israel: Rachel has five children, Aberash and Tsehai each have three. In the interviews, each conducted separately, there was a marked difference between the positive optimistic attitude of Aberash and Tsehai compared with the anger and bitterness of Rachel. The journey and the long separation from her mother were painful formative experiences in her life, Rachel talks as one who sacrificed her childhood to reach Israel, where life has always presented her many challenges.

The Sehalu Family

In the Sehalu family I interviewed the parents Eneye and Fentahun, and five of their six children: Orna and Habtam who were born in Ethiopia, Maayan who was born in Sudan on the journey to Israel, and Sarah and Shimon both born in Israel. There was another daughter who died in Ethiopia.

The family was stuck for nine months in Sudan, when they arrived Orna was ten, her brother (who was not interviewed) six, Habtam two, and Maayan a baby. By the time she was 12 Orna was in a boarding school, her brother was sent to boarding school in the seventh grade. The fact that the two eldest children were sent away had a detrimental effect on the entire family, especially on the relationship between the siblings. All those interviewed talked about this and also mentioned a definitive difference between the children born in Ethiopia and those born in Israel.

Orna is married with four children, Habtam is newly married, the other children interviewed are single. I interviewed Habtam in her home, the others were all interviewed in the living room of the parental home on two separate occasions.

The Anbese Family

I met Dov in one of the schools I visited as a guest author, impressed by him as a teacher I asked if he was willing to be interviewed. He consented, the interview took place in his home (alone), later I travelled halfway across the country to meet his mother, Abigail. She was taking a break in the community centre where she runs workshops for elderly people but was very relaxed and even eager to be interviewed. Abigail spoke a lot about her experiences on the journey to Sudan, her separation from her children, especially Dov, the eldest, and the struggles of the family during their first years in Israel, when two more children were born (six altogether) and also about her eventual divorce.

In Ethiopia, Abigail had returned to the maternal home with two small children to give birth to her third child when her husband announced that they needed to leave urgently for Israel. At this time her two older children, including Dov, were staying with their father's parents. The father went to their village to collect his children before the family left but came back only with the younger one. Dov was left behind to help his grandparents, upon their request, he was eight years old. Abigail and her husband continued to Sudan, where they spent about three years during which she gave birth to the fourth child. The family suffered a great deal in Sudan, during the interview Abigail repeatedly went back to the story of the journey and her traumatic experiences in Sudan, where the family became separated, and the second child was imprisoned with her parents without her knowledge. There are gaps and inconsistencies in the story, for example Abigail says she was separated from Dov for five years, he said it was for three or four, according to the dates they gave it could have been six years. Regardless of the exact time, clearly the separation was experienced by them both as long and painful. And yet soon after being reunited in Israel, Dov was sent away to a boarding school. Abigail becomes flustered and angry when she talks about this, but her strength and resilience are evident throughout the interview. She described her struggle to keep her children alive in the refugee camp in Sudan and her insistence on being involved in her children's lives in Israel despite all the obstacles she experienced.

The Matan Family

The only member of this family I was able to interview was Edna, married with four children, a teacher who spoke eloquently about her life and experiences. When Edna was almost five years old her mother set out with her four children to walk to Sudan to reach Israel. The grandfather, worried for the safety of his grandchildren, went after them and brought Edna back before they crossed the border. Later her father, who had objected to his wife leaving with the children, went himself to Sudan to bring them back. Only the youngest child, who did not want to be separated from her mother, stayed, and later died in Sudan. The quarrel between her parents about the journey to Sudan caused their divorce, the father brought Edna to Israel via Addis Ababa eight years later, in 1991 (Operation Solomon).

Edna's narrative portrays her father as an exceptional man, very devoted to his children and adhering to his own principles regardless of tradition. After he remarried, she continued to live with him until she went to boarding school. In the interview she explains,

> My father remarried twice after my mother; his second wife raised me like a daughter. Today we are not really in touch, just on family festivities, sometimes she asks me advice about her children. I have a very high opinion of her, she taught me a lot of things, like how to cook. My father's third wife is younger, so she is more like a friend, I don't see her as a mother figure.

The Tafere Family

I interviewed two members of this family: Tigist, the second child and eldest daughter of Abynesh. The family arrived in Israel in Operation Solomon and were initially housed in a hotel in Jerusalem that was converted into an Absorption centre. A year later they moved to temporary housing in their current location, a neighbourhood full of Ethiopian immigrants. Tigist was eight when she arrived in Israel, four of her siblings were born here. One of her teenage brothers was in her apartment when I came to interview her, he left to give us privacy, but he obviously treated it as his home too. In her interview Tigist inadvertently referred to her brothers as 'my children'.

As we walked to her mother's apartment after her interview Tigist told me that her mother was fluent in Hebrew. I found this not to be the case, in fact it was very hard to have a conversation with her in Hebrew, as she constantly reverted to Amharic. Her small apartment was full of children, but the atmosphere was very friendly, and everybody seemed happy. It was Abynesh who said to me about her initial years in Israel 'for six years I did not sleep', because she was so worried about her children in this new environment she did not understand, with all it's unknown dangers.

1.7 The Parents Interviewed in the First Study

The parents interviewed in the previous study (Shmuel, 2010) were all Jewish Amharic immigrants from the Gondar region of Ethiopia, who arrived in Israel about thirty years earlier via Sudan, except Takele who arrived via Addis. They are all people I either knew through working with the community or as Emmanuel's relatives.

Musherit was approximately 55 years old when I interviewed her, since births were not recorded in the villages in Ethiopia her age is only an estimation, this applies to most of the first-generation immigrants. Musherit's parents sent her to her husband's village when she was eight, as the intended wife of Emmanuel's eldest brother. The young girl slept in her mother-in-law's bed until she reached puberty, she described herself as growing up with her husband's siblings as if she was one of them, certainly Emmanuel related to her as a sister. In Ethiopia, she gave birth to seven children before they made the perilous journey on foot to Sudan to reach Israel, one of the children died on the way. The family were settled in a small town in the Judean hills in Israel, where three more children were born. Musherit had no formal education and devoted herself to her children and later grandchildren.

Ziv is Musherit's second-born son, he was 40 years old when I interviewed him, married to Bossana with four children and working as a policeman. As a bright and diligent child, Ziv was sent by his father to learn Jewish scripture with a *Kes* (Rabbi) after school hours, while his elder brother was chosen to help with the farming. Ziv was at least partly responsible for the family's journey to Sudan: he left before them when he was just 16 to avoid conscription, later they followed him. It was a long and difficult journey, when he arrived in Israel, he was taken to one of the better boarding schools where he completed his high school education. Being an industrious man, not long before I interviewed Ziv he completed a qualification in engineering.

Bossana is Ziv's wife and the friend who helped in the translation of the interviews in Amharic, she was 36 when I interviewed her. She came from a large and well-respected family in Ethiopia, her father was a *Kes*. Bossana and Ziv were the first marriage of choice in their families of origin, although introduced to each other by Ziv's uncle. Bossana also made the journey to Israel with her friends when she was just 13, the reunion with her parents in Israel took place only several years later. She studied in a religious boarding school, completed community service and achieved an undergraduate degree in education. She works as a home-instructor to parents of blind children.

Takele grew up in the city of Gondar, he was 42 when I interviewed him, we met in a professional capacity. Takele's father was a prominent figure in the Jewish community in Ethiopia and used to take his children to a Jewish village, Wolleka, on a regular basis to inculcate in them Jewish traditions and customs which were not practised in the city. Takele is married to Nava, both academics, they have two children.

Nava, 34, made the difficult journey on foot to Sudan with her family from a small village in the Gondar province, when she was just 11. Resourceful and intelligent, she completed her high school education and went on to study a degree in business. I interviewed Nava and her husband Takele separately and was very impressed by the similarity of their responses on many issues, they were both very eloquent and provided invaluable descriptions of their childhoods in Ethiopia and their analysis of the absorption process in Israel both on a personal and community level.

Rinat was 45 when I interviewed her, married with nine children, she had no formal education but was active in her community assisting new arrivals and initiating local projects to help children who were struggling at school or spending too much time on the streets. Although facing many challenges raising her many children in Israel, I found her always cheerful and optimistic.

Neta, 38, married with four children, was known to me in a professional capacity, she had worked for many years with the new immigrant community. She was studying for her undergraduate degree while working full time and looking after her family, I was surprised by her willingness to spend time telling me her story and sharing her insights from her own experiences.

References

Amit, K. (2018). Identity, belonging and intentions to leave of first and 1.5 generation FSU immigrants in Israel. *Social Indicators Research, 139*(3), 1219–1235.

Backman, K., & Kyngäs, H. (1999). Challenges of the grounded theory approach to a novice researcher. *Nursing and Health Sciences, 1*(3), 147–153.

Boer, E. (2006). *Uncertain territories: Boundaries in cultural analysis*. Rodopi.

Bogale, Y. (1985). The schools of Beta Yisrael in Ethiopia. *Peamim. Ben Zvi Institute, 22*, 89–92.

Bourdieu, P. (1988). *Language and symbolic power*. Harvard University Press.

Briggs, C. (2007). Anthropology, interviewing, and communicability in contemporary society. *Current Anthropology, 48*(4), 551–580.

Dittmann, A. (1962). The relationship between body movements and moods in interviews. *Journal of Consulting Psychology, 26*(5), 480.

Doleve-Gandelman, T. (1990). Ethiopia as a lost imaginary cultural space: The role of Ethiopian Jewish women in producing the ethnic identity of their immigrant group in Israel. In F. J. MacCannell (Ed.), *The other perspective in gender and culture: Rewriting women and the symbolic* (pp. 121–144). Columbia University Press.

Duranti, A. (1997). *Linguistic anthropology*. Cambridge University Press.

Freedman, Y., & Freedman, G. (1987). Changes to Ethiopian Jewry 1974–1983. *Peamim*. Ben Zvi Institute, *33*, 39–128.

Glasner, B., & Strauss, A. (1967). *The discovery of grounded theory*. Aldine.

Goodnow, J. (2006). Cultural perspectives and parents' views of parenting and development: Research directions. In K. Rubin & O. Chung (Eds.), *Parenting beliefs, behaviours, and parent-child relations: A cross cultural perspective* (pp. 35–60). Psychology Press.

Greenfield, P. M., Keller, H., Fuligni, A., & Maynard, A. (2003). Cultural pathways through universal development. *Annual Review of Psychology, 54*(1), 461–490.

Harkness, S., & Super, C. (2006). Themes and variations: Parental ethnotheories in western cultures. In K. Rubin & O. Chung (Eds.), *Parenting beliefs, behaviours, and parent-child relations: A cross cultural perspective* (pp. 61–80). Psychology Press.

Heath, H., & Cowley, S. (2004). Developing a grounded theory approach: A comparison of Glaser and Strauss. *International Journal of Nursing Studies, 41*(2), 141–150.

James, A., & Prout, A. (1997). *Constructing and reconstructing childhood: Contemporary issues in the sociological study of childhood.* Routledge.

Janoff-Bulman, R. (2010). *Shared assumptions: Towards a new psychology of trauma.* The Free Press.

Kaplan, S. (2007). Community organization. In H. Salamon (Ed.), *Ethiopia: Jewish communities in the east in the 19th and 20th centuries* (pp. 43–55). Yad Ben Zvi & Ministry of Education.

Kaplan, S., & Rosen, H. (1998). Ethiopian immigrants in Israel: Between preservation of culture and invention of tradition. In E. Leshem & J. Shuval (Eds.), *Immigration to Israel, sociological perspectives.* Transaction Publishers.

Lam, C. (2005). Chinese construction of adolescent development outcome: Themes discerned in a qualitative study. *Child and Adolescent Social Work Journal, 22*(2), 111–131.

Lieblich, A., Tuval-Mashiach, R., & Zilber, T. (1998). *Narrative Research.* Sage Publications.

McAuley, C., & Rose, W. (2010). *Child Well-being: Understanding children's lives.* Jessica Kingsley Publishers.

Nigusie, A. (2018). An integrated approach to the study of ethnicity and its relevance to Ethiopia. *International Journal of Social Science Studies, 6*(12), 38–46.

Portes, A., Fernandez-Kelly, P., & Haller, W. (2005). Segmented assimilation on the ground: The new second generation in early adulthood. *Ethnic and Racial Studies, 28*(6), 1000–1040.

Remennick, L., & Prashizky, A. (2019). Generation 1.5 of Russian Israelis: Integrated but distinct. *Journal of Modern Jewish Studies, 18*(3), 263–281.

Roer-Strier, D., & Nadan, Y. (2020). Introduction: The Israeli stage for context-informed perspective on child risk and protection. In D. Roer-Strier & Y. Nadan (Eds.), *Context-informed perspectives of child risk and protection in Israel* (pp. 1–12). Springer's Child Maltreatment Series.

Rosen, H. (1985). Falasha, Kyla or Beta Israel? Ethnographic notes on names given to the Jews of Ethiopia. *Peamim.* Ben Zvi Institute, *22*, 53–58.

Rubin, K., & Chung, O. (2006). *Parenting beliefs, behaviours, and parent-child relations: A cross cultural perspective.* Psychology Press.

Sands, R., Bourjolly, J., & Roer-Strier, D. (2007). Crossing cultural barriers in research interviewing. *Qualitative Social Work, 6*(3), 353–372.

Schmidt-Lauber, B. (2012). Seeing, hearing, feeling, writing: Approaches and methods from the perspective of ethnological analysis of the present. In R. Bendix & G. Hasan-Rokem (Eds.), *A companion to Folklore* (pp. 559–578). Blackwell Publishing.

Sharaby, R. (2021). Between cultures and generations: Ethnic activism of 1.5 generation immigrant leaders. *Journal of ethnic and cultural. Studies., 8*(1), 270–290.

Shmuel, N. (2010). *Educational traditions of Ethiopian Jewry: The dynamics of continuity and change.* Master's dissertation. Hebrew University of Jerusalem.

Shmuel, N. (2018). *Family and tradition in cultural transition: From Ethiopia to Israel.* Doctoral dissertation. Hebrew University of Jerusalem.

Swidler, A. (1986). Culture in action: Symbolism and strategies. *American Sociological Review, 51*(2), 273–286.

Tardiff-Williams, C., & Fisher, L. (2009). Clarifying the link between acculturation experiences and parent-child relationships among families in cultural transition: The promise of contemporary critiques of acculturation psychology. *International Journal of Intercultural Relations, 33*(2), 150–161.

Trevisan Semi, E., & Weil, S. (2011). *Beta Israel: The Jews of Ethiopia and Beyond*. Cafoscarina.

Ungar, M. (2003). Qualitative contributions to resilience research. *Qualitative Social Work, 2*(1), 85–102.

Uttal, L., & Han, C. (2011). Taiwanese immigrant mothers' childcare preferences: Socialization for bicultural competency. *Cultural Diversity and Ethnic Minority Psychology, 17*(4), 437–443.

Hebrew References

Kopperberg, E. (2010). The four worlds model for analysing interactive discussion. In L. Kasan & M. Kromer-Nevo (Eds.), *Analysing data in qualitative research* (pp. 155–180). Ben-Gurion University Publication.

Shmuel, N. (2015). Transitions and not gaps: Integrating Ethiopian immigrant children in the education system. *Gilui Daat, Seminar Hakibbutzim*, 137–146.

Weil, S. (1987). Yona Bogale leader of Beta Yisrael. *Peamim. Ben Zvi Institute, 33*, 144.

Chapter 2
Children's Wellbeing in Ethiopia

'I think I had a good childhood, that I had everything I needed', Takele stated with a reflective smile on his face. It is interesting that Takele frames his 'good' childhood through an absence of deficiency and does not once refer to himself as *happy* during his childhood. In fact, some of his stories reflect stressful situations for a young child. But the way he said that his childhood was good, smiling and appearing self-content, seems to indicate an overall positive feeling about it. The absence of the word happiness in Takele's descriptions could be attributed to a general cultural or gender related avoidance of using emotions to frame experiences, or it could be attributed to a specific perception of what is a *good* childhood: as one in which a child's every need is catered for. Weisner (1998) has defined wellbeing in childhood as forged by effective, innovative, and competent participation of children in everyday routines and activities, providing children with a sense of agency and significance in the social environments in which they live. Thus, specific cultural pathways guide children's development, organizing the routines of everyday life through cultural activities shaped by social structures and containing tasks, goals, motives, relationships, and rules of behaviour. Cultural pathways to child development are formed and sustained within the context of community and environmental ecosystems. Where these provide relative stability and predictability for children growing up within supportive functional families children are likely to be able to say, like Takele, that their childhood was good. The cultural pathways for the children growing up in Ethiopia, a collectivistic society, aimed primarily towards interdependence as members of cohesive supportive communities.

In this chapter, the voices of the adults describing their former childhood in Ethiopia will be presented along with other studies on children growing up in Ethiopia. This will give us an opportunity to understand the *settled lives* experience of the participants Ethiopian childhood, and thereby become familiar with the cultural toolkit they brought with them to Israel. Looking at family continuity between the generations as it is framed in the Ethiopian context will help us locate the

© The Author(s), under exclusive license to Springer Nature Switzerland AG 2023
N. A. Shmuel, *Children's Wellbeing in Immigrant Families*, Children's Well-Being: Indicators and Research 26,
https://doi.org/10.1007/978-3-031-31917-4_2

narratives within a cultural conceptual framework defining childhood and adulthood, clarifying both culture-specific norms and practices whilst revealing in-culture diversity and differences.

2.1 Growing Up in a Community

'They raised us like corn' said Yafit, cupping her hands together to illustrate how corn is wrapped from all sides. She smiles, her eyes gleaming. The image fills her with nostalgia for her happy childhood surrounded by many relatives in a small village deep in the Simien Mountains. Corn grows tall and strong on little water and warm sunshine. The analogy is clear: the children in Ethiopia were all equally enveloped and nurtured, but perhaps also without attention to each child's uniqueness. The emphasis was always on the collective, it was clear that the interests of the community preceded those of the individual. Most children felt safe and looked after, they were raised collectively by the whole extended family, and if there was ever disagreement between parents and children, they always had other relatives to turn to: brothers, cousins, grandparents, uncles, and others.

The community was instrumental in educating the children, and every parent knew they could rely on those around them to enforce rules and boundaries, as Takele explained:

> In Ethiopia you have no choice. If the parents don't supervise you then the rest of the family does, or the neighbours, or the community. So, from every direction you have barriers!

The significance of this network of supporting relatives cannot be overestimated. But, aside from supervision, this network provided a close-knit spiritual framework in which children learnt their own self-worth and came to see themselves as part of a community, for which they willingly relinquished personal desires for the good of all.

The children ate their food from a shared plate, they shared responsibility for one another, the older children made sure the younger ones got their fair share. There was generally an adult in the vicinity who observed the children and made sure none of them were too selfish. Sometimes my own children, when they were young, would scoop themselves big helpings from the joint dishes on the table. Their father was quick to scold them, explaining how he and his eight brothers shared their meals in Ethiopia, crouching around one big *engera*[1] with a meat or vegetable sauce on top. This custom of sharing food defined relationships: adults would criticize children who quarrelled with these words: 'but you ate together; you are brothers'! Sharing food created a bond of kinship, thus an adopted child in Ethiopia is called *engera-lidge*—child of *engera*.

---

[1]Traditional Ethiopian flatbread with a spongy texture, generally made from Teff, a fine-grained cereal which grows in Ethiopia.

Similarly, Christian and Muslim children growing up in Addis Ababa who participated in Poluha's study (2004) belonged to collectives: the extended family, the school and their religious groups, which provided them with social, emotional, and economic security. Most of the children came from very poor families with little or no resources, and yet these were generally distributed in an egalitarian manner. Joint responsibility and sharing whatever resources available were concepts the children in Poluha's study spoke about and valued.

2.2 Siblings Cared for One Another

In Amharic there is a saying that if parents raise the first child well, he or she will raise all the others. Thus, as part of a deliberate strategy which contributes to family cohesion, children looked after each other. One of the results was that a great deal of learning happened between children, through play and imitation, as they spent time together. In fact, studies have shown that this is the main way children learn social and cognitive skills, language, and management of emotions in many cultures of the world (LeVine et al., 1996; Maynard & Tovote, 2012; Perner & Ruffman, 1994; Weisner & Gallimore, 2008).

The children in Poluha's study (2004) often referred to siblings as taking care of them, making them study programs, checking their homework or punishing them. When they talked about themselves getting jobs after school, they said it would be their turn to pay for the education of their younger siblings.

Bossana and others described how, in the villages, adults encouraged children to care for one another, and most of the time they did so unsupervised. Sometimes there were adults about, but they did not intervene in the interactions between the children. Learning through spending time in a mixed-age group encouraged children to take on different roles, share responsibility, evaluate situations, to be sometimes considerate, persuasive, or demanding. The culture provided the context and the expected behaviour.

2.3 A Hierarchical Society

Children in Ethiopia knew their place in the social and family hierarchy based on age and gender. From a young age they learnt to differentiate between people according to their social status, above or below them, and to behave appropriately. This behaviour included cultural codes of respect in language used, intonation, and body language. Children were expected not to disturb the adults unnecessarily and to accept adult authority. Children learnt to be quiet when there were adults around. Not following this respectful behaviour was considered rude and punishable (Levine, 1965; Poluha, 2007; Rosen, 1986; Shmuel, 2010). As Ziv explains:

> There is one leader, one decider, one speaker, and that is *father*. He is the one who determines everything, for good or for bad. If Father says *do this* we do it, without needing any explanations. It is not possible to argue with father.

Children did not expect to have things explained to them, from their father's expression they knew what was expected of them, as Takele explains:

> We never waited for Father to say yes or no. We looked at his eyes, we got the message from his eyes, he gave us signs. If he wanted us to leave, he would express it with a look, that was the extent to which his word counted!

The body language, the look, were so powerful that even young children understood what was meant without the need for words. As Rinat put it; 'Mother looked at me, I was always afraid of her eyes'.

The fear Rinat is referring to preserved hierarchy and created a *respectful distance* between parents and children, as Takele describes:

> Father was very authoritarian; he was a respected man. People used to come and seek his advice. I don't remember him ever taking an interest in our schooling.

The children were bound by an obligation to make him proud and not shame him, as Takele goes on to explain:

> It was as if his word was sacred, it must be fulfilled! I needed to achieve things not only for myself, but also for his gratification. This is not a positive memory for me, but because of the culture, the tradition, it was effective!

Parental command in Ethiopia had to be obeyed. There was no place for doubt or argument. Children did not refuse their parents.

Once Bossana's father sent her to guard the crops from scavenging birds. Deep in play the child failed to notice the approaching birds. Her father, watching her from afar, gave her a commanding *look*, but she continued in her play. Suddenly he rose and shouted her name out loud. Bossana 'cried and cried… I was so insulted that he did that'. She knew that she had offended his dignity and was ashamed.

Non-verbal communication, present in every culture, was a potent tool used by Ethiopian parents for gaining compliance (Exline, 1974; Knapp, 1972; Poyatos, 1983). Understanding childhood in Ethiopia means understanding the significance of the social and family hierarchy, based on age, perceptions of child development, education and punishment, family communication, and gender roles. The hierarchy into which every Ethiopian child was born determined everything. Children did not demand explanations, they knew what was expected of them, as Bossnana explains:

> For us a father was a father, he did not need to say anything, mostly he did not intervene, we *knew* what was expected of us.

The respect for parents and other elders, such as the *Kes* (Rabbi) was absolute, and led to complete and unequivocal obedience. Children kept these rules even in child's play, and this respect was never questioned (see the discussion of child's play in the next chapter). This respectful awe towards parents was backed by the belief in their power to bless or curse a child, as Rinat explains:

> In Ethiopia there are a lot of blessings. The blessing from the parents is very important to the child.

The parental blessing had great supernatural power—children wanted to be blessed by their parents and were afraid to be cursed, especially by their father.

These findings all correlate with the descriptions in Poluha's study (2004), in which children's' relationships growing up in Addis Ababa are described as explicitly hierarchical, while age, adult status, physical size, strength, gender, and social status determined super or sub-ordination. The children expected the adults around them to supervise them, according to the children this was the way they expressed their love and care. They expected themselves to be obedient and respectful, these were the most common terms they used describing appropriate *good* behaviour of children. Obedience was not talked about by the children in negative terms, but as natural positive behaviour, the children talked about their parents in loving and respectful terms even if these were harsh with them. Most children were closer to their mothers, who took more of an active role in taking care of them. Girls were expected to be more obedient than boys, and respectful behaviour was expected of both towards all adults. This respect was also expressed verbally, by addressing their elders using the plural *antu* and *irswo*, and physically, by using body language: children stood up when an adult entered a room, bowed their heads and lowered their gaze, let adults walk in front of them, and inadvertently shrunk their bodies in the presence of adults. When guests came to visit children were expected to leave the room, they did so without being told. They also talked about the parent's blessing as being highly valued, although they only expressed this when talking to the interviewer, when receiving the blessing they remained silent and serious. One child mentioned thanking her parents in her stomach, the place containing all emotions.

2.4 Punishment

The parent–child relationship inevitably involves power relations, mediated and shaped by culture, social norms, and the law. Punishment defines the distribution of power and implies guilt. Physical punishment of children has long become illegal in Western countries but is still practiced in many parts of the world especially where the social hierarchy is based on age and gender. Physical punishment is an expression of the existing hierarchy—the strong using force over the weak, keeping the status quo. A study exploring the connection between gender norms and children's experiences of violence in the home in Ethiopia found a distinct correlation between community norms and boys or girls experiences of violence at home (Murphy et al., 2021). This was especially true of rural areas, while in urban areas adolescent attitudes were more influential than community norms, perhaps indicating less cohesive communities. More than half the adolescents in this study reported having experienced physical violence at home during the past year, even more reported experiencing psychological violence (being shouted at or called names) there was little variation between girls and boys. Moreover, this was considered by all the children normal parental behaviour. Girls were more likely to be punished for non-conformity to expected gender roles, which were upheld by female caregivers as much as male caregivers. One of the conclusions was that collective norms are more important and powerful in determining behaviour than individual attitudes.

The participants in my study described punishment of children as a way of gaining obedience, as educational, and as maintaining the existing hierarchy, as Ziv explains:

> My father told me to call my [older] brother with his respect-name. That I should call him Yaye, instead of Baye, something like this. Once I didn't do this and my father came and slapped me. He wanted me to use this respect name, not my brother. My brother never asked for this.

The father tried to coerce his children to obey the rules of the hierarchy based on age, by using the appropriate respect-names—names that the younger child must call the elder as a sign of respect. The parents had not only a right but a duty to use physical punishment in educating their children or correcting their behaviour, this was the expected norm (Ketsela & Kebede, 1997; Poluha, 2007; Shmuel, 2010).

Neta explains how the alternative to physical punishment was verbal abuse:

> But mostly they cursed you, and sometimes, if father came to beat us, our mother would be very protective.

Mother's punishments were more gentle, mostly little pinches, as Rinat explains

> I remember my mother getting very cross with me and giving me lots of *quontats* [pinches].

Some adults hardly used physical punishment at all, and sometimes the gentle pinches from mother could prevent the harsher beatings from father. The degree of punishment differed between different families and could be at differing levels of severity: it could take the form of a *quontat*—a little pinch—which can be almost unfelt, like a symbolic punishment, or it could be a real beating. When the assumption is that children have reason and can understand, things can be explained to them, but here the cultural assumption was often that children are not capable of advanced thought processes and must be educated by force.

The children accepted punishment as legitimate, it was part of the norm and not an exception. Nava explains this:

> Children were not abused; they did not see it like this either. In Israel a child might feel resentment, but in Ethiopia he didn't, because he knew he did something wrong, that his father would not get up to hit him for no reason. It took a long time before the father would actually do that.

These descriptions are similar to those in Poluha's study (2004) which found physical punishment to be the acceptable norm in both home and school, more likely to be given by fathers than by mothers, who were more inclined to slap, pinch, or use words. Older siblings were also entitled to use physical punishment, girls tended to be beaten more often than boys, to whom a certain leniency was often shown when they disobeyed. Children understood and accepted this as the norm and did not complain about being punished, except in instances when the severity of the punishment seemed excessive or unjustified, but the children were powerless to do anything about this.

2.5 Family Behaviour Based on Age and Gender

In every family there are younger and older people, in families with a strict hierarchy based on age and gender the group one belonged to determined one's rights and obligations. Everybody knows that the young will grow to be older, and one day it will be their turn to receive the respect they give to their elders. In family meetings such as the *Kiddush* (traditional Jewish blessing to receive the Sabbath) it is the eldest person present who says the blessings, and it is obvious to all that the *Dabbo* (traditional *Halle*, bread for the blessing) be distributed according to age—from the elder to the younger. Food is distributed in the same way; children are familiar with this custom and respectfully wait their turn. As Ziv explains:

> Children do not eat with adults. The adults eat first, and only afterwards the children. Not only on the Sabbath, this applies all the time.

This was a custom which not all families adhered to, for example Rinat, Edna, and Takele all described having joint meals with their parents as children in Ethiopia.

Age was based on conjecture, most people did not know their accurate date of birth, since births were not registered in Ethiopian villages and birthdays were not celebrated. From the descriptions of the participants, a child of four or younger was considered small—Nava talks of herself at age seven as small. Children were expected to know how to behave by the time they were six, after which children were expected to help in the home according to their abilities and gender. Bossana describes her desire to help as a little girl, and how this made her feel grown up:

> It was fun to feel one can do things, and you wanted to be part of the grown-up world. When you reach seven or eight you are already expected to do things, to participate, to take part.

Her words stress the desire and motivation of the children to participate, to reach adult status. In Ethiopia, to tell someone they are *young* was an insult implying inability, and not at all complimentary.

The division according to age is emphasized by Bossana's description of family life:

> During *Buna* [coffee] all the adults sit around and talk on a high level, they don't include the children. The children stay outside, they play, all the children together, laughing and telling stories. So, the children and the adults are separate. It was not acceptable for them to mix.

This division was absolute: children and adults did not converse together. Children learnt their roles according to gender from a young age, mostly through spending time with the parent of the same gender. As Rinat explains:

> In Ethiopia girls help the mothers, watch what she did, while boys help the fathers, outside, in the fields, tending the sheep or the goats.

Bossana gives examples of this:

> I was at home a lot, with my mother. I used to help with the babies, to put them on my back.

Nava also recalls:

> Helping to make food, grind the flour, helping to cook things, or watch the food that was ready, so the birds didn't eat it, on the days when I wasn't in school.

Girls were expected to know household chores when they were very young, as Rinat explains; 'if they marry you off early, you need to know how to make stuff'.

The only gender categories people referred to are male and female, homosexuality in Ethiopia and amongst the Ethiopian Jewish community in Israel was a taboo subject that was never mentioned.

Parents needed working hands in the fields and at home, and did not consider schooling more important than this, especially not for girls, who were often told; 'if a girl studies or not is unimportant in her life' (Poluha, 2007). Bossana remembers her father's words when he saw she was sad because she was not allowed to go to school, which was far away from her village:

> It's not so bad if you don't study—what do you think will happen to you? If it works out you will study, and if not—so what? You will get married like your mother, and have a home like your mother, why should you be sad?

Poluha's study (2004) reiterates these findings, in which she analyses how children talked about *good* or *bad* behaviour of boys or girls. The fact that the children's rhetoric mixes gender stereotypes with ideals, in other words stating the same qualities as existing and desirable, shows that they have internalized societal norms about gender and try to abide by them. Although girls and boys were both expected to be obedient, respectful, and hardworking, these expectations from girls were more restrictive and misbehaviour more likely to be regarded severely as opposed to a certain mischievousness almost expected from boys. When talking about *children* both adults and children were referring to *boys*, thus the male gender became the norm, the female the exception. Speech, body language, use of space, and attitude to time were ways in which the division between male and female was socially expressed and overtly perpetuated. Thus, deference was shown by girls to boys and women to men using the appropriate address and subservient body language. Girls were expected to spend more time inside the home, available to do chores and comply with requests, than boys who could play outside or in the street, out of reach. Even in the school yard girls clustered near the wall, while boys spread their play all over the school compound. These arenas thus became social constructs of inequality.

2.6 Women's Status in Ethiopia

In 2018, Sahle-Work Zewde became the first woman president of Ethiopia and prime minster Abiy Ahmed formed a cabinet in which half the ministers were women. While these changes are impressive, women's status in Ethiopia has always been much more complex than it appears. On the one hand, women were considered weak and men ruled them. On the other hand, they were appreciated as powerful and strong, and within the social rules and restrictions they had a degree of independence. Ethiopian patriarchy is different from that in Arab or Muslim countries: Ethiopian women are part of the public sphere, entitled to talk to men and do not cover their bodies completely (Weil, 2005; Rosen, 2009 unpublished). Girls were expected to be virgins when they married, but this was not expected of boys. Sometimes men were allowed to marry more than one wife.[2] Young girls were married by pre-arrangement, after which they generally set up home near the husband's family.

To understand fully the complexity of relations between the genders in Ethiopia, we will examine firstly the terminology for gender and relations, according to Rosen's explanations (2009 unpublished). In Amharic there is no connection between the word 'man'—*wand*, and 'woman'—*seyt* as there is in the Hebrew—*Ish* (man) and *Isha* (woman). The word *seyt* has negative overtones and is used to denigrate—for example *ye-seyt-lidge* means boy of a woman—meaning a boy who is rude or impolite. The expression *ye-seyt-maret* means the soil of a woman and refers to infertile soil. While the phrase *ye-wand-maret*—man's soil—refers to valuable and fertile land. A married couple is called in Amharic *ballena-mist*—the word '*mist*'—wife—is considered more respectful than '*seyt*'. The terminology depicts the social hierarchy—as a boy is considered less than a man, so a woman is considered less than a man, and in addition her sexuality and menstruation make her dangerous. Having said this, the wife has respect—for example as *balebet*, the woman of the house—this does not express ownership of property, but her traditional role. If a man calls his wife *balebetey*—owner of my house—this is a term of appreciation.

Elderly men were at the head of the hierarchy in Ethiopia. They sat at the head of the table; the women served them. But the balance of power between the sexes is much more subtle than meets the eye. For example, women in Ethiopia did not relinquish their father's name after marriage. When Yafit wanted to come to Israel her father did not try to stop her, but he did not allow her to take her child with her. Abigail's father-in-law refused to let her son Dov (his grandson) leave with them for Israel. Rachel did not get along with her stepfather and ran away from home to her grandparents, after which her mother sent her to Israel. Edna's grandfather followed her mother to Sudan and brought the child back, probably saving her life. These examples illustrate power relations and who decides at critical times. Freedom is relative—within the constraints of the culture.

[2] See the Desta family.

In Ethiopia, men and women were expected to bring equal quantities of cattle and land to finalize their wedding, a woman was not sold to her husband for a price. If they divorced, the woman received half of the land and the cattle. There is an expression *be-ikul gabbicha*—of equal status in marriage. This indicates economic equality (Rosen, 2009, unpublished). It was also acceptable in Ethiopia that men punish their women physically, but they could not do as they wished—the woman could always complain to her relatives, who could shame the husband or help her leave him.

It is important to understand that Ethiopian women did not gain their independence in Israel—they were strong and independent in Ethiopia, and in some ways safer because of their family's support (Rosen, 2009 unpublished; Edelstein, 2014; Eyal-Assael, 2014).

Abigail recalls 'my mother always did what she wanted, in Ethiopia and in Israel'. Genet's mother was a midwife and *mohel*;[3] she says about her that she was always the dominant one and 'an amazing woman who took the idea of knowledge and turned it into power'. Naama explains that her mother Yafit took part in a government initiative traveling around local villages in Ethiopia to encourage young girls to study. Women's power in Ethiopia was hidden by respectful gestures so that it would not be a threat to men, sometimes deliberately creating the illusion that they had no power. This is how Habtam describes her mother:

> Sometimes you think she is being trodden on, but she knows exactly what she is doing.

2.7 Child Marriage

Naama said about her mother:

> The fact that her parents married her off, that was no small crisis. It was common practice. It was a crisis for a lot of Ethiopian women. They were girls, not even women.

Naama's mother Yafit was seven when she came to live with her husband's family, Musherit was eight, in both cases the husbands were allowed in the wife's bed only after menstruation. Yafit as a little girl ran away from her husband's village several times before she accepted her fate. This was the reality for girls in Ethiopia: Fasika was 12 when she was married, Abynesh 13, Tareke married his wife when he was 18 and she was 8. Emebet's mother-in-law died soon after her wedding, so that at a very young age she became responsible for the whole household including her husband's younger brothers who were not much older than her.

Child brides had no prior acquaintance with their grooms, and were generally tutored by their mother-in-law, who taught them how to run a household and care for the children. Often, she became a very significant person in their lives. It was

[3] The person who performs the Jewish custom of circumcision for boys (traditionally eight days after the birth).

acceptable that young girls went back to their own mothers to give birth, and that the grandparents on both sides took a significant role in raising the first child. (For further reading on Jewish women in Ethiopia, see: Salamon, 2007; Shavtai & Kasan, 2005).

Parents-in-law, and especially mothers-in-law, became important and influential in the lives of many young brides in Ethiopia. Thus, Worknesh spoke proudly of her mother-in-law teaching her hygiene, especially in relation to carrying babies on her back:

> No baby would take a wee on *her* back! Everything was kept clean, like in Israel.

This cleanliness included high moral standards and purity of speech:

> My mother-in-law was very clean, and I learnt from her, like all her brides. We did not curse, we did not shout, because our mother-in-law did not curse or shout. If we told a child, *you are edgy like a dog*, she told us *don't talk like that, don't tell him he is like a dog, use nice words*. I don't curse my children, others say they are spoilt, but I learnt this from my mother-in-law.

This woman was respected by her daughters-in-law, who wanted to be like her. She taught them standards of hygiene and educational methods which were exceptional in rural areas, thus wisely shaping reality for the next generation.

On the African continent child brides are common, 40% of girls are married before they are eighteen.[4] Amongst the Amhara population in Ethiopia, primarily Orthodox Christians, the figure was 58% in 2016.[5] In a comprehensive study on the subject in Niger and Ethiopia, by John et al. (2019), combining quantitative and qualitative methods, researchers found significant negative associations between very early marriage (before the age of 15) and overall psychological wellbeing. Early marriage was associated with depression and anxiety, many child brides reported suffering emotional distress associated with the burden of handling marital responsibilities. Other major factors found to affect the psychological wellbeing of child brides were intimate partner violence, diminished decision-making ability, and reduced access to financial and social resources. Another study by Gage (2013) among Amhara adolescent Ethiopian girls found increased odds of suicide among girls who were ever married, promised in marriage, or had received marriage requests when compared to unmarried girls.

Yafit explained the folk-logic behind the early marriage of girls: a young unmarried, widowed, or divorced woman was considered unprotected, vulnerable to rape or unwanted pregnancy. Early marriages were meant to protect the girls from these dangers. Genet's mother chose to be the second wife (while her husband was still married) to be protected, but she lived separately from her husband who was a well-known *Kes* [Rabbi] and she kept herself by working as a midwife and *mohel*, and by selling her own pottery.

---

[4] United Nations Children's Fund. Ending Child Marriage: Progress and prospects. New York: UNICEF; 2014.

[5] Ethiopian Demographic and health survey.

Effectively, traditional power relations creating and upholding the hierarchy of Ethiopian society leave young girls vulnerable and unprotected. The women in my study who shared their stories spoke about this openly, this was the norm in the society they came from. Girls who were lucky, such as Musherit, were absorbed into their husbands' families as children and protected, others were less fortunate. There is a related issue which I find important to mention even though it was a taboo subject which did not come up in the interviews: female circumcision. It is mentioned by participants in Poluha's study (2004) as a possible reason given for girls to be badly behaved—if they had *not* been circumcised. This practice was also common amongst the Jewish community, although few women are willing to talk about it.

2.8 The Menstruation Hut *Mergem Godjo*

The practice of separating women from their home and community during menstruation and after childbirth (forty days for a boy and eighty days for a girl) was a Jewish custom based on biblical scripture[6] and the premise that during this time women were *impure* (Anteby, 1999). It is an example given by Avi when describing his mother as

> a very smart girl who soon understood what was expected of her [...] she was taken there [the menstruation hut] the first time, after that she went on her own.

Many women described this as a time they could rest, while in the hut they were free of their household duties. Other women in the family (mothers, sisters, mothers-in-law, elder daughters) took responsibility for the household and brought food to the women in the hut. Worknesh described at great length the many preparations for her absence from home, and how difficult it was for her to be separated from her other children. The ostracism of women to these huts was hard on their children, who were not prevented from joining their mothers but knew that if they did so they too would be considered impure and required to wait until sundown to bathe in the cold river before they could return home or enter the village. Worknesh recalls how her daughter Lee, then four years old, ran to her furtively and 'stole a hug' early in the morning before anybody could see her.

2.9 Communication in the Family and Emotional Expression

> Us girls were always on the margin, but you hear things, you cannot intervene, but you can listen.

[6] Book of Leviticus, Parashat Tizria, Chapter 12, Verses 1 to 5.

This is Rinat's description of the position of children in Ethiopia as external to adult discussions, not allowed to interrupt conversations or ask questions, but able to listen attentively and observe what was going on around them. The time children spent in proximity to adults created strong intuitive communication without the need for words, and yet this also might lead to misunderstandings and children feeling confused or left out. An example of this is the time Rinat's father died, when she was four. Nobody came and told her explicitly, she understood through the events that followed:

> A lot of people came, and they were all crying. These are signs [for death] you know from birth. Then relatives and friends came and took us children and looked after us and our mother and all her family sat *shivah* [seven days of mourning]. You see that and you know there was a catastrophe. But nobody came to tell us, to explain. That was missing. I would have liked somebody to explain.

Rinat recounts the visible signs for an event of death, signs that every child can identify. She describes the treatment of the children, they were not ignored, but nobody explained anything to them. Suddenly she found herself moving to a new village and being expected to accept a stepfather, but even this was not explained to her:

> It bothered me that nobody talked about it. I didn't call him *father*. When he called me, I came, I knew what my mother wanted, but it was hard for me. It bothered me.

Emotions were not communicated verbally, it was assumed Rinat would adjust herself to this new situation, there was no legitimacy for children to complain about or question adult decisions.

Rachel describes a similar experience soon after her biological father died, when she was suddenly faced with a stranger as a stepfather:

> Nobody prepares you. Nobody gives you the news. They don't say—this and this is going to happen in your family. There is going to be a change. There is no such talk. The parent makes the decision and everybody else must adapt themselves.

But Rachel was incapable of adapting to this, she did not get along with her stepfather, which led to her mother sending her with an uncle to Israel when she was just eight years old. She grew up in an orphanage and foster homes until her grandmother arrived.

As children, Rinat and Rachel were not able to express in words what bothered them. Nava also talks about this:

> Maybe as children we were silent because that is what we were taught, to be quiet. But not because nothing bothered us. Things bothered us, but we kept silent. That is one of the things we still do.

Learning to keep silent is such a deeply rooted part of the culture, that even if they want to, many people find it difficult to say what they feel or what they want, or even to recognize these feelings inside themselves, as Nava explains:

> Because this is something that is embedded in us, in our community, you don't say what you feel, because if you did it would be considered rude or abnormal, it is forbidden.

Every culture has forged a *normal* acceptable way of behaving, especially regarding public expression of emotions. Thus, in Ethiopia, the norm was not to show emotions at all, as Bossana explains:

> With parents you can see their appreciation, their worry, their heart… but it is not out in the open, it is not expressed by words—how are you? What have you been doing?—it's all inside.

The parents did not show an active verbal interest in their children or verbally express their love for them. Restraint, saving on words, keeping emotions bottled up—these were considered virtues. The expectation was that children know how to cope with life's disappointments, that they too act with restraint and do not express their frustrations out loud. Additionally, in Ethiopia, it was common practice not to praise a person directly, so that children became used to hearing their praises through a third person—in other words parents spoke *about* the children to other people, but not directly to the children themselves.

In the framework of a cohesive community there is a general desire to keep harmony. To do so people must avoid outright conflict. Nava says about her mother that she

> never complained, or cursed, or got upset with anyone. She was always patient, she always got along. So, if we went anywhere, we were like that too, we always got along. Nothing ever happened, wherever we went we got along, that is what she taught us. If there was a conflict, she never let it develop, she immediately put a stop to it. We learnt this from her.

Avoidance of conflict, emotional restraint, and concise verbal communication were thus the norm, within families as well as in society in general. A study on sixteen-year-old children in two government high schools in Addis Ababa (Bireda & Pillay, 2018) heightens the importance of open parent–child communication for the wellbeing of adolescents. In this study, there was a direct correlation between perceived maternal and paternal communication and children's wellbeing as measured by self-reported scores of depression, school adjustment, substance use, and self-esteem. This study found that female participants perceived the nature of communication with both parents as more open than boys did.

2.10 Ambiguous Multi-messaged Communication

Language both creates and reflects reality. Children who grow up in a certain language learn to represent their surroundings verbally, these verbal definitions shape the way we think about everything. Language weaves connections between people, which in turn teach us about the world and our place in it through culturally formed concepts we come to see as natural. Language is simultaneously our means of learning about reality and acting upon it (Burr, 1995; Burr & Dick, 2017).

Language is one of culture's most potent tools: growing up in a specific culture we learn to think through its channels, which influence the way we see the world.

Language forges our experiences through definitions and descriptions, and each language does this differently (Vygotsky, 1978; Ochs, 1996).

The Amharic language is both gender-specific and contains honorific morphology, meaning that certain words and expressions create and back up authority. Thus, a book teaching Amharic (Appleyard, 2013) explains:

> In the informal register, which you use when talking to someone whom you either know well and are close to, or with someone of lower status than yourself such as a child or a servant…

Hence, the language itself carries terms that classify people according to relative status. Respectful address includes using a *respect name* or a special term denoting respect or using plural rather than singular as a sign of respect.

But this is not all, inter-personal communication in Ethiopia was envisaged and constructed in a unique and mystifying way, as Takele explains:

> If somebody wants to jibe you or comment on something you did, maybe a mistake you made, or what they think is a mistake, they can't just come and say, look you made this and this mistake and it's your fault. They will tell you a proverb and let you work it out for yourself. Why did this person tell me this proverb? And if you can't understand—and not everybody does—then you need to go and ask someone else. If this person understands, then they tell you what the proverb means, while being careful not to assign malice, they will give you a positive interpretation.

What Takele is describing is *double talk*, known as 'the wax and the gold'—*Sen-ena-Werq*—common in Ethiopian, especially Amharic, culture. This means a saying that has a double meaning, concealed and opposite, creating a sophisticated and complex form of communication. The figurative meaning of the word is the wax, while the concealed important essence is the gold (Levine, 1965). Messay (1999) calls this a double entendre. The result is a hide and seek of words and meanings, creating an ambiguous multi-messaged communication. According to Girma (2011), the origins of the wax and gold tradition lie in theological teachings of the Ethiopian Orthodox Church, stemming from a differentiation between the literal, material (considered evil), and what is hidden and spiritual (considered superior). Basing their authority on the latter, both political and religious leaders in Ethiopia have historically positioned themselves beyond the realm of criticism and thus safeguarded the status quo. Although there is disagreement between scholars such as Levine (1965), an American sociologist, and Messay (1999) an Ethiopian philosopher, on the significance of the wax and gold tradition, both accept its distinctive contribution to Ethiopian culture (Girma, 2011). Levine saw wax and gold as a form of communication enabling the transferal of covert messages, the criticism of a person higher up in the hierarchy while being respectful, the maintenance of privacy by avoidance of direct answers to personal questions, and the diffusion of social pressures by using humour in a society where hierarchy can be humiliating. In contrast, Messay perceived Levine's analysis as a misrepresentation of Ethiopian culture, missing the deep religiosity of the people, and the use of wax and gold as a sophisticated process of thought similar to ancient Greek philosophy. Messay contends that authority in Ethiopia was obviously prevalent and enforced, and that wax and gold was not about protecting the individual sphere as Levine suggested.

Girma (2011) has another explanation for the wax and gold tradition as having paradoxical significance, on the one hand contributing to shaping Ethiopian identity, creating a unique national metanarrative that is 'religiously tinged', overriding the divisive nature of Ethiopian ethnic diversity. On the other hand, it provides a delicate means of both coping with and rebuffing change, by adapting new ideas to preexisting conceptions without changing the overriding paradigm.

For the context of this book, the historical political aspects of the wax and gold tradition are less relevant, what is important is understanding the nature and consequences of this form of communication *within the family*. Now we can return to Takele's description and imagine a child trying to decipher what a parent or another adult relative is trying to convey via a proverb or metaphorical story. According to Takele's narrative, reiterated and confirmed by other participants of my study, turning to other adults or an older sibling for help decoding such a message may produce several differing or even conflicting results. A child's ability to rise to the challenge and understand such aphorisms will gain appreciation and respect, it is through such everyday casual parley that he or she are being socialized into their cultural world. While inter-personal communication is indirect, filled with hidden content, ambiguous statements and circuitous talk that never cuts to the chase. If the truth were told directly, most likely it would not be accepted *as is*, on the assumption that something else lies behind it. As in many cultures based primarily on verbal rather than written communication, where few people were literate, the manipulative use of language becomes a valued art, considered as reflecting high capability and intelligence. Spoken words are carefully considered, nothing is said lightly, since words carry consequences—statements can be sharpened like swords or soft like feathers, but they are never neutral, they are always of great impact (Fuglesang, 1982).

Thus, children grow up in a world of infinite meanings, created by proverbs, stories, metaphors, and sayings formulated in the *wax and gold* tradition. This form of dialogue contributes to creating the social hierarchy, to weaving family connections and personal status in a certain way, pre-defining people's position in relation to one another. Children are not excepted, their education within the family is based on this.

2.11 Learning Through Observation and Imitation

> When I was little, I watched what my mother did and always tried to do the same, (Rinat).

Children in Ethiopia learnt from adults primarily via observation and imitation; they were motivated to do so because they wanted to be a part of village life. Children's desire to imitate adults came from an identification with them. Children took upon themselves activities which became part of their perspective on life, turning them into partners in the real world. To accomplish this, they developed learning competencies based on observation. The adults encouraged this, expecting children to take on responsibilities befitting their age, gender, and abilities. As is common in many non-Western cultures, children initiated the learning process, which was not dependent on adult intervention or explanation. Children were busy internalizing what they saw daily, and since they initiated the process they learnt quickly, with great attention to detail, collecting a vast amount of information (Gaskins & Paradise, 2012).

What and from whom children learnt was based on gender, as Rinat explains:

> I watched my mother as she cooked, not like here—where everything is explained, or you open a book to tell you how to do things—in Ethiopia you looked and learnt, you wanted to do the things yourself, because most of the time, especially women, need to know how to do housework.

This type of learning is an automatic intrinsic part of family life and is based on the adult's assumption that children will take responsibility for their own learning process, and it is not necessary to add detailed explanations. As the participants in both my studies describe their childhood—how they knew what was expected of them, how they learnt their Jewish identity—the same expressions are used repeatedly by different people: 'it was natural learning, there was no formal instruction', and:

> I don't remember being told, I understood from what was going on around me.

While the children growing up in the Jewish villages did not all attend school on a regular basis, the children growing up in Addis Ababa who participated in Poluha's study (2004), especially the girls, combined school and home chores. Poluha stresses the context in which these children were growing up, shaped by poverty, a hierarchy based on age and gender, their social status and religion. Their schooling was adapted to these contexts, they were expected to be obedient, polite, and studious, to conform to gender appropriate behaviour, and to learn by repetition and memorization. They were not encouraged to be inquisitive, to ask questions and to think critically about knowledge or life. The 'habitus' as Bourdieu (1988) called it, is the practice of everyday life, shaping people's ways of thinking and acting until these are internalized to seem 'natural'. Children expressed a deference to authority not only verbally, through the appropriate greetings and respect names, but physically, by body movements such as bowing their heads, lowering their eyes and shrinking their bodies. Thus, the status quo gains legitimacy during childhood and is reinforced both by home and school, with limited room for change.

2.12 Ethiopia-Utopia

All the participants in my studies described their childhood in Ethiopia through the prism of Israeli reality today, and the picture created is full of longing for the past. As Nava said: 'We had a really good life'. Their childhood as they remember it was filled with family and relatives, a vast network of people embedded in a rich cultural tradition who cared for and nurtured them.

This idyllic representation of village life, with obedient children who never quarrelled with their parents and always did what they were told, is at least to some extent a result of nostalgia. Creating a perfect past is in part an effort to negate the difficulties of the present (Schwarz, 1998). The memories are formed in comparison to current reality in Israel, which is complex and hard for the parents, Dolve-Gandelman (1990) called this a *lost imaginary cultural space*. To these parents, the world they have lost was stable and safe, parent–child relationships were harmonious, everybody knew their place in the family and in society. These descriptions suggest that the opposite may be true in their current families, forged on the intercultural divide, in which parental authority is often questioned, gender roles are changing, and life in Israel presents many challenges. When talking about their Ethiopian childhoods they are omitting the challenges their parents probably faced, such as high rates of child mortality, lack of available medical care and accessible education, and other stressful issues related to the political regime, conscription, female circumcision, and child marriage. In the literature available on children's wellbeing in Ethiopia today much of the focus is on child survival, health issues, sanitation, poverty, and access to medical care and education in the peripheral areas. All this needs to be considered when listening to the narratives in my study.

References

Anteby, L. (1999). There's blood in the house: Negotiating female rituals of purity among Ethiopian Jews in Israel. In R. Wasserfall (Ed.), *Women and water: Menstruation in Jewish life and law* (pp. 166–186). University Press of New England Brandeis University Press.

Appleyard, D. (2013). *Colloquial Amharic* (p. 23). Routledge.

Bireda, A., & Pillay, J. (2018). Perceived parent–child communication and well-being among Ethiopian adolescents. *International Journal of Adolescence and Youth, 23*(1), 109–117. https://doi.org/10.1080/02673843.2017.1299016

Bourdieu, P. (1988). *Language and symbolic power*. Harvard University Press.

Burr, V. (1995). *Where do you get your personality from? An introduction to social constructionism* (pp. 17–94). Routledge.

Burr, V., & Dick, P. (2017). Social constructionism. In *The Palgrave handbook of critical social psychology*. Palgrave Macmillan. http://eprints.hud.ac.uk/id/eprint/26455

Dolve-Gandelman, T. (1990). Ethiopia as a lost imaginary space: The role of Ethiopian Jewish women in producing the ethnic identity of their immigrant group in Israel. In J. MacCannell (Ed.), *The other perspective in gender and culture: Rewriting women and the symbolic* (pp. 121–144). Columbia University Press.

Edelstein, A. (2014). Intimate partner femicide against Ethiopian women in Israel. In E. Witztum & N. Grisaru (Eds.), *Social and clinical aspects of Ethiopian immigrants in Israel* (pp. 249–278). The Jewish Agency and Ben Gurion University of the Negev.

Exline, R. (1974). Visual interaction: The glances of power and preferences. In S. Weitz (Ed.), *Non-verbal communication: Readings with commentary* (pp. 65–98). Oxford University.

Eyal-Assael, V. (2014). Misunderstandings, conflicts and domestic violence among rural Ethiopian immigrants (offspring of Beta Israel) awaiting immigration in Ethiopia and after arriving in Israel. In E. Witztum & N. Grisaru (Eds.), *Social and clinical aspects of Ethiopian immigrants in Israel* (pp. 211–248). The Jewish Agency and Ben Gurion University of the Negev.

Fuglesang, A. (1982). *About understanding: Ideas and observations on cross-cultural communication* (pp. 104–110). Dag Hammarskjold Foundation.

Gage, A. (2013). Association of child marriage with suicidal thoughts and attempts among adolescent girls in Ethiopia. *Journal of Adolescent Health, 52*(5), 654–656.

Gaskins, S., & Paradise, R. (2012). Learning through observation in daily life. In D. Lancy, J. Bock, & S. Gaskins (Eds.), *The anthropology of learning in childhood* (pp. 85–118). Alta Mira Press.

Girma, M. (2011). Whose meaning? The wax and gold tradition as a philosophical foundation for an Ethiopian hermeneutic. *Sophia, 50*, 175–187.

John, N., Edmeades, J., & Murithi, L. (2019). Child marriage and psychological well-being in Niger and Ethiopia. *BMC Public Health, 19*, 1–12. https://doi.org/10.1186/s12889-019-7314-z

Ketsela, T., & Kebede, D. (1997). Physical punishment of elementary school children in urban and rural communities in Ethiopia. *Ethiopian Medical Journal, 35*(1), 23–33.

Knapp, M. (1972). *Nonverbal communication in human interaction* (p. 1–25; 19–168). Holt, Rinehart and Winston.

Levine, D. (1965). *Wax and gold: Tradition and innovation in Ethiopian culture*. The University of Chicago Press.

LeVine, R., Dixon, S., LeVine, S., Keefer, C., Richman, A., Leiderman, P., & Brazelton, T. (1996). *Child care and culture: Lessons from Africa*. Cambridge University Press.

Maynard, A., & Tovote, K. (2012). Learning from other children. In D. Lancy, J. Bock, & S. Gaskins (Eds.), *The anthropology of learning in childhood* (pp. 181–206). Alta Mira Press.

Messay, K. (1999). *Survival and modernization: Ethiopia's enigmatic present: A philosophical discourse*. The Red Sea Press.

Murphy, M., Jones, N., Yadete, W., & Baird, S. (2021). Gender-norms, violence and adolescence: Exploring how gender norms are associated with experiences of childhood violence among young adolescents in Ethiopia. *Global Public Health, 16*(6), 842–855. https://doi.org/10.1080/17441692.2020.1801788

Ochs, E. (1996). Linguistic resources for socializing humanity. In J. Gumperz & S. Levinson (Eds.), *Rethinking linguistic relativity* (pp. 407–434). Cambridge University Press.

Perner, J., & Ruffman, T. (1994). Theory of mind is contagious: You catch it from your siblings. *Child Development, 65*, 1228–1238.

Poluha, E. (Ed.). (2007). *The world of girls and boys in rural and urban Ethiopia*. Forum for Social Studies.

Poyatos, F. (1983). *New perspectives in nonverbal communication: Studies in cultural anthropology, social psychology, linguistics, literature, and semiotics* (Vol. 5). Oxford Pergamon Press.

Schwarz, T. (1998). *Ethiopian Jewish immigrants in Israel Living well and "becoming deaf" in the homeland: This study elucidates the meanings of two apparently contradictory ascriptions which the Ethiopian Jewish immigrants make about themselves: 'being well' and 'becoming deaf'*. Doctoral dissertation. Department of anthropology, LSE University of London.

Vygotsky, L. (1978). *Mind in society: The development of higher psychological processes* (p. 10–16; 19–51). Harvard University Press.

Weisner, T. (1998). Human development, child well-being and the cultural project of development. *New Directions for Child Development, 81*, 69–86.

Weisner, T., & Gallimore, R. (2008). Child & sibling caregiving. In R. LeVine & R. New (Eds.), *Anthropology and child development: A cross-cultural reader* (pp. 264–269). Blackwell Publishing.

Hebrew References

Rosen, H. (1986). *Questions and answers about Ethiopian Jewish cultural behaviour*. Hadassah Women and the Ministry of Absorption.

Salamon, H. (2007). The life circle. In H. Salamon (Ed.), *Ethiopia: Jewish communities in the east in the 19th and 20th centuries*. Yad Ben Zvi and the Ministry of Education.

Shavtai, M., & Kasan, L. (Eds.). (2005). *Mulualem: Ethiopian women in spaces, worlds and journeys between cultures* (pp. 24–29). Lashon Zaha.

Shmuel, N. (2010). *Educational traditions of Ethiopian Jewry: The dynamics of continuity and change*. Master's dissertation. Hebrew University of Jerusalem.

Weil, S. (2005). Jewish Ethiopian women in transition. In M. Shavtai & L. Kasan (Eds.), *Mulualem: Ethiopian women in spaces, worlds and journeys between cultures* (pp. 24–29). Lashon Zaha.

Chapter 3
Learning Jewish Culture and Identity in Ethiopia

How do children acquire, internalize, and negotiate cultural knowledge? In the previous chapter, we have seen how childhood itself is rooted in culture, how children learn in culturally specific ways enabling their active participation in family and society. Many participants in my study spoke of *knowing* what was expected of them as children in an intuitive way, by observing what was going on around them. The narratives reflect children as active participants in the acquisition of knowledge, building on their experiences in the primordial family and village surroundings as they become increasingly socially active (Weisner, 1998). In the context of the cohesive community children unfold their cultural pathways, acquiring cultural knowledge through attentiveness to their surroundings, mimicking in play the world of adults. Using Boer's paradigm (2006), in the space between generations children negotiated their budding adulthood, and in the space between their own community and their Christian neighbours children gave meaning and significance to their Jewish identity. This chapter details these processes, beginning with parental perspectives on childhood and adulthood, education and child development. Followed is a discussion on verbal and non-verbal communication in the family, the world of play, and a brief discussion of cultural acquisition and in-culture diversity in settled lives.

3.1 Education According to Parental Perspectives

Parenting and family management are intimate private acts and yet take place in social and cultural contexts (Goodnow, 2006). In other words, parental behaviour is a cultural practice shared by cultural groups who have specific expectations about normative parenting. Parents have culturally based assumptions about desired qualities for children to grow into capable adults. These assumptions contain a culturally

© The Author(s), under exclusive license to Springer Nature Switzerland AG 2023
N. A. Shmuel, *Children's Wellbeing in Immigrant Families*, Children's Well-Being: Indicators and Research 26,
https://doi.org/10.1007/978-3-031-31917-4_3

specific world view which guides parents and other caregiver's educational strategies. There is a cultural concept of the *ideal child* which drives parenting decisions with a great deal of emotional investment (Carlson & Harwood, 2014). This is a sort of automatic parental pilot forged by cultural concepts of what is right or wrong, good or bad—also known as *parental ethnotheories* (Roer-Strier, 2001; Harkness & Super, 2006).

In collectivistic hierarchical societies the values on which these are based include respectfulness and obedience as well as gender and age specific behaviour. Poluha's study (2004) found that girls were more likely to be punished for gender inappropriate behaviour than boys. In individualistic democratic societies the emphasis is more on personal expression, creativeness, and self-fulfilment, and even being free spirited (Carlson & Harwood, 2014). The cultural toolkit of every parent contains values alongside strategies of action, these are intertwined in daily life to form behaviour and expectations. Berhanu (2005), who did research with parents of Ethiopian origin in Israel, found that qualities considered desirable in children do not change after emigration, in other words parents continue to educate according to these culture-specific norms. The parents he interviewed defined the following qualities as desirable in children: patience, respectfulness, obedience, respect for parents, fear of God, work ethic, the desire to study, sociability, politeness, and emotional restraint (described as keeping feelings in the stomach).

Every society constructs their own concepts of *childhood* and *adulthood* based on time and place (Lancy, 2014). In Western society there is a clear division between these two worlds; children are seen as dependents and adults as responsible providers. Children are not expected to work, and for most hours of the day children and adults do not spend time together (James & Prout, 1990). In contrast, in participants descriptions from my studies of childhood in the Jewish villages in Ethiopia, children and parents spent most of their days together, most child-learning was a result of this proximity. Children were motivated to learn from the adults around them because they wanted to be useful, because it was expected of them to help, and because they wanted to make their elders proud of them.

The concept of the child as distinct from the adult is a social, culture-specific construct. Thus, children are perceived as inferior to adults, in the process of becoming adults themselves, or as people in their own right, this latter more common in societies striving for egalitarianism and concerned with children's rights. In collectivistic societies, geared towards the wellbeing of the community above individual needs and desires, children are expected to adjust themselves to the adult world rather than the opposite. In most Western societies, it is common for adults to play with children as part of an educational and a bonding process, but in many cultures in the world, especially where there is a clear hierarchy based on age such as Ethiopia, adults do not play with children (Maynard & Tovote, 2012). There are even proverbs in Amharic that justify this, indicating that playing with children is a source of trouble and may be humiliating for the adults. For example, 'playing with a child is like racing a dog' since eventually the dog will bite (Berhanu, 2006) or 'do not play with a child, who will poke you with a stick' (Poluha, 2007).

In other words, adults should maintain deference, a *respectful distance* between themselves and children to avoid being humiliated.

3.2 Perceptions of the Parental Role in Education and Child Development

Parental roles in child development are socially constructed, studies have shown significant differences in parental behaviour towards infants when comparing African and European or American parenting (Harkness & Super, 2006). The primary differences stem from cultural goals and perceptions expressed through the degree of active intervention in educating children, for example Western parents tend to spend time playing with and reading to their children. In contrast, African parents are more inclined to address their children verbally with instructions on how to behave, expecting compliance and not a verbal response. This indicates a different purpose of communication—to direct behaviour rather than forge bonds. In many African cultures as children grow up parents *decrease* verbal communication, often limited to criticism, scolding, and threats. The parental expectation is that children be obedient, not communicative. Children are expected to be quiet around adults, to internalize and maintain a respectful distance between adults and children. By the age of three or four children are supposed to know their position in the social hierarchy and act accordingly (Harkness & Super, 2006). As they grow older children spend more of their time in interaction with other children, especially siblings and cousins who look after them, it is in this context that children learn language and socially acceptable behaviour (Weisner & Gallimore, 2008; LeVine et al., 1996). These children enter society at the lowest level of the hierarchy, facilitated by siblings and cousins, who are the first people they learn to listen to and obey. Thus, it is not the parents in these societies who carry the primary role of socialization or even education. In Poluha's study (2004), there are many examples of this, as siblings and cousins took an active role in supervising children's homework or administering their schedule and generally looking after them. While there are examples of the abuse of this power, these were exceptions. In my study, Bossana explained how children were give autonomy over their relationships with one another, although there were usually adult figures in proximity keeping an eye on what was going on, it was rare for them to intervene between the children.

Learning takes place in context which gives meaning to the process and is socially channelled according to cultural values and goals (Lancy et al., 2012). Thus, children are encouraged towards individualism and independence, self-expression and self-fulfilment or alternatively collectivism and inter-dependence, joint responsibility respect and loyalty (Greenfield et al., 2003). Every society encourages varying degrees of all these qualities, but the overall cultural and educational messages, both overt and covert, tend towards one of these pathways. For example, in individualistic societies cooperation between siblings is encouraged, but generally seen as a choice, not an obligation (Greenfield et al., 2003).

The Ethiopian Jews came from a collectivistic society, most of the children grew up in socially cohesive villages with their extended families. Babies were usually breast-fed until they grew out of infanthood, internalizing in their bodies family proximity, intuitive care, and reciprocity. Their sibling and cousin carers introduced them into the social world where they gradually learnt the language and cultural codes of behaviour, as well as what was expected of them as boys and girls. In contrast, Western society mostly encourages children's independence from birth—with separate sleeping, prams and pushchairs as opposed to baby carriers, surrounding infants with objects rather than people. These differences are forged into the course of life; in Ethiopia, the predominant values were reciprocity, obedience, and maintaining social harmony, while Western cultures tend to value independence, personal choice, and initiative. Western education is based on Piaget (1951) with an emphasis on analytical, scientific knowledge, and man in relation to objects. In African and Asian societies, social-emotional intelligence, understanding people, is valued above scientific knowledge and theories. These background ideologies have far-reaching consequences for the learning process, parental behaviour, expectations from children, and self-perceptions—people who are raised to make decisions as part of a social or familial entity or as motivated by personal desires and interests. Obviously, the differences noted here are not absolute and child-rearing practices are constantly changing everywhere, but they indicate general cultural-geographic tendencies. There is diversity within cultures as well as between them, it is recognized today that many Western assumptions considered universal concerning human behaviour and development, psychology, and attachment are culture-specific and have many more variations (Weisner, 2014; Carlson & Harwood, 2014).

In Ethiopia, as in many African countries, parents expected children to learn of their own volition, through observation, imitation, and improvisation, with little need for direct adult intervention. Acquiring knowledge was the prerogative of the child, seen as responsible for his or her own learning, since it facilitated their ability to be a part of what was going on around them. As Bossana stated:

> you don't wait to be told what to do, you watch what others are doing and you want to help, to be a part of it.

As in Poluha's study (2004), even children who went to school still participated in household chores. But the cultural continuance between home and school provided a constant that children could negotiate, if not always comfortably then at least without stress.

Traditionally in Ethiopia, fate and not parents are perceived responsible for child development. Children who do not develop healthily are considered cursed (Poluha, 2007). A recent study on perceptions and experiences of stigma among Amhara parents of children with developmental disorders in Ethiopia (Tekolaa et al., 2020) found that many parents perceived and experienced different forms of stigma, directed towards their child or themselves, resulting in some families self-isolating to avoid this. Supportive attitudes and social acceptance came from those who had some understanding of developmental disorders and rejected traditional assumptions that attributed autism or intellectual disability to supernatural causes such as possession by evil spirits, curses, and punishment from God for the sins that the child's family may have committed. Their recommendations include targeting communities to raise awareness and focusing on the wellbeing of the family rather than on individuals. In my study, there were two families with children with severe mental disorders, the Gedamu family and the Demse family. In neither case were these children discussed directly during the interviews, and when discussed indirectly mental illness was never specifically mentioned. In the Demse family both mother and daughter spoke extensively around the issue, with much contention between them as to the causes which led to this situation.

If tradition places child development in the realm of fate, then parents cannot be held responsible for how their children develop, thus the proverb *bedilu yadigal* meaning that fate dictates how a child will grow. On the other hand, the proverb 'a tree must be straightened when it is young' suggests that parents are responsible in guiding and moulding their children. There are other proverbs which strengthen this attitude, such as 'the child will grow to the father's design' and 'patience is bitter but it's fruit is sweet'. Proverbs with conflicting messages exist in all languages, they reflect multiple perspectives on an issue. This seems to suggest a recognition of a degree of parental responsibility for children's development, which is also regarded as dependent on fate and wider social influences (Berhanu, 2006).

3.3 Verbal and Non-verbal Communication

Language is not only a reflection of reality but an active means of shaping that reality, through directing thoughts, creating and maintaining hierarchies, social status, and meaning (Duranti, 1997; Heath, 1983; Sterponi & Bhattacharya, 2012; Wexler, 2006). Different societies construct adult–child communication according to cultural goals; in many cultures' words directed at children are aimed to guide behaviour or initiate a practical response (such as obedience), not to invite conversation or encourage free thought, since children are not expected to understand.

As children grow up, their understanding of the world is not based on objective reality, but on the interpretation of reality created by people past and present—made accessible by language containing culture-specific concepts and categories (Burr, 1995). Thus, children are constantly learning simultaneously language and social constructs (Ochs, 1996; Vygotsky, 1978).

Hierarchical societies such as Samoa (Platt, 1986), the Philippines (Rosalso, 1982), and Ethiopia (Shmuel, 2010) use honorific morphology, a respectful terminology to denote relative status in the family and society.[1] Thus, language both creates and perpetuates social structure, age and gender differences. Children watch,

[1] Discussed in the previous chapter.

listen, learn, and internalize these constructs as they learn the language of communication, which is also the language of socialization directing behaviour.

The participants in both my studies all described another, very powerful form of communication, prevalent in all societies and shaped by culture, based on facial expressions and body language. As Takele explained:

> We never waited for father to tell us yes or no, only his eyes gave the message, there were signs, if he wanted us to leave…this was the meaning.

Children learnt to read these non-verbal ques from a very young age, they were predominant over words, which were used sparingly, often in intricate and creative ways such as through proverbs and stories. Rinat described being 'afraid of my mother's eyes, the way she looked at me'. Rinat understood what her mother expected of her through the expression in her eyes, effective in lieu of words.

3.4 Stories and Proverbs

Cultural narratives are passed on to children through the powerful medium of stories and proverbs, creating meaning, shaping perception, forging gender and group identity, and defining acceptable morality. The stories told to children were aimed to inculcate ethics and values, often using examples of what negative things can happen to people who do not follow societies rules and expectations. Stories and proverbs contain collective knowledge passed between the generations; this form of inter-generational communication is common in many cultures (Lancy et al., 2012).

There are many examples in my research of parents remembering being told stories as children, but none of them could remember a specific example to recount in an interview and attributed this cultural knowledge to the older generation. In Ethiopia, the elders of the community were the knowledge-bearers, their life experiences and wisdom were greatly valued. Thus, stories and proverbs were interwoven into everyday life as a narrative passed between the generations (examples appear in Berhanu, 2006; Salamon, 1995; Dereje, 1996; Rosen, 1989). A study of Oromo speakers in Ethiopia (Tadesse, 2014, 2018) demonstrates the significance of stories and proverbs as a means of inter-generational transferal of important cultural knowledge. Tadesse concluded that children's participation in the re-telling of folktales is a creative expression through which they are learning and affirming survival skills and cultural values as active agents able to draw analogies between the imaginary and the real. These children are talented and creative participants in the adult world, to the extent that what might appear to Western eyes as play-acting is in fact much more than this, as it embodies children's active participation in cultural creation, transferal, and renewal.

Amongst the Jewish Amhara community, a popular character in folktales is Gebre Hana. Rosen (1986) makes an interesting observation that many of these stories are ethically problematic, since the hero repeatedly wins through cheating, deception, and manipulation rather than hard work, diligence, and education. In this connection it is interesting to note that in Ethiopia, people who do not abide by social norms are known as *shifta* (Horowitz & Mosher, 1997), although rejected by society at large there are those who admire them for their courage and manliness (Rosenblum et al., 2008). As in many cultures of the world, society provides mixed messages, on the one hand, upholding cultural norms and rules whilst simultaneously developing a folk culture which admires those who dare to break them and even sees them as heroes (for example, Bonnie and Clyde).

The narratives of folklore are created and passed on in a specific time and place which gives them meaning and includes local symbolism. Changing the context of the story may distort the meaning or make the messages blurred or incomprehensible (Bauman, 2004). Every society constantly contains a mix of past sayings and new additions, as texts are passed between the generations and renewed, maintaining, and re-forming traditional cultural heritage. Ethiopia was no exception to this, many stories have multiple versions, with much in common and unique differences, just as not all 'traditional' customs are practised in the same way in each region, language group, or family. These variations lead Edna to say 'there are many different types of Ethiopians', stressing the diversity within an ethnic group which often might be overlooked, especially after immigration.

3.5 Learning Jewish Identity

Jewish children in Ethiopia learnt their identity through biblical stories and tales of Jerusalem, as Bossana describes:

> To the light of the moon they [the adults] told us *terat terat* [stories] especially on the Sabbath about Jerusalem… what Jerusalem is, full of Jews, and spiritual learning, Hebrew and the bible!

Nava described how the adults:

> talked about coming to Israel, and we asked why are we in Ethiopia? And mother answered that God has scattered our people [around the globe] because of something that happened, and that one day we would all be reunited in Jerusalem, which is like paradise on earth.

Jewish children learnt stories depicting characters from biblical times, as Bossana explains:

> I knew biblical stories before we came to Israel, many stories, about Abraham and Lot and Sdom… my father told us these stories, all sorts of stories about what it means to be Jewish. In the evenings we often had *terat terat* and *unkoklish* [riddles].

These stories, often told by adults on Friday evenings (the onset of the Sabbath), on Sabbath and on special occasions when the whole village gathered to mark a Jewish festival or holy day, perpetuated Jewish traditions, and defined the community, creating cohesion and distinguishing them from their Christian neighbours. Bossana's father was a *Kes* (Rabbi and spiritual leader), his daughter has great admiration for him:

> It was not easy to be a *Kes*, to keep the Jewish observances in a Christian environment, where you have no control of the place…the town or any other place… my father used to set out on long journeys and he never ate until he came home or arrived in a Jewish home…this is tremendous self-control…I would not want to break the chain—to lose what my father always valued and kept.

Bossana's words reflect the power of action—how one man's deeds become the duty of the community to keep tradition, in this case to adhere to the rules of Kosher food. To this day Bossana's actions are guided not only by her faith, but by her deep respect and loyalty to her father as she maintains a religious household. The younger generation absorb and perpetuate ancient traditions by example, the bond between people fuels their commitment to do so.

Participants in my studies described their experiences during Jewish festivals, the weekly gathering in the sanctity of the Sabbath day, prayers, stories, special clothing and food suited to each event in line with convention. These are Ziv's words:

> We celebrated all the Jewish festivals. At Pesach [Passover] we ate *Kita* [unleavened bread]. I knew I was Jewish because my parents and the Kessim [Rabbis] told us about the Shabbat, about Judaism, about Jerusalem. I can still remember the stories about Ethiopian Jewry from my childhood.

Ceremonies and traditional customs during childhood were adorned with symbolism which acted on the five senses, creating powerful memories linking personal and collective identity. As Takele describes:

> *Berekete* [special bread made for the Sabbath], every feast, all these things, like fasting for a whole day [the Day of Atonement]—I never managed to do that, always ate before the end! But listen, these are all good memories, that strengthen my personal identity.

The most mentioned festivals were Passover, the Jewish New year, and the Day of Atonement. This is how Nava described the preparations for Passover:

> I especially remember the communal preparations, taking all the kitchen utensils down to the river to make them Kosher for Pesach.

The memories are embedded in ceremonial acts, specially cooked meals and preparations in which children were often assigned tasks. The festivals themselves often involved visiting the local synagogue, participating in prayers, and listening to stories told by the Kes. Nava continues:

> We children especially loved the New Year, because you had to collect plants, usually the leaves from palm trees, and you spread them on the floor to symbolize renewal, like you made a new surface… and there was the special coffee ceremony, when we ate bread and butter for the New Year, like here we eat apples with honey…and the week before we had to get up in the middle of the night and purify our bodies in the stream… as children we loved these ceremonies.

Ceremonies were full of mystery and symbolism, joint preparations and participation, in rhythm with the changing seasons, repeated on a yearly basis thus engrained in personal and collective memory, linking the younger generation to cultural and spiritual traditions.

Ziv describes the special ceremony associated with the Day of Atonement:

> They took a sheep through the village, round and round, all day long, and then slaughtered it and burnt it, the skin and the meat, and everybody came to taste it, to bear their iniquities…

In this description, the whole village is part of the ceremonial act and the preparations leading up to it, the expectation of renewal and the concluding ritual, binding community and creating meaning embedded in sensual experience.

Family folklore was intertwined with cultural, ethnic, and religious traditions, bonding the community, creating order and meaning in people's lives (Bynum, 1987). Inherited traditions and family stories, jokes, names, ways of doing things, all became part of the family assets passed between the generations, creating collective identity. Shared history forges belonging, family and group mythology is built by the narratives passed from one generation to the next. The children born into this on-going story become part of the continuing narrative, their legacy creates meaning to their existence and forges a sense of belonging to something greater than themselves (Keith & Whitaker, 1988). Thus, ceremonies and rituals become the fabric of continuance, creating and perpetuating culture and traditions in memorable and meaningful ways, expressed according to context of time and place (Salamon & Goldberg, 2012). In times of crisis, repeating familiar rituals assigned magical or spiritual powers can be a source of comfort and group cohesion.

Other traditional Jewish customs mentioned by participants centre around food and a constant reminder of their differentiality from their surroundings. For example, Ziv describes how it was forbidden to eat meat outside the family home:

> We were told explicitly—*they* [the Christians] *have other blessings, we have our own blessings, you cannot eat their meat*—and really we didn't.

When Ziv was a student in the town his family brought him food from home:

> we could not eat their meat, so I used to take food from home, we could sit with the Christians at the same table, we could eat together, but we had separate food.

Children were aware of Kosher observances, their practical behaviour was guided by these, even if they did not always respect them. For example, Takele, who grew up in the town of Gondar surrounded by Christians, says:

> I was told at home not to eat their meat, but when I went to the neighbour's house and they were eating I joined in and ate everything!

Jewish children knew their distinct identity from a very young age, the rules and restriction defined them, as Bossana describes:

> There was always a difference. You know you are Jewish, you cannot do what other children outside are doing.

But they were allowed to play with Christian children, as Nava explains:

> we knew they were Christian, and we were Jewish. But we were not prevented from playing together. They respected us and we respected them.

Mutual respect enabled each to live according to their beliefs, the villages themselves were separate, each child knew what community they belonged to, but they were able to play together (for further reading on Jewish customs of Beta Israel, see:

Ben-dor, 1985; Ziv, 2017; Corinaldi, 1988; Shalom, 2016). In settled lives, socially and religiously defined boundaries are clear, even if they were crossed sometimes (for example, by eating forbidden food) identities remained distinct, children were firmly rooted in family and community.

3.6 The World of Play

In all societies children participate in meaningful social contexts which ease them into community cultural values and norms (Lancy et al., 2012). But children are not simply passive in cultural acquisition, they are active participants in creating and maintaining culture and customs (Fung & Smith, 2012). The realm of the village was the children's play-space, re-defined to recreate socially acquired meaning, as Nava describes:

> Each child chose a tree, then we created our pretend houses and marked them with lines of stones, inside these areas we did what was expected—*this place* was for adults and *this place* was for children [she indicates assigning spaces with her hands] and we had the *mergem godjo* [impurity hut], and pretend marriages, and defined families… all in play…

The sphere of play provided the context for events created by children, perceived social boundaries became separated spaces in the children's play area. Thus, stones and trees defined the limits of appropriate conduct, recreating social and family hierarchy, including gender roles. Rinat also recalled such play:

> We built… you know, with natural things, like leaves we placed on the floor and sticks and stones for boundaries… we built our house, and brought water from the well, and in play we girls did what our mother's did…

Girls stayed at home, boys went out to the fields, the existing social order was accurately copied in play. Space was pre-defined as belonging to specific age groups (adults or children), houses as belonging to specific families (parents or newlywed offspring), outside the mock village was an impurity hut and a well. Nava tells how the children recreated and adhered strictly to the social order, thus social rules and gender roles were not challenged even in play:

> We did exactly what the adults did, the parents decided for the children, the children were not allowed to intervene or be rude, not at all, not even in pretence.

But children could be adults, girls could be boys, while maintaining the hierarchy: the young were obedient, respecting the old, women remained at home and cared for the house and children, as Nava continues:

> We divided up naturally, those who were suited to play the adults, like me [laughter], I played the adult, and those suited to be the daughter or the son, a girl could play the son if she wanted…[implying that the opposite was not acceptable]. I never wanted to be anybody's wife, so I always chose to be the *shmagele* or something like that, just not to be a wife! Then the father and some of the children would go to look after the sheep and the mother would do housework. I loved this game!

Through this game those of lower status temporarily gained higher status, thus a girl could play a boy, a young child an adult, but not the other way around. The *Shmagele* was an adult intermediary concerned with keeping the peace (usually older men, but it could also be a woman). I asked Nava what the *Shmagele* did:

> If a couple quarrelled, then the Shmagele was called. I had to ask them what happened, and explain to them, solve their problem so that they would not be quarrelling, make peace so everything is back to normal.

Social order requires that disputes are amicably settled, taking responsibility for this is a form of leadership, conferring much greater status than being anybody's wife. Child's play recreated the adult world, emphasizing rules and expected behaviour, gender roles and social order. Play enabled children to practise different social and familial roles within the confines of accepted role-playing that did not challenge the status quo. Rinat described how the girls played at being mothers:

> We made dolls from material and leaves, or one of the smaller children played the daughter, that's how we played. We pretended to breast-feed, and to carry the baby on our backs, in the *unkulba* [baby-carrier], the girls always wanted to be better mothers… better than their own mothers, better means not to be cross, or to talk to the baby that cries… we did what mothers do—making *engera*, braiding our daughter's hair, or making cotton threads… we copied what mothers do…

The children tried to be an improved version of their own parents, always attentive and nurturing, within the confines of culturally expected familial roles. Just as their division of space marked social boundaries, so their awareness of time, seasons, and festive days adhered meticulously to cultural-religious dictates. Thus, the children respected the sanctity of the Sabbath in play and did not even pretend to work, as Nava explains:

> On Sabbath we sat and talked, we did not *do*. On regular weekdays we *did things* like grinding flour or working with clay or fetching water from the well, but on Sabbath—no. On Sabbath we just sat, this is the difference.

The children copied adult behaviour with great accuracy, including avoiding what was prohibited and fulfilling adult duties. Nava explains that on the Sabbath:

> All the elders of the village sit on the grass, they talk while the children play. On the Sabbath it is forbidden to wash, you are not even allowed to go near the river, not even to stick your foot in the water, it is forbidden! We knew what our parents did, and this is what we did too.

Children's play replicated the adult world in perfect imitation, guided and structured along culturally and religiously acceptable pathways forged by adults. Rules and regulations were internalized down to the last detail, children refrained from doing anything that was forbidden even in play. For example, Nava says:

> On the Sabbath morning our family ate, after the *Kiddush* [blessing]… which we did in one of the houses… we kept some of the *Dabbo* [bread] and we pretended this was an adult's house and the oldest child repeated the blessing and then we all ate…

3.7 Culture in Settled Lives

The narratives in this chapter have shown children's active agency in acquiring cultural knowledge as they became increasingly active participants in family and community life in Ethiopia, recreating adult conceptual structures in play. The language learnt throughout their childhood, both spoken and unspoken, provided the building blocks for the knowledge filling their cultural toolkits. Their cultural pathways unfolded in the context of time and place, anchored in family and community. In the space between the generations the conceptual framework organizing values and patterns of action was transmitted and negotiated. Settled lives provided the continuity to enable this as a natural process, containing both the dynamics and intricacies of culture in all its overt and covert forms. Thus, culture was internalized as a spontaneously acquired 'theory of practice' which may come into question only in an inter-cultural context (Bourdieu, 1988). This does not mean there was no change or diversity in traditions in Ethiopia, rather it suggests that such change and diversity was contained and absorbed without rocking the boat.

When I finished interviewing Liora's 85-year-old father I was amazed to see his young granddaughter climb onto his lap, gently grab his chin with one hand and with the other insist on pouring water from a bottle into his mouth saying, 'Grandad you mustn't get dehydrated'. The elders I knew in the community all strictly observed a *respectful distance* between themselves and the younger generation and would never have permitted such behaviour. I commented on this to Liora and she laughed, saying that the granddaughter's behaviour was typical to her family, who never worried much about maintaining reverence between the generations. The grandfather, Tareke, had told me in the interview that Yona Bogale was his uncle, proudly recalling how:

> He taught us to educate our children without hitting or cursing them, to teach them as one does in Israel. I learnt this from him.

Diversity within cultures develops because of personal and group innovation as well as external influences. Yona Bogale studied in Jerusalem, Germany, Switzerland, and France before returning to Ethiopia, founding and managing the Beta Yisrael schools. He was a well-known educator and popular leader active in the emigration of Ethiopian Jewry, many changes in the villages were initiated by him (Weil, 1987; Bogale, 1985).

Another example of diversity within Ethiopian culture is the tradition that dictated children should be fed *after* adults, yet there were many exceptions to this rule. Edna described how her father always fed his children first, even presenting them with the finest cuts from slaughtered sheep to the dismay of his guests. 'It was very clear to him that the children came first', says Edna. In villages with no electricity children were expected to stand holding the lamp when it was dark, yet Edna reminded her brother

> I don't remember you ever picking up a book to read without father being there next to you, holding the lamp.

This blatant role reversal was very exceptional behaviour, in total opposition to family hierarchy, and yet this is how Edna's father raised his children in Ethiopia.

In every society time brings change, the inevitable inter-generational clash is always there, forging a certain conflict between conformism to tradition and acceptance of innovation. People's ability to cope with this dissonance amicably is dependent on a certain sense of stability, on viable community leadership and optimism about the future. These are the prerogatives of settled lives, brought into question in the turmoil of transition. Sometimes the resultant generational rift is simply unbearable (Wagaw, 1993).

References

Bauman, R. (2004). *A world of others words: Cross-cultural perspectives on Intertexuality*. Blackwell Publishing.

Berhanu, G. (2005). Indigenous conceptions of intelligence, ideal child, and ideal parenting among Ethiopian Jews in Israel. *Journal of Cognitive Education and Psychology, 5*(1), 47–71.

Berhanu, G. (2006). Parenting (parental attitude), child development, and modalities of parent-child interactions: Sayings, proverbs, and maxims of Ethiopian Jews in Israel. *Journal of Cognitive Education and Psychology, 5*(3), 266–287.

Boer, E. (2006). *Uncertain territories: Boundaries in cultural analysis*. Rodopi.

Bourdieu, P. (1988). *Language and symbolic power*. Harvard University Press.

Burr, V. (1995). Where do you get your personality from? In V. Burr (Ed.), *An introduction to social constructionism* (pp. 17–94). Routledge.

Bynum, J. (1987). Folklore in the family. *ETC: A Review of General Semantics, 44*(4), 408–411.

Carlson, V., & Harwood, R. (2014). The precursors of attachment security: Behavioural systems and culture. In H. Otto & H. Keller (Eds.), *Different faces of attachment: Cultural variations on a universal human need* (pp. 278–307). Cambridge University Press.

Dereje, G. (1996, August). Proverbs on children in Amharic, Oromo, and Tigrinya. In H. Wondimu (Ed.), *Research papers on the situation of children and adolescents in Ethiopia: Proceedings of the conference on the situation of children and adolescents in Ethiopia*. Addis Ababa University Printing Press.

Duranti, A. (1997). *Linguistic anthropology*. Cambridge University Press.

Fung, H., & Smith, B. (2012). Learning morality. In D. Lancy, J. Bock, & S. Gaskins (Eds.), *The anthropology of learning in childhood* (pp. 261–286). Alta Mira Press.

Goodnow, J. (2006). Cultural perspectives and parents views of parenting and development: Research directions. In K. Rubin & O. Chung (Eds.), *Parenting beliefs, behaviours, and parent-child relations: A cross cultural perspective* (pp. 35–60). Psychology Press.

Greenfield, P. M., Keller, H., Fuligni, A., & Maynard, A. (2003). Cultural pathways through universal development. *Annual Review of Psychology, 54*(1), 461–490.

Harkness, S., & Super, C. (2006). Themes and variations: Parental ethnotheories in western cultures. In K. Rubin & O. Chung (Eds.), *Parenting beliefs, behaviours, and parent-child relations: A cross cultural perspective* (pp. 61–80). Psychology Press.

Heath, S. B. (1983). *Ways with words: Language, life and work in communities and classrooms* (pp. 1–14). Cambridge University Press.

Horowitz, T. R., & Mosher, N. (1997). Achievement motivation and level of aspiration: Adolescent Ethiopian Immigrants in the Israeli Education System. *Adolescence, 32*(125), 169–180.

James, A., & Prout, A. (1990). *Constructing and reconstructing childhood: Contemporary issues in the sociological study of childhood* (p. 3–15; 28–37; 66). Falmer Press.

Keith, D., & Whitaker, C. (1988). The presence of the past: Continuity and change in the symbolic structures of families. In C. Falicov (Ed.), *Family transitions: Continuity and change over the life cycle* (pp. 431–448). Guildford Press.

Lancy, D. (2014). Babies aren't persons. In H. Otto & H. Keller (Eds.), *Different faces of attachment: Cultural variations on a universal human need* (pp. 66–113). Cambridge University Press.

Lancy, D., Bock, J., & Gaskins, S. (Eds.). (2012). *The anthropology of learning in childhood*. Alta Mira Press.

LeVine, R., Dixon, S., LeVine, S., Keefer, C., Richman, A., Leiderman, P., & Brazelton, T. (1996). *Child care and culture: Lessons from Africa*. Cambridge University Press.

Maynard, A., & Tovote, K. (2012). Learning from other children. In D. Lancy, J. Bock, & S. Gaskins (Eds.), *The anthropology of learning in childhood* (pp. 181–234). Alta Mira Press.

Ochs, E. (1996). Linguistic resources for socializing humanity. In J. Gumperz & S. Levinson (Eds.), *Rethinking linguistic relativity* (pp. 407–434). Cambridge University Press.

Piaget, J. (1951). 6. Principal factors determining intellectual evolution from childhood to adult life. In *Organization and pathology of thought* (pp. 154–175). Columbia University Press.

Platt, M. (1986). Social norms and acquisition: A study of deictic verbs in Samoan child language. In B. Schieffelin & E. Ochs (Eds.), *Language socialization across cultures* (pp. 127–165). Cambridge University Press.

Poluha, E. (Ed.). (2007). *The world of girls and boys in rural and urban Ethiopia* (p. 69–90; 134–197). Forum for Social Studies.

Roer-Strier, D. (2001). Parental ethnotheories. Socialization in changing cultural contexts: A search for images of the 'Adaptive Adult'. *Social Work, 46*(3), 215–228.

Rosalso, M. (1982). The things we do with words: Ilongot speech acts and speech act theory in philosophy. *Language in Society, 11*(2), 203–237.

Rosen, C. (1989). Getting to know the Ethiopian Jews in Israel by means of their proverbs. *Social Sciences Information (SAGE, London), 28*(1), 145–159.

Rosenblum, S., Goldblatt, H., & Moin, V. (2008). The hidden dropout phenomenon among immigrant high-school students: The case of Ethiopian adolescents in Israel - A pilot study. *School Psychology International, 29*(1), 105–127.

Salamon, H. (1995). Metaphors as corrective exegesis: Three proverbs of the Beta-Israel. *Proverbium, 12*, 295–313.

Salamon, H., & Goldberg, H. E. (2012). Myth-ritual-symbol. *A Companion to Folklore, 37*, 119.

Shalom, S. (2016). *From Sinai to Ethiopia: The Halachic and conceptual world of Ethiopian Jewry*. Gefen.

Sterponi, L., & Bhattacharya, U. (2012). In Hymes' footsteps and beyond: Language socialization studies. *Language et Société, 1*, 67–82.

Tadesse, J. (2014). Positive parenting: An ethnographic study of storytelling for socialization of children in Ethiopia. *Storytelling, Self, Society, 10*(2), 156–176.

Tadesse, J. (2018). Folktales, reality and childhood in Ethiopia: How children construct social values through performance of folktales. *Folklore, 129*, 237–253. https://www.tandfonline.com/doi/full/10.1080/0015587X.2018.1449457

Tekolaa, B., Mersha, K., Fikirte, G., Charlotte, H., & Hoekstraa, R. (2020). Perceptions and experiences of stigma among parents of children with developmental disorders in Ethiopia: A qualitative study. *Social Science and Medicine, 256*. https://doi.org/10.1016/j.socscimed.2020.113034

Vygotsky, L. (1978). *Mind in society: The development of higher psychological processes* (p. 10–16; 19–51). Harvard University Press.

Wagaw, T. (1993). *For our souls: Ethiopian Jews in Israel* (p. 81). Wayne State University Press.

Weisner, T. (1998). Human development, child well-being and the cultural project of development. *New Directions for Child Development, 81*, 69–86.

Weisner, T. (2014). The socialization of trust: Plural caregiving and diverse pathways in human development across cultures. In H. Otto & H. Keller (Eds.), *Different faces of attachment: Cultural variation on a universal human need* (pp. 263–277). Cambridge University Press.

Weisner, T., & Gallimore, R. (2008). Child and sibling caregiving. In R. LeVine & R. New (Eds.), *Anthropology and child development: A cross-cultural reader* (pp. 264–269). Blackwell Publishing.

Wexler, B. (2006). *Brain and culture: Neurobiology, ideology and social change*. MIT Press.

Hebrew References

Ben-dor, S. (1985). Sacred places of Ethiopian Jews. *Peamim. Ben Zvi Institute, 22*, 32–52.

Bogale, Y. (1985). The schools of Beta Yisrael in Ethiopia. *Peamim. Ben Zvi Institute, 22*, 89–92.

Corinaldi, M. (1988). *Identity and traditions of Ethiopian Jews*. Reuven Mass.

Rosen, H. (1986). *Questions and answers about Ethiopian Jewish cultural behaviour*. Hadassah Women and the Ministry of Absorption.

Shmuel, N. (2010). *Educational traditions of Ethiopian Jewry: The dynamics of continuity and change*. Master's dissertation. Hebrew University of Jerusalem.

Weil, S. (1987). Yona Bogale leader of Beta Yisrael. *Peamim. Ben Zvi Institute, 33*, 144.

Ziv, Y. (2017). *Festival and holiday in the Ethiopian Jewish tradition of Beta Israel*. Ben Zvi Institute.

Chapter 4
Children's Wellbeing and Immigration

My sister and I were once immigrant children.[1] Did this experience change us? Definitely. Would our lives have been better or worse if we had never been immigrant children? Nobody can answer this, it is the proverbial path not taken. Perhaps it is a question all parents ask at one time or another: if we had done things differently… if we had gone somewhere else or stayed put… then what? Possibly these questions arise because immigration is never the child's choice, it is the responsible adults who decide, often with their children's future in mind, but with no guarantees. Undoubtedly the transition changes the child's life, it also changes families and their functioning in intricate and complex ways.

It is the changing context which is unsettling. Immigration, at whatever age, is forged into a child's life story as a defining event separating both time and space, indelibly marking the before and after. It is the precipitous transformation from settled to unsettled lives, disrupting cultural pathways, and presenting new challenges. Transition rocks the family boat, as family members react differently to their new surroundings. The cultural toolkit available may provide helpful means for coping with all this, at the same time certain culturally woven paths of action may be obstructive to integration (Swidler, 1986). It may take a lifetime to sort between them, understanding through trial and error what is effective and what is hindering to individual and family wellbeing in the new context. In the process of doing so the children of the second generation are growing up on unsteady ground, their moorings to the historical and cultural heritage of generations often effectively tethered. Circumstances will determine which cultural elements will survive in the long run, providing anchors into the future, what will be preserved or discarded in the new context. These circumstances include specific geographical, socio-political, and economic locations, local hierarchies and sub-cultures. Individuals and communities negotiate their new surroundings in the grey area between cultures

[1] My personal story is detailed in the foreword.

© The Author(s), under exclusive license to Springer Nature Switzerland AG 2023

N. A. Shmuel, *Children's Wellbeing in Immigrant Families*, Children's Well-Being: Indicators and Research 26,
https://doi.org/10.1007/978-3-031-31917-4_4

which includes perceptions of past and present, there and here, which can be more or less optimistic and empowering. These perceptions themselves are forged by experiences in the new surroundings, which can be welcoming and accepting of pluralism and difference or (more often) harshly rejecting all that is foreign.

This chapter will discuss firstly the diversity in the immigration experience and the idea of segmented assimilation. Afterwards follows a look at the nature of receiving contexts as amicable or hostile to newcomers, with an emphasis on the school context, followed by a brief discussion on the overrepresentation of immigrant children in special education. Finally, I will look at the family in which children of immigrants are growing up as the primordial context, using examples from research on various immigrant communities.

Before this it is important to relate to the context of migration itself, whether the family transition is voluntary (for whatever reasons) or forced by extenuating circumstances such as war, local conflict, man-made and natural disasters creating refugee populations. In the latter case, the transition seldom leads to a stable permanent new home, as issues of documentation, legal status, and local policy often create quite the opposite: a perpetual vulnerability and impermanence. The discussion in these pages is limited to voluntary legal migration and does not encompass the issue of refugees, which requires special consideration beyond the scope of this book.

4.1 Diversity in the Immigration Experience

While framing the immigration experience in context, it is useful to use the paradigm of segmented assimilation (Zhou, 1997; Portes et al., 2005; Alba & Foner, 2015) with the addition of the parameter of gender (Bueker, 2021), for better understanding the complexity of immigrant lives and opportunities in their host countries. Segmented assimilation focusses on the variability of the host society, specifically the socioeconomic hierarchy, and the potential for immigrants to integrate into different rungs of the ladder. Alba and Foner (2015) define integration as:

> entailing a variety of processes that both enhance the life chances of immigrants and result in increased levels of acceptance by the members of the receiving society.

In other words, the trajectory following immigration is dependent both on the host society's reaction towards and assistance to the immigrants, as well as their own individual and group agency. Thus, immigrants might integrate into the higher levels of society (upward mobility), or into marginal groups (downward mobility), or they might be absorbed into the comfortable middle class (Zhou, 1997). Which one of these scenarios is likely to apply to any specific family depends both on the receiving context, social and economic opportunities and individual capabilities such as levels of education, language proficiency, and aspirations.

Studies have shown a disproportionate representation of people of colour in marginalized groups, including second-generation immigrants whose ethnicity marks them as different even when born in the host country (Portes et al., 2005). An important part of segmented assimilation theory involves recognizing the structural variables that affect immigrant integration in the host countries (Zhou, 1997), which are themselves constantly changing, and include increasing internal divisions between rich and poor, peripheral and central areas, levels of educational and employment opportunities available, as well as often increasing xenophobia and overt or covert discrimination on the basis of colour, ethnicity, and gender. Both Zhou (1997) and Portes et al. (2005) have pointed out the significance of cohesive supportive communities to buffer both the effects of such discrimination on the second generation and the common inter-generational crisis which often accompanies immigration and subsequent role reversal and breakdown of parental authority. Such communities can provide valuable resources, encourage school attendance and positive expectations, as well as resilience and ethnic pride (Bueker, 2021).

Unsettled lives involve enhanced risks in which the stakes are high, and neither family nor community can definitively determine the outcome. In the positive trajectory, segmented assimilation may lead the second generation to educational accomplishments, gainful employment, and a bright future. In the negative trajectory the downhill spiral includes dropping out of school, premature childbearing, and altercations with the law which may result in imprisonment. These alternatives are not deliberately chosen paths, but the consequences of various constraints, limited opportunities, and misfortune (Portes et al., 2005).

The importance of segmented theory is in viewing the complexity of immigrant experiences, their pathways constricted and limited by historical, economic, and contextual factors. My personal immigrant experiences and my academic research with immigrants have taught me that any attempt to compartmentalize these experiences distorts their complexity. In other words, life is messy, perhaps especially so after immigration, and there are multiple ways in which people negotiate transition. One might say that the cultural mix in people's lives creates an intricate mesh of meanings and interpretations, that it can take a lifetime to situate oneself and organize strategies for action in dynamic, often confusing and overwhelming contexts in which newcomers are inevitably to some extent lost or likely to misread the map.

4.2 The Receiving Context

National immigration policies, local circumstances, and attitudes towards immigrants provide the new contexts into which immigrant families must settle and build their new lives. These new contexts vary between and within nations, and can be amicable or hostile, providing practical help and support or presenting challenges and obstacles in the path of acculturation and adjustment.

A recent study addressing these issues (Marks et al., 2018) found strong connections between macro-level contexts of multicultural policies and positive local integration approaches with overall wellbeing for G1.5 and G2 children. This study also mentions the evidence demonstrating that in many cases this wellbeing decreases over time spent in the United States or Canada (but not necessarily in Europe), perhaps contrary to the expectation that with time in the new country things get better rather than worse, especially for the new generation. The country with most positive multicultural policies and favourable attitudes towards immigrants was Sweden, also rated highest for children's wellbeing (of both native and immigrant children). The detrimental effects of perceptions of discrimination on the wellbeing of G1.5 and G2 children were also noted.

Discrimination and xenophobia can be powerful overt and covert forces in the lives of young immigrants, at the critical time when they are forming their own self-image and learning their place in society. Many studies have shown that more inclusive social attitudes, specifically appreciation and value of human diversity, create a social climate in which G1.5 and G2 children can develop viable hybrid identities which are conducive to their own wellbeing (for example: Marks et al., 2013; Dimitrova et al., 2015).

Many studies have shown a connection between immigrants' wellbeing and identity, for example Phinney et al. (2001) who discuss the balance between ethnic identity (based on the culture of origin) and national identity (of the receiving country) as forged by an interaction between the attitudes and characteristics of immigrants and the responses of the receiving society. They also conclude that a bicultural or hybrid identity is generally associated with higher levels of overall wellbeing, and that attaining such an identity is strongly influenced by the degree of pluralism accepted in the receiving institutions, especially the schools. While many countries seem to favour multicultural policies, these are not always implemented at the local level, where frequently an assimilationist attitude still prevails. An example of this is provided by Bitew and Ferguson (2011), who investigated the effect of cultural differences on sixteen secondary school students of Ethiopian origin from various schools in Melbourne, also interviewing parents and teachers in a qualitative study. Multicultural inclusive education has been the official policy in Australia since the 1970s, however its specific implementation may vary between different schools, and possibly not all teachers have sufficient training in this (McInerney & McInerney, 2003). Most of the students felt a significant cultural difference between school and home, primarily related to different cultural expectations. For example, the students were taught by their parents to be polite and obedient and not to speak unless spoken to, but at school they were expected to speak up in class and express their opinions. The ability of students to negotiate these differences was enhanced by flexible parental attitudes and by school environments appreciative of diversity. Part of the conclusion was that such contexts enable students to develop viable hybrid identities, and thus cope better both academically and socially. To be effective in the school context, this inclusive attitude must permeate all curriculum, multiculturalism being explicitly present as a positive theme in the school. Schools in which cultures are celebrated once a year do not fulfil this need, since on a day-to-day basis immigrant children are still struggling with the culture clash (Bitew and Ferguson).

The school context is instrumental in shaping the experiences of both immigrant children and the children of immigrants, as providing an environment inherently appreciative of diversity or intolerant and even hostile towards visible and expressed differences. Schools are social institutes which effectively encourage assimilation or biculturalism (Marks et al., 2019). The resultant experiences are instrumental in shaping children's educational prospects and wellbeing, which are more likely to be affirmative when hybridity is a viable option. This is dependent on both state or local policy and staff attitudes towards these issues. The question of teacher training arises; does this include anti-bias education and an awareness of how to create a classroom welcoming a heterogenous community? Is this dependent on local initiative or part of declared state policy? It also includes the question of attitudes towards immigrant parents, and efforts made by the school to facilitate communication despite possible language difficulties and differing cultural perceptions and expectations of parent–school relations. Children easily pick up on covert messages, respecting and including immigrant parents as part of the community of a school sends a clear message to the children on the value of their culture and traditions. It also helps create a passable bridge between home and school. A good example of this is the study by Delgado-Gaitan (1993), reflecting conflicting cultural values of Mexican immigrant families in America. The immigrants came from a cooperative traditional society where children were expected to be obedient and respectful to adults, very similar to the expectations of Ethiopian immigrant parents in Israel. Similarly, a child who expressed independent ideas was considered rude, children were not expected to enter adult conversations. But at school in America children were encouraged to use critical thinking, to express their opinions and ask questions based on knowledge and not age. Delgado-Gaitan found that parents who had participated in parenting classes were enabling their children to voice opinions and even argue with them, since they realized that these were skills their children needed to learn to compete with their peers at school.

Visibility is a powerful factor in school dynamics (Lomsky-Feder & Rappaport, 2010) providing extra challenges for dark-skinned children. There are subtle ways in which ethnicity and colour influence children's self-perception and define identity for the second generation struggling to belong. One example is provided by a study on immigrant children in a privileged white school in America (Bueker, 2021). Two of the G2 participants passed amongst their classmates as white (one the daughter of a North African immigrant, the other the daughter of an immigrant from Central America). In fact, this is a reminder that socially defined boundaries are often unclear, and as suggested by Boer (2006) people are in constant negotiation with them. The educational policy which entitled the girls in Bueker's study to attend a privileged white school, was less explicitly discussed by the children than internal school policies that might encourage an appreciation of diversity. Raising the question of general awareness to public policies shaping people's lives and their significance at the macro and micro levels.

Another example is a study on middle school children from Chinese immigrant families in America (Chen et al., 2019) which shows that by middle childhood children seemed to have partially internalized stereotypes of white Americans as societal ideals. Learning to position themselves in the social context they are growing up in—learning to understand social status—is an instrumental part of children's self-perception. The study concluded that children's awareness of their own social status and self-evaluation of this as low may be associated with negative feelings such as loneliness. A child's sense of self-worth and feeling of belonging are crucial factors influencing both their wellbeing and ability to learn. Support networks formed by peers and school staff can greatly contribute to this, as illustrated by a study on Chinese Canadian youth (Gagné et al., 2014).

The complexity of the immigration experience and its many variations requires a comprehensive look at multiple aspects of children's wellbeing and an ability to see children both in the context of transition and as agents in their own process of adjustment. To illustrate this, it is interesting to look at Sharples (2017) case study of one Ethiopian immigrant student in a London school. His analysis reflects how the primary problem seems to be conflicting mutual expectations (between teacher and student) rather than the often-assumed issue of language knowledge. To view the student's coping mechanism as an attempt to make sense of his new reality through past experiences, allows a perception of him as a person in transition who has not fully understood the subtle cultural codes of his new classroom. This proves much more helpful in finding solutions than any pre-defined knowledge about him as an immigrant or as an Ethiopian. This is an important message for teacher training programmes, to prepare educators with the professional and institutional ability to work with diversity and embrace it, to see immigrant children as people in the context of change, and not as representatives of an immigrant group. All these studies would suggest that national and school policies regarding multiculturalism and diversity, as well as teacher knowledge on coping successfully with a heterogenous classroom, are powerful factors shaping the experiences of immigrant children in schools.

4.3 Overrepresentation of Minority Students in Special Education

Many years ago, I remember reading the impressive research of Igoa (1995) encouraging educators to avoid testing and streaming children during their first year in a new country, with valuable practical insights for helping their adjustment. And yet decades later studies still suggest that this issue has far from been resolved. Dyson and Berhanu (2012) examined the overrepresentation of minority students in special education in Europe. Their findings indicate that children of minority ethnic groups, especially new immigrants, are more likely to be identified as in need of special education, especially if they are of poor socioeconomic status and male gender. Additionally, cases of children with general learning or social difficulties may often lead to referral to special education.

The issue of the overrepresentation of minorities in special education seems to be a problem in many countries. For example, Tefera and Fischman (2020) found an over-identification of students of colour in special education and overrepresentation of students of colour with disabilities being disciplined in the United States. Their findings stress the need to address wider contexts to understand this phenomenon, including historical legacies of inequality, education policies, and sociocultural contexts.

In Swedish schools the overrepresentation of minority students may not be a national phenomenon but is evident in large cities with a concentration of immigrant children (Berhanu, 2008). The reasons were found to be multiple, including the assessment procedures and criteria for referral and placement, which often include a cultural bias, language problems, lack of parental participation in decision-making, power relations, and institutional intransigence and prejudices.

With its diverse population, including many immigrants and children of immigrants, the Israeli educational system is extremely challenged to distinguish between cultural and linguistic differences, underachievement and learning difficulties (Gumpel & Sharoni, 2007). This is especially so with communities such as the Ethiopian Jews, many of whom arrived in Israel with little or no schooling and are often also of low socioeconomic status. Parents from this community tend to be suspicious of testing and categorization following past tendencies to label children struggling at school as ‘special needs’ or suffering from a ‘cultural deficit’.

It seems that often children from minority groups, especially immigrants and dark-skinned children, are more likely to be regarded as less capable or at risk and in need of institutional intervention. Engdau-Vanda (2020) explored the perceptions of risk as applied to children by social workers of families of Ethiopian immigrants in Israel. The findings indicate that the risk posed to children from the Ethiopian community, as perceived by the social workers charged with their treatment, tends to emerge at the intersection of four main contexts: the societal, the neighbourhood, the education system, and the welfare system. Like the cycle of poverty, children from minority groups are often caught in a perpetual cycle of risk. Engdau-Vanda suggests changing perspectives to break this cycle, taking into consideration other contexts forming the reality for these children who have become part of an immigrant minority, creating an awareness of institutional, political, historical, and social contexts as well as changing power relations.

In Israel, there have been many recent changes related to the inclusion of children with disabilities in the regular educational system (following an amendment to the law in 2002) and from 2018 parents have the right to choose the type of learning setting (regular class, special education class in a regular school or special education school) for a student who is eligible for special education services. Today there is an attempt to reduce the number of students in special classes and special schools and to increase the inclusion of children with special education needs in regular settings, not entirely without difficulties of implementation. This issue deserves more detailed consideration, which is out of the scope of this book, and has been presented briefly as an example of the intersection of educational policies, possible inherent bias, social power structures, and the vulnerability of children of minority groups, especially immigrants and their offspring.

4.4 Family Context

However well prepared for, emigrating with a family is a leap of faith. Of course, settled families also face uncertainties and surprises (pleasant and otherwise), the difference is primarily that being anchored in a community and having a cultural toolkit to fit the context makes coping with everything that much easier. Family members respond differently to the process of adjustment in their new society, during which time they may be more or less capable of being supportive to one another, sometimes overwhelmed by culture shock, separations, losses, the difficulties of the journey, and the struggle to survive economically and socially. How the adults in such situations manage the transition and negotiate between cultures sets the context for the incoming (or recently arrived) generation. The heterogeneity of the family itself expands to contain not only different generations, genders, ages, temperaments, and whatever cultures and languages they already possess, but also a new language and culture (and often sub-cultures) with all intricate accompanying baggage. The very fabric of family life, the intricacies of relationships, the form and effectivity of interpersonal communication, the prospective viability of intergenerational transferal, the extent of family cohesion, and coping methods for challenges and conflicts are all rattled, sometimes undermined, in the aftermath of immigration.

To illustrate this, it is interesting to look at a study on Korean immigrant families in America (Ben Park, 2003) which found that it was not the inter-generational conflict itself that was damaging to the children as much as the fact that it was prologued and unresolved. The children found this stressful, leading to depression and low self-esteem. Like my findings with the Ethiopian immigrants in Israel, the second generation had little communication with their parents and tended to either suppress their needs or do as they please without consulting their parents. The gap between the generations was forged out of different life experiences after immigration. One of the examples given in this study is different world views based on collectivist as opposed to individualistic outlooks, coupled with the change from a hierarchical to a democratic society. Differing and often clashing values and expectations make communication between the generations difficult, this varying with the parents' levels of education, employment, knowledge of English, and general adaptation to the new cultural context. Like my own findings, it seems that the more culturally flexible the parents, the more likely it is that the children can adopt hybrid identities, more beneficial to their own wellbeing.

The divide between collectivist as opposed to individualistic outlooks has come up in many studies of immigrant families from Latin America, Asia, or Africa, residing in the West (for example, Chao, 2001; Lim & Lim, 2004; Driscoll et al., 2008; Jambunathan et al., 2000; Roopnarine et al., 2006). Families from these countries are usually used to a culture of community-based child raising, based on cooperative rather than individualistic ideologies and enhanced by hierarchical relations defining relative status in society and in the family. Families in such cohesive communities benefit from multiple caregivers, enhancing shared values and traditions as collective heritage, while children learn their sense of worth, identity, and belonging as part of the collective.

In most of these communities parenting styles tend to be authoritarian—stressing obedience and coercion (parental authority based on status), rather than authoritative—stressing autonomy and self-regulation (parental authority based on connection). The transition of such families to Western countries brings two opposing value systems into direct conflict, how each family copes with this dilemma and the resulting context for the G2 children is of the utmost importance for their development and wellbeing. Let us look at some examples from these countries.

In a study on Arabic speaking migrant families in Melbourne (Renzaho et al., 2011), parents continued to expect obedience from their children and complained that Australian children had too much freedom. Their attempts to limit their children led to frequent conflict, sometimes to the point of disconnection. The parents felt they were losing control of their children yet fear of Australian law against corporal punishment prevented them from taking action. An alternative often chosen was an attempt to regain control through material means, such as giving presents. In another study, on West Indian immigrants in America (Waters & Sykes, 2009) found that authoritarian parenting, corporal punishment, and expectations of children to be respectful and obedient were common practice regardless of social class. Even the second generation expressed an acceptance of corporal punishment as part of their child-rearing practices, but many also said they would 'tone it down', communicate more with their children, and show more affection than their parents had. The researchers concluded that the second generation are more likely to combine parenting methods from both cultures.

Both these examples seem to indicate that parents are seeking solutions from within a hierarchical paradigm in which parental authority is based on status, without examining the basic premise that children should be obedient, and adults should have ultimate control. An alternative model for parental authority, based on connection, does not seem to come into consideration. Parental interpretation of children's behaviour based on culturally specific parental ethnotheories determines parental reactions. This can be clarified by another study (Trommsdorff, 2006) comparing Japanese parenting with German parenting, in which disobedience was regarded by the German parents as a threat to their authority and led to conflicts between parents and children. Whereas Japanese parents interpreted disobedience as immaturity and reacted with leniency. Parental goals in the two cultures were also different: the Japanese parents emphasized family harmony, while the German parents emphasized independence and maturity. Often the contradiction between an expectation of obedience and independence leads to increased conflicts as children get older.

There is a large population of Chinese immigrants in America. Vu et al. (2019) found greater behavioural participation in American culture was associated with more positive psychological wellbeing, which was associated with less reported engagement in authoritarian parenting and more authoritative parenting. In other words, the ability of mothers to adopt a hybrid, American Chinese identity, gaining competence and efficacy in both cultures, has positive outcomes for their wellbeing and subsequently their parenting capabilities. In comparison to American parents,

Chinese immigrant parents in America are often considered strict, expecting obedience and frequently using punishment. And yet their children do very well in school. Gorman (1998) set out to understand this paradox and discovered that although Chinese parents did have high expectations of their children, they also gave them autonomy in making decisions. Chinese mothers based their parenting on traditional values but were flexible and considerate of the children's new environment. Gorman found that contrary to common perceptions, Chinese parents were involved and affectionate, often using covert means for passing on their beliefs or guidance to avoid direct cultural conflict. The parents spoke to the child's logic rather than using force, they were encouraging them to function effectively in two cultures. In another study of Chinese immigrants in Canada, Lam (2005) found that the parents raised their children to collective responsibility and encouraged them to see their good grades at school as beneficial to the whole family. In this case, traditional values were harnessed for successful acculturation. Many immigrant parents are aware of the need to be flexible, to integrate elements of the two cultures, for example in a study of educated Chinese mothers in America (Cheah et al., 2013) they were found to use less punishment and more conversations, encouraging independence.

These examples demonstrate how immigrant parents are often able to harness specific cultural strategies and find creative solutions to maintain influence in their children's lives while avoiding direct conflict, perhaps having accepted that children adjusting to a new environment require different, more flexible, and supportive parenting. There are more examples of this, for instance in a qualitative study of Mexican immigrants in America (Perreira et al., 2006) the narratives revealed the creative means used by families to create inter-generational communication and empathy as joint pathways for solving together the challenges of adolescents after immigration. Similarly, qualitative research on families of Japanese origin in America (Usita & Blieszner, 2002) found that there were many coping mechanisms used by Japanese immigrant mothers and daughters to maintain their relationship after immigration, such as using humour, or a third party, or girls who actively taught their mothers English or repeated things that they said to make sure they had understood each other. In all these families both parents and children are active agents in maintaining inter-generational connection.

A supportive community provides a sense of protection and reciprocity (Maholmes, 2014) but it can also be an 'immigrant island' in which the opportunities for integration are limited and immigrants feel marginalized. Bueker (2021) talks of the immigrant family and community as an asset, providing support and enhancing resilience, but also as potentially limiting, as cultural expectations may restrict opportunities for girls. Thus, concentrated communities of immigrants provide advantages and disadvantages, as illustrated by a study on Chinese immigrants in America (Zhou, 2009) which found that while ethnic social and cultural institutions reinforce traditional parental expectations, they also enable immigrant youth to interact and share their frustrations in a protective, supporting environment.

Immigrant families might be struggling, but are also resourceful, and it might be wise not to forge generalizations about parenting based on culture, but to remember that there is variety and change within and not only between different cultural groups. This has been stressed by Lau (2010) who studied Chinese immigrants in America and warns of the misconceptions caused by generalizations about culturally based parenting, since each family is different and forges their own coping methods, sometimes using cultural values to protect their offspring and not necessarily endanger them. It seems essential to consider multiple contexts influencing immigrant children and the children of immigrants, and not make assumptions based on limited information and characterization of parenting methods according to cultural traditions. If children are struggling, more often than not the reasons are embedded in a combination of factors within and outside the home.

References

Alba, R., & Foner, N. (2015). *Strangers no more: Immigration and the challenges of integration in North America and Western Europe* (p. 5). Princeton University Press.

Ben Park, B. C. (2003). Intergenerational conflict in Korean immigrant homes and its effects on children's psychological Well-being. *Journal of Intergenerational Relationships, 1*(3), 73–93.

Berhanu, G. (2008). Ethnic minority pupils in Swedish schools: Some trends in over-representation of minority pupils in special educational programs. *International Journal of Special Education, 23*(3), 17–29.

Bitew, G., & Ferguson, P. (2011). The Ethiopian adolescent and the effect of cultural difference on immigrant students' learning. *Diaspora, Indigenous, and Minority Education, 5*(1), 1–16. https://doi.org/10.1080/15595692.2010.534398

Boer, E. (2006). *Uncertain territories: Boundaries in cultural analysis*. Rodopi.

Bueker, C. (2021). "It's Because You Don't See Yourself as Unequal to Anybody": Exploring the segmented assimilation model in the experiences of 1.5- and 2nd-generation women in an Elite Public High School. *Journal of International Migration and Integration, 22*, 791–807.

Chao, R. K. (2001). Extending research on the consequences of parenting style for Chinese Americans and European Americans. *Child Development, 72*(6), 1832–1843.

Chen, S. H., Gleason, T. R., Wang, M. M., Liu, C. H., & Wang, L. K. (2019). Perceptions of social status in Chinese American children: Associations with social cognitions and socioemotional well-being. *Asian American Journal of Psychology, 10*(4), 362. https://doi.org/10.1037/aap0000161

Cheah, C. S., Leung, C. Y., & Zhou, N. (2013). Understanding "tiger parenting" through the perceptions of Chinese immigrant mothers: Can Chinese and US parenting coexist? *Asian American Journal of Psychology, 4*(1), 30.

Delgado-Gaitan, C. (1993). Parenting in two generations of Mexican American families. *International Journal of Behaviour Development, 16*(3), 409–427.

Dimitrova, R., Aydinli, A., Chasiotis, A., Bender, M., & Van de Vijver, F. J. (2015). Heritage identity and maintenance enhance well- being of Turkish- Bulgarian and Turkish- German adolescents. *Social Psychology, 46*(2), 93–103.

Driscoll, A. K., Russell, S. T., & Crockett, L. J. (2008). Parenting styles and youth well-being across immigrant generations. *Journal of Family Issues, 29*(2), 185–209.

Dyson, A., & Berhanu, G. (2012). Special education in Europe, overrepresentation of minority students. In J. Banks (Ed.), *Encyclopedia of diversity* (pp. 2070–2073). Sage Publications.

Engdau-Vanda, S. (2020). The circular construction of "risk" for children of oppressed groups: Israeli social workers' perspectives on children of Ethiopian origin. *Child and Family Social Work, 25*(3), 602–610.

Gagné, M., Shapka, J., & Law, D. (2014). Moving beyond grades: The social and emotional well-being of Chinese Canadians at School. *Asian American Journal of Psychology, 5*(4), 373–382.

Gorman, J. (1998). Parenting attitudes and practices of immigrant Chinese mothers of adolescents. *Family Relations, 47*(1), 73–80.

Gumpel, T., & Sharoni, V. (2007). Current best practices in learning disabilities in Israel. *Learning Disabilities Research and Practice, 22*(3), 202–209.

Igoa, C. (1995). *The inner world of the immigrant child.* Laurence Erlbaum Associates Publishers.

Jambunathan, S., Burts, D. C., & Pierce, S. (2000). Comparisons of parenting attitudes among five ethnic groups in the United States. *Journal of Comparative Family Studies, 31*(4), 395–406.

Lau, A. (2010). Physical discipline in Chinese American immigrant families: An adaptive cultural perspective. *Cultural Diversity and Ethnic Minority Psychology, 16*(3), 313–322.

Lam, C. (2005). Chinese construction of adolescent development outcome: Themes discerned in a qualitative study. *Child and Adolescent Social Work Journal, 22*(2), 111–131.

Lim, S. L., & Lim, B. K. (2004). Parenting style and child outcomes in Chinese and immigrant Chinese families-current findings and cross-cultural considerations in conceptualization and research. *Marriage and Family Review, 35*(3–4), 21–43.

Maholmes, V. (2014). *Fostering resilience and wellbeing in children and families in poverty: Why hope still matters*. Oxford University Press.

Marks, A., Godoy, C., & Garcia Coll, C. (2013). An ecological approach to understanding immigrant child and adolescent developmental competencies. In L. Gershoff, R. Mistry, & D. Crosby (Eds.), *The contexts of child development* (pp. 75–89). Oxford University Press.

Marks, A., McKenna, J., & Garcia Coll, C. (2018). National immigration receiving contexts: A critical aspect of native-born, immigrant, and refugee youth well-being. *European Psychologist, 23*(1), 6.

Marks, A., Woolverton, G., & García Coll, C. (2019). Children's migratory paths between cultures: The effects of migration experiences on the adjustment of children and families. In R. Parke & G. Elder Jr. (Eds.), *Children in changing worlds: Sociocultural and temporal perspectives* (pp. 112–130). Cambridge University Press. https://doi.org/10.1017/9781108264846.005

McInerney, V., & McInerney, D. (2003). Multiculturalism in New South Wales Australia: A retrospective and prospective view. In *Teaching, learning and motivation in a multicultural context* (pp. 193–222). Information Age. http://handle.uws.edu.au:8081/1959.7/22078

Perreira, K. M., Chapman, M. V., & Stein, G. L. (2006). Becoming an American parent: Overcoming challenges and finding strength in a new immigrant Latino community. *Journal of Family Issues, 27*(10), 1383–1414.

Phinney, J., Horenczyk, G., Liebkind, K., & Vedder, P. (2001). Ethnic identity, immigration, and well-being: An interactional perspective. *Journal of Social Issues, 57*(3), 493–510.

Portes, A., Fernandez-Kelly, P., & Haller, W. (2005). Segmented assimilation on the ground: The new second generation in early adulthood. *Ethnic and Racial Studies., 28*(6), 1000–1040.

Renzaho, A., McCabe, M., & Sainsbury, W. (2011). Parenting, role reversals and the preservation of cultural values among Arabic speaking migrant families in Melbourne, Australia. *International Journal of Intercultural Relations, 35*(4), 416–424.

Roopnarine, J. L., Krishnakumar, A., Metindogan, A., & Evans, M. (2006). Links between parenting styles, parent–child academic interaction, parent–school interaction, and early academic skills and social behaviours in young children of English-speaking Caribbean immigrants. *Early Childhood Research Quarterly, 21*(2), 238–252.

Sharples, R. (2017). Local practice, translocal people: Conflicting identities in the multilingual classroom. *Language and Education, 31*(2), 169–183.

Swidler, A. (1986). Culture in action: Symbolism and strategies. *Americal sociological review, 51*(2), 273–286.

Tefera, A. A., & Fischman, G. E. (2020). How and why context matters in the study of racial disproportionality in special education: Toward a critical disability education policy approach. *Equity and Excellence in Education, 53*(4), 433–448.

Trommsdorff, G. (2006). Parent-child relations over the life span: A cross-cultural perspective. In K. Rubin & O. Boon Chung (Eds.), *Parenting beliefs, behaviours, and parent-child relations: A cross cultural perspective* (pp. 143–184). Psychology Press.

Usita, P. M., & Blieszner, R. (2002). Immigrant family strengths: Meeting communication challenges. *Journal of Family Issues, 23*(2), 266–286.

Vu, K., Castro, K., Cheah, C., & Yu, J. (2019). Mediating and moderating processes in the associations between Chinese immigrant mothers' acculturation and parenting styles in the United States. *Asian American Journal of Psychology, 10*(4), 307.

Waters, C., & Sykes, J. (2009). Spare the rod, ruin the child? First and second generation West Indian childrearing practices. In N. Foner (Ed.), *Across generations immigrant families in America* (pp. 72–97). NYU.

Zhou, M. (1997). Segmented assimilation: Issues, controversies, and recent research on the new second generation. *The International Migration Review., 31*(4), 975–1008.

Zhou, M. (2009). Conflict, coping and reconciliation: Intergenerational relations in Chinese immigrant families. In N. Foner (Ed.), *Across generations immigrant families in America* (pp. 21–46). NYU.

Hebrew References

Lomsky-Feder, E., & Rappaport, T. (Eds.). (2010). *Visibility in immigration, body, outlook, representation* (pp. 43–67). Hakkibutz Hameuchad and the Van Leer Institute.

Chapter 5
The Israeli Context

Israel is a very small country, about the same size as the fourth smallest American state New Jersey. Israel has existed for only 74 years, during which it has suffered eight wars with neighbouring states, two major Palestinian uprisings, and constant terrorist attacks. The historical narratives to explain all this are far beyond the scope of this book, but there are aspects of Israeli reality that are important to understand before discussing the experiences of Jewish Ethiopian immigrant families in Israel. This chapter will give the background on Israeli demographics, previous immigrations, and the sub-cultures of Israeli society to clarify the complicated context into which these new immigrants arrived.

5.1 Israeli Demography

Israeli society is extremely diverse, containing about 70% Jews, 23% Muslims, 1.5% Christians, 1.6% Druze, and 3% not classified by religion (Roer-Strier & Nadan, 2020). The Jewish population into which the Ethiopian Jewish immigrants have been received comprises national religious, orthodox, ultra-orthodox, and secular people, some of them native Israelis[1] others new immigrants or the offspring of immigrants. The educational system in Israel is tailored to cater for these different groups, in the Jewish sector parents can choose schools based on geographic location and religious or other preferences, thus the schools are national religious, orthodox, ultra-orthodox, secular, or private (such as anthroposophical, democratic, or bilingual schools). Israel has one of the highest concentrations of boarding

[1] The term 'native Israelis' is used throughout the book to denote children born in the host country. Children of immigrants are referred to as second generation or G2.

© The Author(s), under exclusive license to Springer Nature Switzerland AG 2023

N. A. Shmuel, *Children's Wellbeing in Immigrant Families*, Children's Well-Being: Indicators and Research 26,
https://doi.org/10.1007/978-3-031-31917-4_5

schools and educational institutions, including youth villages, agricultural and technical schools, and yeshivas (Roer-Strier & Nadan, 2020).

Aside from the country's political and security issues, Israel suffers from extreme overpopulation (Alon, 2016), and in the long term this very small country will not be able to sustain its inhabitants comfortably. Israel's current population is 9.5 million (according to the Central Bureau of Statistics 2022), making Israel significantly more congested than other OECD[2] countries. The population has increased tremendously both through immigration and high birth-rates (in most Western countries, this is 1.6 children per family, in Israel this is 3). As Alon (2016) explains, this is a very difficult topic to talk about in Israel for various reasons. Firstly, large families (with 4–10 children) are very common in certain communities—ultra-orthodox Jews, Arabs, and Bedouins—but to mention this is often considered cultural bias or discrimination. Secondly, history makes this a very sensitive point, as many Jews feel an obligation to produce more Jews in place of those killed in the Holocaust. Thirdly, having many children is a highly valued prerogative with deep religious and political implications for many Jews in Israel. Fourthly, Jewish immigration, termed in Hebrew *Aliyah* which literally means ascent, has been positively encouraged since the forming of the state.

But overpopulation has very damaging long-term ecological and sociological results, which Alon (2016) has detailed, and I will be briefly outline here. Overpopulation increases existing inequalities and enhances poverty. The average percentage of people under the poverty line in developed countries according to the OECD is 13.3, in Israel this is over 20%, and 28.8% of Israel's children. A series of social problems detrimental to people's standard of living is affecting all Israelis. Road congestion which creates long, annoying traffic jams costing both time and money, an acute housing shortage and a reduction in the quality of public services. The medical system has undergone various crisis exacerbated by the Covid pandemic; hospitals are consistently working over-capacity reducing the quality of care. Children are attending schools in classrooms with 28–40 pupils, reducing their level of education, increasing levels of violence in schools and generally damaging the learning experience of many children. The courts are so clogged that it may take people years to get responses to appeals or resolutions for court cases. The damaging effects of overpopulation are already keenly felt by everyone.

Since the founding of Israel in 1948, the country has been struggling with the intricate often volatile friction between its diverse communities, to which can be added socioeconomic inequalities as well as the tension between official and fringe cultures. Political struggles reflecting different opinions primarily on the desired nature and borders of Israel, as well as economic strategies and the relations between state and religion, coupled with constant terrorist threats and attacks on Israel's borders, have created great rifts in the fabric of Israeli society.

To better understand the context into which the Ethiopian immigrants have arrived, what follows is a brief historical overview of previous immigrations and the

[2] The Organisation for Economic Co-operation and Development.

dominant policies in their integration. After this will come an explanation on the various divisions and sub-cultures of Israeli society, and a short discussion on racism in Israel.

5.2 Immigration to Israel

Historical context to immigration in Israel provides valuable insights into the formation of the various segments of Israeli society and the subsequent interaction between them. This not precluding the indigenous populations living in Israel before the formation of the state: Palestinians (mostly Muslim), Christians, Druze, and mostly Sephardic Jews. The first Aliyah (1882–1903) were Zionist immigrants from Russia, Eastern Europe, France, and Germany, and a small group from Yemen. Most of these immigrants settled primarily in Jaffa, Jerusalem, and Haifa as well as establishing twenty new Hebrew agricultural settlements (Ram, 2016). The British who occupied the Land of Israel between 1917 and 1948 were very influential in shaping the political and judicial systems. The second Aliyah (1904–1914) brought 40–50,000 Russian, Lithuanian, and Polish Jews, about 16% of these Zionist pioneers eager to set up new settlements and revive the Hebrew language. About half of these immigrants did not remain in Israel, where conditions at the time were very challenging (Alon, 2016). The Third Aliyah (1917–1923) came from Eastern Europe with a predominantly socialist and nationalist disposition. Following this came the Fourth Aliyah (1924–1928) with 60,000 Jews from Poland, and Fifth Aliyah (1929–1939) with 300,000 Jews from Europe, many of them escaping Nazi persecution. Between 1948 (the establishment of the State of Israel) and 1950, a further one million Jews from the Middle East and North Africa (Morocco, Algeria, and Tunisia) arrived in Israel, many of them being settled in development towns and makeshift immigrant camps in peripheral areas (Ram, 2016). The documentary film 'Salach here is the land of Israel' directed by David Deri (2017) uncovers the blatantly racist and paternalistic attitude of the establishment towards the immigrants from these countries, who were seen as culturally inferior.

During the following years, the Ashkenazi-Sephardic divide would become acutely prevalent (Ashkenazi being Jews of European origin and Sephardic being Jews of Middle Eastern or North African origin) based on the lethal combination of discrimination, inequalities, and politics. Dahan-Kalev (2001b) details her own experiences growing up as the daughter of Moroccan immigrants, and the extent to which her culture of origin was undervalued by the mainstream, which blatantly rejected her rich cultural heritage, absent from school textbooks, and detrimentally misrepresented in academic studies on which absorption policies were based.

The melting-pot ideology was inherently biased to mould the new Israelis in the image of the Ashkenazi white secular Jews who were in power at the time (Ben-Eliezer, 2008). The idea that in the long run ethnic differences would disappear has been thwarted by reality, in which a common essentialist perspective often diminishes identity into a narrow definition of origins. In 1971, second-generation immigrants from North Africa and Middle Eastern countries founded the Black Panther Movement, protesting discrimination against their families and communities. Research by Sagiv (2014) with the offspring of Ashkenazi-Sephardic bi-cultural marriages, based on life narratives, includes painful accounts of the struggles experienced today in Israeli society. One of her conclusions is that Israeli society is still often bound by dichotomous distinctions, struggling to accept the intricacy and dynamics of diversity *within* people's identities.

Absorption policies in Israel have never been uniform for all immigrants but adapted to each group according to a local perception of their capacity to stand up for their rights coupled with assumptions on their resources and ability to cope. Thus, in the 1950s, immigrants from North Africa were sent to development towns which until today remain somewhat neglected peripheral areas, Russian immigrants arriving in the 1980s and 90s were given absorption basket grants for 'direct absorption', while Ethiopian immigrants arriving during those same years were set for a track of centralized absorption. This latter meant being allocated homes in absorption centres which monitored and assisted in their process of integration (Ben-Eliezer, 2008). This differentiation was officially justified as necessary because of the limited resources of the immigrants coming from Africa, but it was often associated with a basic premise of their inherent inability to negotiate their own absorption because of cultural inferiority. Ben-Eliezer (2008) describes many hair-raising examples of institutional and daily racism against Ethiopian immigrants, not as a consorted plan but as an effective reality. This is an important distinction, since I personally worked in both the Jewish Agency and the Ministry of Absorption, I find it necessary to say that there were many good, honestly caring people who went out of their way to help immigrants and make them feel welcome, regardless of where they came from.

An overwhelming majority of the immigrant youth from Ethiopia were sent to vocational religious boarding schools, separated by gender, irrespective of their abilities or wishes. They were introduced to one version of being Israeli, patriotic and religious, although many boarding schools were overwhelmingly occupied by Ethiopian immigrants and therefore not a platform for intermingling. Ben-Eliezer (2008) cites the Brookdale report from 1998 in which 6.2% of the Ethiopian immigrant youth aged 14–17 were not attending school, twice as many as in the general population, with 20% dropping out during middle school. The actual figures are probably much higher.

The Rabbinical establishment in Israel initially did not accept the authority of the Kesouch as spiritual leaders, undermining their status and contributing to the unravelling of community support networks. Recently,

> After over three decades of struggle, Israel has decided to recognize the Kessim as spiritual leaders and accept them into the religious establishment. Ethiopian Rabbis will thus be merged into local religious councils and given the authority to provide religious service. (Ynet 19.2.2018, my translation).

Ben-Eliezer (2008) cites other examples of government policies with long-term detrimental effects on the Ethiopian community. The special mortgages including partial grants to enable families to become homeowners effectively facilitated the purchase of apartments mostly in poor, peripheral areas, some of which soon became predominantly Ethiopian. The humiliating symbolic conversion expected of Ethiopian immigrants due to 'doubts' about their Jewishness was never expected of Russian immigrants, 30% of whom were not considered to be Jewish.

The crux of discriminatory behaviour towards Ethiopian immigrants came in 1996 with the uncovering of the Ministry of Health policy of discarding blood donated by Ethiopian immigrants and their descendants on the pretext that they might have aids. This was a definitive break in confidence between the Ethiopian community and the Israeli establishment, leading to violent public demonstrations.[3]

Ethiopian Jews arrived in Israel to meet both a very diverse and conflictual society, in which the general image of people from Africa was forged by popular stereotypes of naïve, overly sensitive immigrants (Salamon, 2003; Bar-Yoseph, 2013). Some of the common reactions to the protests against racism by younger Ethiopian Israelis reflect the perception of losing innocence and authenticity (Noyes, 2012).

5.3 Sub-cultures in Israel

The segmented parts of society are not mutually exclusive but overlap and interact with one another, thus ethnicity, gender, and poverty when combined enhance experienced bias and inequality. This has been widely discussed as *intersectionality* (Crenshaw, 1989a, 1989b; McCall, 2005). In Israeli society this has been described eloquently by Dahan-Kalev (2001a) regarding daughters of immigrants from Islamic and Arab countries and their experiences as women in the predominantly Ashkenazi feminist movement.[4]

Dichotomous paradigms distort the compelxity of reality, in which identities are both multiple and dynamic. For example religiosity and secularism in Israel have fuzzy boundaries, although as Shavit and Shavit (2016) describe, they represent specific subcultures. The difference between them rests not only on the priority given to religion or state, but the function of these and the existence of other elements specific to each sub-culture, defined as Israeli-Jewish or Jewish-Israeli. These sub-systems are each in themselves dynamic, with their own values and group narratives. In fact, the very definition of what it means to be Jewish or to be Israeli are constantly undergoing changes and subject to volatile public debate. Part of this involves disagreements regarding the actual and desired relationship between Jewish law and civic law. The very definition of the purpose and desired form of the Jewish State is often brought into question in these arguments. As Shavit and Shavit point out, there is no central Jewish authority that all Jews in Israel agree upon

[3] More on this in Chap. 14.

[4] To be discussed further in the chapter on gender.

regarding questions of Jewish Halacha or definitions of desirable cultural practices. While the two sub-cultures—Israeli-Jewish or Jewish-Israeli—exist apart from one another they are in a constant struggle for spheres of influence. Not only this, but in-between the two are many people who appropriate elements from both sub-cultures and often call themselves *traditionalists*. For many secular Israelis, Jewish culture devoid of religious content is a viable entity based on a shared narrative, history, and affiliation, appropriating components of traditional Judaism and adding new elements. Most specifically during the creation of the nation this was the vision to forge a new *Israeli* cultural identity. Reviving the Hebrew language was part of this process. Thus, being Israeli encompasses a vast array of identities and affiliations, which cannot be reduced to definitive qualities or characteristics.

In June 2015, President Reuven Rivlin gave his famous 'four tribes' speech at the 15th Annual Herzliya Conference, in which he urged all Israelis to recognize the reality of what he called 'the new Israeli order' of the country reflected in its demography: 38% secular Jews, 15% national religious Jews, and roughly 25% Arabs, and 25% Ultra-orthodox. Rivlin said that effectively Israel no longer has a clear majority or minority, but these four 'tribes' that must find a way to reconcile their differences and share the land for Israel to be economically viable and secure its future.

> The 'new Israeli order' is not a creative sociological differentiation; it is, rather, a reality with far-reaching consequences for our national strength, for the future of us all. (Rivlin speech).

The four tribes must find a way of getting to know and trust one another to share accountability, provide security to each sector (none need relinquish their identity), share responsibility, and strive for equity and equality. In Rivlin's vision, only together can they create a new *Israeliness*.

Epstein (2016) has described Israel as 'an archipelago of isolated communities' each connected to 'different centres of influence' outside of Israel. He also states the obvious fact that Israel needs something more to unite its population than a common enemy, and proposes a common culture, citing some interesting examples of 'mutually enriching dialogue' between communities.

People who live in Israel are used to rapid drastic daily changes, alternately bearing hope or depair, depending on one's perspective. In 2018, the Israeli parliament approved a law officially proclaiming Israel as the Nation-State of the Jewish People. What upset many people, especially Druze and other minorities, was that this statement felt like a way of officially shutting them out of the mainstream and was not affiliated with an obligation to the equal rights of all citizens, as appears in the declaration of independence.

When leaving office, Rivlin accentuated his message:

> I say today: the different tribes of Israeli society are here to stay. We must always ensure that in the natural tension between statehood and tribalism it is the state, the republic, which prevails over cultural autonomy and communal tribalism. (Rivlin speech in the Knesset July 2021).

Unfortunately, in the current political climate it appears that quite the opposite is happening. Shenhav and Yona (2008) provide plenty of examples of all forms of racism in Israeli society, institutional, cultural and in public interactions, questioning the lack of academic discussion on this. Perhaps this latter stems from the unease of admitting that the Jewish state, created on the embers of the Holocaust, contains overt and covert racism. Certainly, the current Israeli reality (January 2023) in which the recently formed Government had to circumvent the 1985 law prohibiting political parties which incite to racism so it could include explicitly racist and homophobic candidates, racism in Israel can no longer be denied or explained away as temporary pathologies (Ben-Eliezer, 2008).

References

Alon, T. (2016). *The land is full: Addressing overpopulation in Israel*. Yale University Press.

Crenshaw, K. (1989a). *Demarginalizing the intersection of race and sex: A black feminist critique of antidiscrimination doctrine, feminist theory and antiracist politics* (pp. 139–167). University of Chicago Legal Forum.

Crenshaw, K. (1989b). Mapping the margins: Intersectionality, identity politics, and violence against women of color. *Stanford Law Review, 43*, 1241.

Dahan-Kalev, H. (2001a). Tensions in Israeli feminism: The Mizrachi Ashkenazi rift. *Women's Studies International Forum, 24*(6), 669–684.

Dahan-Kalev, H. (2001b). You're So Pretty—You Don't Look Moroccan. *Israel Studies, 6*(1), 1–14.

Epstein, A. (2016). Israeli culture(s) today: Globalized Archipelago of isolated communities. In E. Ben-Rafael, J. H. Schoeps, Y. Sternberg, O. Glöckner, & A. Weberling (Eds.), *Handbook of Israel: Major debates* (pp. 77–86). Walter de Gruyter GmbH & Co KG.

McCall, L. (2005). The complexity of intersectionality. *Signs, 30*, 1771–1800.

Noyes, D. (2012). The social base of folklore. In R. Bendix & G. Hasan-Rokem (Eds.), *A companion to folklore* (pp. 15–39). Blackwell Publishing.

Ram, U. (2016). Hebrew culture in Israel: Between Europe, the Middle East, and America. In E. Ben-Rafael, J. H. Schoeps, Y. Sternberg, O. Glöckner, & A. Weberling (Eds.), *Handbook of Israel: Major debates* (pp. 60–74). Walter de Gruyter GmbH & Co KG.

Roer-Strier, D., & Nadan, Y. (2020). Introduction: The Israeli stage for context-informed perspective on child risk and protection. In D. Roer-Strier & Y. Nadan (Eds.), *Context-informed perspectives of child risk and protection in Israel* (pp. 1–12). Springer's Child Maltreatment Series.

Salamon, H. (2003). Blackness in transition: Decoding racial constructs through stories of Ethiopian Jews. *Journal of Folklore Research, 40*(1), 3–32.

Shavit, Z., & Shavit, Y. (2016). Israeli culture today: How Jewish? How Israeli? In E. Ben-Rafael, J. H. Schoeps, Y. Sternberg, O. Glöckner, & A. Weberling (Eds.), *Handbook of Israel: Major debates* (pp. 22–38). Walter de Gruyter GmbH & Co KG.

Hebrew References

Bar-Yoseph, A. (2013). *Villa in the jungle: Africa in Israeli culture*. Van Leer Institute and the Kibbutz Hameuchad.

Ben-Eliezer, U. (2008). Cushi sambi bilibilibambo: How a Jew becomes black in the promised land. In Y. Shenhav & Y. Yona (Eds.), *Racism in Israel* (pp. 130–159). Van Leer Institute and the Kibbutz Hameuchad.

Sagiv, T. (2014). *On the fault line: Israelis of mixed ethnicity*. Hakibbutz Hameuchad.

Shenhav, Y., & Yona, Y. (2008). *Racism in Israel* (pp. 13–47). Van Leer Institute and the Kibbutz Hameuchad.

Chapter 6
The Journey from Ethiopia to Israel

I once took my youngest son and his cousin to a play depicting the journey of the Ethiopian Jews from Ethiopia to Sudan to reach Israel. Both children were about eight years old and very moved by the play. As we came out of the theatre, I heard my son telling his cousin that his father also made this journey by foot. She looked at him in awe, 'your mother too', I told her, to which she answered astonished '*really*'?

Every immigrant family and community have a story about their journey, where they came from and why. In the case of the Ethiopian Jews, it is often a tale of heroism and loss, Zionism and the sacrifices made to arrive. The story includes the children born on the way or just after arrival, family history now being split between *before* Aliyah and *after* Aliyah, as definitive periods of time denoting the transformative power of transition. Children of the second generation will only have knowledge about this if they are explicitly *told* or the narrative of the journey is shared in family gatherings. The way it is told, or the absence of the story altogether, shapes their understanding of the world and of their parents and other family members. This is the historical context of their childhood, at a fragile meeting point with other contexts now forged by the country they are living in. As I shall explain in this chapter, these changing contexts, and the way the adults caring for them negotiate them, will form the soil in which they grow.

6.1 Immigration from Ethiopia

The chronology of immigration from Ethiopia to Israel has been detailed in Chap. 1. Each wave of immigration was characterized by a unique set of circumstances creating the context for leaving and the context of arrival. Only three families in my study arrived in Israel directly via Addis: Desta, Solomon, and Teferra. All the other

© The Author(s), under exclusive license to Springer Nature Switzerland AG 2023

N. A. Shmuel, *Children's Wellbeing in Immigrant Families*, Children's Well-Being: Indicators and Research 26,
https://doi.org/10.1007/978-3-031-31917-4_6

participants arrived during the first wave, their courageous journeys were harrowing formative events, the memory of these mark a division in their lives separated by time and place. For many the terminology for this was referring to their lives *before* and *after* Sudan. Implicit in their narratives is the fact that the changes accompanying their adjustment to Israel were forged on the scars left by their journey to arrive. Every family found their own way of coping, re-grouping after prolonged separations and losses, their pain and grief often absorbed into the fabric of everyday life unspoken.

In many instances, asking people to describe their families resulted in a prolonged recounting of their journey to Israel and those who did not survive. And so Modesh spoke of her two small children who died, Edna of her little sister, Yaniv of his uncle, Abraham of his grandfather. Yafit was separated from her infant child, Naama, for almost two years, and from her husband Mahari for about 10 years. Lee arrived in Israel alone at the age of 13, she was only reunited with her parents after a year. Edna was almost five when she was separated from her mother for seven years, never to see her younger sister again. Rachel arrived in Israel with her uncle when she was only eight, it was another eight years before she saw her mother again. Dov was eight when his parents left Ethiopia and he stayed behind with the grandparents, arriving only five years later. In Sudan parents were incarcerated with their children, in the refugee camps many children became ill and hardly survived. Abigail described how her eight-year-old son saw his escort to Sudan slaughtered in front of him (For further reading on the journey, see Ben-Ezer, 2002; Salamon, 2007; Finklestein & Solomon, 2012; Edga, 2000; Ingedaw-wanda, 2019; Meiri & Elazar, 2001; Feldman, 1998; Shmuel, 1995; Parfitt, 1985).

6.2 The Family Immigration Story

Shy was amazed when his son, a combat soldier in the army, told him:

> I volunteered to a combat unit because of my grandparents, because of you, you all suffered so much in Sudan to come to this country, how can I not protect it?

People who grow up knowing the family immigration story have inbuilt as part of their collective identity 'knowing that we are part of something really big' as Habtam put it.

They look up to their parents and see them as heroes. Often the story is told as part of the Passover festival, alongside reading the *Haggadah*[1] and recounting the exodus the people of Israel made in Biblical times out of Egypt, the elders of the family are called upon to tell of the Ethiopian exodus. Habtam distinguished between the narrative told to children at school that emphasized the Israeli initiative to bring the Ethiopians to Israel, and the narrative she heard at home that emphasized the heroism of her parents who set out on this incredible journey (this

[1] Jewish text that tells the story of Passover.

distinction is also discussed in Shatu, 2011). To rectify this, since 2003, the Israeli Knesset marks a Memorial Day for those who perished in Sudan. The national ceremony is held at a memorial site completed in 2000 on Mount Herzl, also known as Mount of Remembrance, where the leaders of the nation are buried.

Abigail, during her interview, repeatedly returned to the challenges she faced in Sudan, saying 'the difficulties I overcame will always accompany me'. Recounting how she saved her children from death during a landslide, Abigail sees this as proof of her ability to overcome any future difficulties she may face through faith, resourcefulness, and resilience. The survivor's narrative of triumph is both inspiring and affirmative of personal and community strength—implying their ability to overcome whatever challenges they face as immigrants in Israel. The aptitude to prevail over traumatic experiences is both personal and collective: being part of something 'bigger than themselves' is an invisible inter-generational lifeline that can give the younger generation fortitude to cope with the challenges they face. But this only works if there is sufficient communication between the generations to enable the older generation to share their stories and the younger generation to attentively hear them.

In Landaus' (2007) study of Hispanic women at risk, she found knowing grandparents' stories and contact with extended family significantly reduced risk for young women. She defined trauma as upsetting inter-generational continuance, while stories from the past were a means to reconnect and build resilience. Newman (2007) reached a similar conclusion discussing stories Ethiopian grandmothers told their daughters in Israel. In a study on women suffering from depression in a mental health clinic Landau also found that familiarity with family stories related to vulnerability and overcoming had a protective effect on patients. In other words, stories and rituals repeated from the past can assist those living in the present, passed on from one generation to the next they enhance the younger generations self-image and may act as a buffer against self-endangering behaviour. Yisrael provides a good example of this:

> every situation I found myself in, if I quarrelled with my father or was rude to my mother, if I was punished in the army, whatever happened I told my grandfather, and he always had a story for me, an allegory about what had happened to me and how to get out of it.

Despite the vast differences between their lives, the grandfather managed to relate to his grandson through stories from the past that helped him in the present.

But as illustrated in the opening paragraph of this chapter, not all families share stories. Naama heard no stories from her mother Yafit, who explicitly said she never told her children anything about Ethiopia or the journey. Her son Yisrael heard the family story from his uncle. In fact, most of the second generation in my study did not know their parents' immigration story, some of them (Yaniv, Shimon, Matan, Avi, and Addis) took responsibility for this in their interviews, saying 'I never asked'. Noa explains her parents silence as a reflection of the cultural attitude towards children: 'they don't think these are important things to pass on to the children'.

There may be a multitude of reasons why parents do not tell children; the type of connection between them that does not encourage open direct communication, the fact that the stories are sad, often tragic, and parents wanted to save their children the pain of knowing, and that, as Noa said, they did not think it important for them to know these things. Whatever the reasons, their silence shapes their children's lives with a certain emptiness where the absent knowledge could build connection and inspire them. Moreover, studies have shown that not speaking about traumatic events does not prevent their transferal to the next generation, quite the opposite: silence fosters an emotional legacy of trauma that effects the next generation in complex encumbering ways (Atlas, 2022).

6.3 The Changes Accompanying Immigration

The context into which the new generation is born and raised in Israel can best be understood by examining the many changes facing their families after immigration. These include seven simultaneous transitions, each of which carries far-reaching consequences:

- Changing definitions of the family
- The transition from a collectivistic society to an individualistic society
- The transition from a hierarchy to a democracy
- Life as a continuum vs a reality in which adults and children live in separate worlds
- Changing communication patterns
- Changes in women's status and gender relations
- Visibility, difference, and finding a new identity

Together these changes forge new *unsettled* lives, the in-between spaces in which transitional change is negotiated. All these issues are further discussed in detail in the chapters of this book, I will give a brief overview here.

6.4 Changing Definitions of the Family

The cultural definition of a family, the proximity and form of connection to different relatives, their relevance and availability in the lives of children—are all crucial to understanding children's experiences.[2] Every child in Ethiopia was able to recount the name of their father together with the male ancestral line seven generations back. This was mentioned repeatedly by all the grandparents in the study, to them this defined identity—genealogy linked the younger generation to their roots and

[2] A brief description of the Amharic terminology for family appears in the preface.

defined them as family, embedded them as members in the community. But the grandparents were equally aware that this knowledge is lost in Israel, with sadness and sometimes anger they recounted how the younger generation do not know the names seven generations back and take no interest in family genealogy. Many young people relate their elder's obsession with this to the issue of arranged marriages, which to them is obsolete and irrelevant in the Israeli context. In the Jewish community in Ethiopia, the adults counted seven generations back to preclude marriage between distant relatives. But to the older generation this knowledge is crucial to the community's continuity: knowing one's ancestors, threading each new child on the endless chain of the generations, is the very foundation defining personal and community identity, without which all are lost, untethered from the moorings of their ancestral birthright.

Aside from this, the transition from a vast extended family to a nuclear family which functions as an independent unit changes the context of existence for all the generations, suddenly forced to redefine their connection in both time and space. New young families no longer automatically set up home adjacent to the husbands' parents as they would have done in Ethiopia. Even if they live in the same city or town, they are no longer visibly present in each other's daily lives but separated by walls, streets, and neighbourhoods. Suddenly young couples oversee their own lives, can choose to live further away from their parents, or adjacent to the wife's parents. As the balance of power between the sexes and between generations shifts, and the very concept of family undergoes transformation, the whole process of decision-making, responsibility, and connection changes, open to negotiation or reappraisal. Large extended families in small villages formed a cohesive, supportive community. Separation and disintegration into small, nuclear family units has isolated young parents as solely responsible for their children, often without the supportive network of grandparents and other relatives. The communal shared space of the village where much of family life was public has disappeared, behind closed doors separated by stone and concrete family life becomes private. Physical and conceptual changes intertwine, the elders are no longer the primary source of knowledge. Raising children, marital relations, formative life decisions as well as everyday acts of living have all moved from the public sphere to the private, the intricate fabric of extended family living thus unravelled, collectivism has effectively been replaced by individualism. This disintegration infiltrates the perception of self, from significance as part of a whole to the insignificance of the individual, as one of the elders said about himself: 'here I am nothing and nobody' (Mamu). Moreover, children raised in Ethiopia by multiple caregivers learnt connection through trust—the basis for cooperative living. This is common practice in most African countries (LeVine et al., 1996). Children were bonded to the community through participation, which put less emphasis on the specific emotional connection to a mother or a father. As immigrant families adopted normative Israeli practice and parents sought employment to support their families, infants and children joined day-care, kindergarten, and school. Thus, child-care became the shared responsibility of parents and institutions, while grandparents, siblings, and other relatives became less available to compensate for the emotional deficit of overworked parents struggling with the many challenges of acculturation.

6.5 The Transition from a Collectivistic Society to an Individualistic Society

Immigration brought two opposing cultural systems into direct conflict: the cooperative tradition valuing collectivism and community versus individualism stressing free choice and personal gratification. Of course, most societies contain an element of both, but generally one predominant ideology creates a certain predefined social and family order. Metaphorically akin to a sudden earthquake, the changes accompanying immigration restructured entire families, creating new rifts and reshaping power relations. This was expressed in the interviews as liberalism versus conservatism, traditional roles and behaviour versus new perceptions of responsibilities and acceptable conduct. Added to the inter-generational gap was a cultural chasm familiar from the experiences of other immigrants from collectivistic societies entering individualistic societies (Greenfield et al., 2003) as two opposing conceptual paradigms guiding towards differing cultural pathways—interdependence or dependence—come into direct head on collision (to be discussed in detail in the following chapters).

The new generation are born into this divide, without being enveloped and nurtured by community while at the same time lacking their own individualistic backbone of personal identity connecting them to any clear goals and aspirations for their future. This is part of the meaning of detachment, which is both external and internal, creating an inbuilt alienation from self and society.

6.6 The Transition from a Hierarchy to a Democracy

In Ethiopia, children were not expected to verbally demonstrate their knowledge, express curiosity or take initiative, all of which are normative and expected behaviours for children in Western countries. Moreover, Western families are child-centred; children are considered dependents, they are not expected to contribute to the upkeep of the household, however they are often asked for their opinion and their wellbeing generally precedes the needs of adults. This model is contradictory to the hierarchical model of the traditional Ethiopian family, in which children are expected to demonstrate their subservience to adults, to be obedient and respectful. Parental perceptions and expectations do not change with immigration (Roer-Strier, 2001). Members of the G1.5 generation know intuitively what is expected of them and act accordingly, most of them develop viable hybrid identities over time and remain respectful and reverent to their elders in the Ethiopian community. But the younger G2 generation find it hard to meet these expectations, which they do not always understand, and find themselves in frequent conflict with their elders.

In a hierarchical adult-centred society such as Ethiopia, roles are designated according to status and relationships are shaped accordingly, with clear cultural codes for respectful and polite behaviour which are common knowledge from a young age. These form the basis for cultural authority as well as parental authority. In a democratic, often child-centred society such as Israel, authority is based on knowledge and relationships, it may vary between different cultural groups, but the basis for parental authority is generally the establishment of a bond enabling effective mutual communication. Going back to the metaphor of the earthquake, after immigration each family realigns itself on the axis of communication to contain the changes, or alternatively clings to the traditional hierarchy and is overcome by chaos, as traditional methods become ineffectual and the necessity for change is more powerful than the desire for continuity. As shall be demonstrated in the following chapters, paradoxically, the continuity of the family, the ability to retain and preserve cultural traditions, is dependent on flexibility to adapt and change in the new context.

6.7 Life as a Continuum versus a Reality in Which Adults and Children Live in Separate Worlds

Where children actively participate in village life, their transition to adulthood is gradual and unceremonious. In Ethiopia, children were effectively an asset to their families, being useful and appreciated built their self-image as valued members of the community, aware and confident of their own abilities. The separation between the world of adults and the world of children which occurs after immigration to Israel, where children go to school and adults go to work, has two significant outcomes. Firstly, the continuum of connection and resultant intuitive communication between adults and children is effectively severed. In the new reality a great deal of effort is necessary to bridge between their separate worlds, something it takes many parents a long time to realize, if at all. Secondly, children's learning in Israel is no longer based on observation and imitation, moreover *what* they learn is not obviously connected to their immediate reality.

Where children are part of the adult world as apprentices and assistants, they learn from a young age to be aware of what is going on around them. This attentiveness enables them to internalize information and retain knowledge even before they fully understand it. In contrast, in the Western world, where 'childhood' has evolved as a distinct time in life unconnected to 'adulthood', children's learning has become the responsibility of adults. Thus, children are less attentive, for shorter periods of time, and tend to wonder in thought to imaginary worlds and miss what is going on around them (Gaskins & Paradise, 2012).

6.8 Changing Communication Patterns

The very building blocks of connection between the generations, between people—spoken and unspoken language—undergo an indelible transformation with immigration. This reformation of the most valuable asset in the cultural toolkit has dire consequences.

Most of the G2 generation from my study stated that their parents do not understand them most of the time, some of them went so far as to say their parents did not really know them at all. Most participants from the G2 and G1.5 as children did not confide in their parents or ask them for advice. Many of the G1.5 parents mentioned listening to their children as important to them because nobody listened to them when they were children.

The interviews reflect a very somber picture of the lack of communication between the generations, and the resultant isolation and frustration of both adults and children. At the same time there are striking examples of parents who make great efforts not to lose their children by adopting new and alternative modes of communication with them, and families in which siblings are supportive to one another after the total breakdown of communication with their parents (discussed in Chaps. 7 and 12).

6.9 Changes in Women's Status and Gender Relations

One of the most significant and complex changes to the Ethiopian community following the transition to Israel is changing gender relations, reflected both in roles taken and in gender expectations and status. These changes are inseparably linked to the transition from a hierarchical cooperative society to a democracy individualistic society. As the balance of power changes, and men and women experience the transition differently, inevitably conflicts arise. These changes have an immense impact on family functioning and the ability of the family unit to survive and adapt jointly to the new reality. Since the changes are both overt and covert, mostly without any mechanism to openly discuss and negotiate them, as the delicate balance between the sexes prevalent in Ethiopia is broken, chaos often takes over. These issues are discussed in detail in Chap. 11.

6.10 Visibility, Difference, and Finding a New Identity

Perhaps the single most significant change that Jewish immigrants from Ethiopia must cope with after immigration to Israel is the attitude of Israeli society to their culture and background. The issue of visibility and representation comes up in all the interviews, not only of the G1 and G1.5 participants but also of the G2, painfully aware of being constantly differentiated by their colour. This issue has drastic consequences for both their sense of belonging and their self-perception, compounded by segmented assimilation, together leading to an inevitable reappraisal of identity. If this was forged in Ethiopia by genealogy, status, and community membership, the sudden transition to an individualistic Western, predominantly white society containing many versions of *Israeliness* raises difficult personal questions and on-going self-reflection on the whole issue of identity and belonging. Perhaps the confusion of the G1 and G1.5 immigrants is inevitable, but the fact that the same applies to their offspring, the G2, requires further explanation. What appears evident from this study is that this confusion is fuelled both by their experiences within the family and in Israeli society. These issues are discussed in detail in Chap. 13.

References

Atlas, G. (2022). *Emotional inheritance. A therapist, her patients, and the legacy of trauma*. Little Brown Spark.

Ben-Ezer, G. (2002). *The Ethiopian Jewish Exodus: Narratives of the Journey*. Routledge.

Finklestein, M., & Solomon, Z. (2012). Trauma and loss among Ethiopian immigrants in Israel. In E. Witztum & N. Grisaru (Eds.), *Social and clinical aspects of Ethiopian immigrants in Israel* (pp. 279–310). The Jewish Agency and Ben Gurion University of the Negev.

Gaskins, S., & Paradise, R. (2012). Learning through observation in daily life. In D. Lancy, J. Bock, & S. Gaskins (Eds.), *The anthropology of learning in childhood* (pp. 85–118). Alta Mira Press.

Greenfield, P. M., Keller, H., Fuligni, A., & Maynard, A. (2003). Cultural pathways through universal development. *Annual Review of Psychology, 54*(1), 461–490.

Landau, J. (2007). Enhancing resilience: Families and communities as agents for change. *Family Process, 46*(3), 351–365.

LeVine, R., Dixon, S., LeVine, S., Keefer, C., Richman, A., Leiderman, P., & Brazelton, T. (1996). *Child care and culture: Lessons from Africa* (pp. 247–275). Cambridge University Press.

Meiri, B., & Elazar, R. (2001). *A dream behind bars, prisoners of Zion from Ethiopia*. Gefen.

Newman, R. (2007). Ethiopian Israeli Grandmothers' Stories. *Journal of Aging, Humanities, and the Arts, 1*(3–4), 211–219.

Parfitt, T. (1985). *Operation Moses: The story of the exodus of the Falasha Jews from Ethiopia*. Weidenfeld & Nicolson.

Roer-Strier, D. (2001). Socialization in changing cultural contexts: A search for images of the 'Adaptive Adult'. *Social Work, 46*(3), 215–228.

Hebrew References

Edga, A. (2000). *Journey to dream* (self-published).

Feldman, M. (1998). *Coming out of Ethiopia*. Bialik and Jewish Agency.

Ingedaw-wanda, S. (2019). *Resilience in immigration*. Resling.

Salamon, H. (2007). The life circle. In H. Salamon (Ed.), *Ethiopia: Jewish communities in the east in the 19th and 20th centuries*. Yad Ben Zvi and the Ministry of Education.

Shatu, S. (2011). *The different narratives of the journey made by Ethiopian Jews.* Master's dissertation. Hebrew University of Jerusalem.
Shmuel, Y. (1995). *The way to Jerusalem, the first immigration from Ethiopia (1980).* Reshafim.

Chapter 7
Language, Communication, and Wellbeing in the Family

Words are the building blocks for human interaction, coupled with gestures, facial expressions, and body language. Together these form the verbal and non-verbal language through which cultural knowledge is preserved, organized, and transmitted between the generations. Cultural knowledge is constructed and classified using language, creating epistemes that define the association between things (Foucault, 1980, 1982). Communities create historical narratives and shared traditions which form tangible links to the past and serve current social processes. Social power structures determine what becomes heritage (Swidler, 1986).

Transition involves two important processes in relation to all this: firstly, a changing context in which previous forms of communication may have different effects, as we shall see in this chapter. Secondly, learning a new language as a new immigrant is effectively crossing a cultural boundary, stepping out into that in-between grey area defined by Boer (2006) between cultural epistemes in which definitions and associations are re-examined and re-negotiated in the new context both consciously and subconsciously through language. The process of appropriation and ownership of the new language (and with it a new culture) involves a revision and reorganization of knowledge which if completed to the full paves the way to bilingualism and biculturalism in which structures of knowledge are retained and processed by differing (sometimes opposite) cultural and linguistic frames (Bennet-Martinez et al., 2002, 2006). This process has far-reaching consequences for adaptation and integration into a new unfamiliar environment. However, it seems that many immigrants remain somewhere in-between two cultures and languages, stuck in the 'grey area', incorporating into their repertoire elements of both but never becoming equally culturally competent in both. As we shall see in this chapter, this has significant consequences for family communication and intergenerational relations.

© The Author(s), under exclusive license to Springer Nature Switzerland AG 2023

N. A. Shmuel, *Children's Wellbeing in Immigrant Families*, Children's Well-Being: Indicators and Research 26,
https://doi.org/10.1007/978-3-031-31917-4_7

7.1 Families in Transition

The children born in Israel to Ethiopian immigrant families are growing up in a new reality, in which new patterns of verbal and non-verbal communication are shaping their experience of family and self. Yaniv, a recently discharged soldier, describes his relationship with his father:

> I don't really feel his presence. He's there, in front of the television. A total lack of communication. I say A, he understands B. [....] In my friends' houses... they go out to work, and when they come back, they pass their mother in the living room, and this is the extent of their relationship with her. This lack of communication in our community is very hard. Everybody is afraid to talk.

Many young Ethiopian Israelis are growing up in an atmosphere at home that precludes communication, distancing them not only from their parents but also from their cultural heritage and from themselves. The son passing his mother in the living room, the son who says A while his father understands B, *effectively live in different conceptual worlds*. The painful truth, as Maayan says, is that:

> In some families there is simply no longer a connection between parents and their children.

Ester, an undergraduate student, says that in her family 'there is no such thing as *let's talk about it*'. Traditional restraint combines with the growing rift between the generations following immigration and results in many families being engulfed in painful silence.

A preliminary necessity for effective communication is having a shared reality, but sometimes when cultures meet within the family this is not the case (Wynne, 1988). Avi describes it like this:

> You can see internal conflicts in many families, between parents and children. To the extent that the kid leaves home as soon as he can support himself and comes back infrequently. There is a disconnection between parents and children because they don't have a common language. They look at things differently.

Note that Avi is referring to both language and *perspective*. Another condition for good communication is the ability to perceive another person's outlook (Blaker, 1984; Hong et al., 2003). Beyond language itself, the capacity to understand local logic is an important part of acclimatizing to a new place (Shany, 2006). Thus, the inter-generational rift is forged throughout childhood, insomuch as parents and children interpret reality differently and act according to different and often opposing cultural values and strategies of action. These obstacles to viable communication are further compounded by a language barrier, together all these often-thwart efforts to create meaningful interaction between the generations (G1 and G2). This frequently results in the older new immigrants barricading themselves into their traditional cultural perspective and becoming defensive, as they feel that the new culture which enters their home via their children is threatening the very foundations they are attempting to preserve.

7.2 Verbal Communication

Children in immigrant families may often answer their parents in the new language, but they understand their parent's language when it is spoken. In many families of Ethiopian origin in Israel, the children have limited understanding of their parent's language. If the parents have not mastered Hebrew, this seriously limits the communication between them. In every society a common language between parents and children is a given basis for family communication. What is happening in the Ethiopian immigrant community in Israel is exceptional and requires special attention, having ramifications not only for family communication but also for child language development (see Shany & Geva, 2012).

Shany (2006) found children from the Ethiopian community to have only basic knowledge of Amharic, and since their parents did not know Hebrew concluded that in many families children and parents were not actually talking to one another. It seems that the children's reports of talking Amharic reflected hearing this language at home but not using it for communication. This can be explained as children being told what to do in Amharic, so they acquire a very basic knowledge of various commands such as eat, bathe, look after your brother, or do your homework, but not much more than this. Another study (Berhanu, 2005) on Ethiopian immigrant families in Israel, found that parents did not take an active initiative to teach their children Amharic, they simply spoke the language daily. When asked if they wanted their children to speak Amharic they answered affirmatively, but said the children already spoke in Hebrew. The growing rift between themselves and their children did not concern the parents or arouse them to action. Contrary to this, in my study some of the parents took the initiative to have their children taught Amharic (further details later in this chapter. This issue has also been discussed by Shuster, 2012).

Out of the 19 G1 participants in my study, all were fluent in Amharic but only six people could converse in Hebrew. All 15 G1.5 participants were fluent in Hebrew, but the majority admitted that they were not fluent enough in Amharic to talk to their children in this language. Seven of the 16 G2 participants knew Amharic well enough to have a conversation in it, but most of the children and grandchildren in most families knew no Amharic at all. Without a shared language, most of the grandparents and grandchildren are unable to communicate properly, the children request translation, and the adults express their frustration.

Many of the parents interviewed saw themselves responsible for their children not knowing Amharic, regretting that they never insisted on talking to them in their own language. As Danny put it:

> The problem is that they [his children] don't speak Amharic, but I think this was our fault, because we didn't speak to them, we wanted to learn Hebrew.

The parents wanted to acclimatize to Israel, speaking Hebrew was an expected way of doing this. As new immigrants they were not aware of the price of losing Amharic, they were busy attempting to adapt and prepare their children for life in Israel. Whether the parents did not consider it important to teach the children

Amharic or whether they did not believe it in their power to do so, the result is the same.

In addition, Israeli society at large did not encourage the immigrants to preserve their language, as Tigist says:

> When we got here, they said *now you are in Israel, no more Amharic*!

This attitude fits the *melting-pot* ideology common in Israel in the 1950s when to create a unified state, immigrants were encouraged to discard their language and culture as part of the assimilation process. Despite the common use of the term *multiculturalism* today, in practice many people continue to hold this perspective (Sever, 2001, 2004). The assumption is often still that new immigrants are the ones who must make the effort to adjust to life in Israel, primarily by learning Hebrew and adopting local customs.

Naama talks of her father having 'crooked, broken, inarticulate and unclear Hebrew' and yet he 'insists' on speaking Hebrew with the children. Abigail noted that many parents speak 'incorrect Hebrew' to their children. Several of the younger people interviewed told me I could interview their parents in Hebrew but when I met them, I discovered this was not possible as they quickly reverted to Amharic. All these parents are examples of immigrants stuck in the grey area between cultures, in the sense that they literally pay lip-service to the new language (and by extension also cultural perceptions) but are not fluent or even eloquent enough to be clearly understood by their own children or grandchildren.

7.3 Language and Culture

Addis describes how in his family when his parents had 'something important' to say they spoke in Amharic. Maayan and Tigist said that their parents spoke in Amharic when they were angry. Thought constructs related to cultural perceptions are anchored in the language, which diverts emotional reactions according to culturally acceptable paths. Thus, the parents of Addis, Maayan, and Tigist reverted to Amharic when they wished to convey cultural authority enhancing their traditional place at the top of the family hierarchy. The language acts to trigger cultural associations and elicit an appropriate response from the children—obedience. This is called cultural priming (Mok & Morris, 2009; Oyserman & Lee, 2008). Shy, a member of the first generation although fluent in Hebrew, admits that

> sometimes I think in Amharic, it reminds me of the culture I grew up in, so that I do not disconnect.

Thinking in Amharic is like a journey through childhood, it awakens ways of being that perhaps assimilation into the new culture has made him forget—hence the sense of disconnection. From the interviews it seems that often parents interweave phrases in Amharic into their children's daily lives as reminders of the obedience expected of them. But children who have learnt to function in Hebrew have not internalized these culturally specific codes of behaviour, thus a few words in a language they barely understand is unlikely to bring them to order.

The loss of language, coupled with the fact that traditional Ethiopian culture does not encourage spontaneous open conversations between adults and children, often leaves the Ethiopian Israeli youngsters alienated both within and outside their families: disconnected from their ancestral heritage while not yet connected to the local scene. In effect, many of these children have grown up without linguistic competence in any language, which has dire consequences for their educational development. Shany (2006) reported that a developmental delay in language acquisition was already evident in children of Ethiopian origin in pre-school.

The lack of language skills is confounded by an absence of cultural knowledge, normally learnt alongside language (Duranti, 1997). Language represents the world in certain culturally and historically specific ways, shaping the perception of reality through classification and categorization (Burr & Dick, 2017). The new generation (G2) do not internalize their place in the hierarchy through the appropriate use of courteous terminology, in effect the respectful distance between themselves and their elders is not embedded in them through linguistic morphology as it was in Ethiopia.

7.4 Language and Status

Linguistic fluency, eloquence, and accent are social markers which determine status and belonging. Ester and Tigist reported attending parents' evenings at school as children, their teachers talked to them rather than their parents.[1] They could not translate what was said, since they did not know Amharic, they simply repeated it to their parents in simple Hebrew. This experience is embedded in their memory as degrading to their parents and embarrassing to themselves. Tigist, who works as a nurse in a hospital, recalls medical staff ignoring patients who could not explain themselves in Hebrew:

> This is how they, the society at large, how people relate to those who don't know the language. It is beyond the lack of knowledge of the language—it is the attitude towards those who *don't know*... I find it very frustrating; one would expect after so many years of absorbing immigrants that there would be ways of coping with this. [Patients] who have no family to translate for them and can't express themselves—nobody even looks at them to see if they can be helped. They just say—*doesn't know Hebrew*.

Tigist has observed that despite being a nation absorbing immigrants for many years, there is still often a certain *disrespect* for people who do not speak the language, thus many immigrants find themselves ignored. Tigist cannot understand why people do not try to help by using simple Hebrew:

---

[1] Discussed also in Chap. 10.

When you go to schools or hospitals people don't use simple Hebrew, and I can't understand why not? You can explain anything calmly and quietly so a person can understand.

In other words, language is not just a means of communication, it also denotes social status, legitimacy of presence, degree of knowledge, and the right to belong. At significant junctions in family life the children born in Israel enter the scene not as translators of a language but as *interpreters of a culture*—they explain Israeli reality to their parents, who often find this experience demeaning. The status of being in-between languages and in-between cultures is effectively a no-man's land.

7.5 Emotional Expression and Non-verbal Language

In my first job in an Absorption Centre in Israel many years ago I was struck by the lack of faith the Ethiopian immigrants showed towards words spoken by *Ferunge* (white people), and the distinction made between statements which came *from the throat*—meaning words spoken frivolously, or *from the stomach*—the storage place of deep emotions. Empathy and inter-personal understanding are based on the communication of emotions. There is great potential for misunderstandings between people of cultures which define differently—almost conversely—when and how it is socially acceptable to express emotions. When such misunderstandings are experienced *within* the family, between generations who have adopted different cultures, the natural expectation of being understood at home is seldom realized.

Emotional expression is rooted deep in cultural conditioning, in perceptions of what is normal or abnormal, which guide and limit personal practice. Genet explains:

For people from Ethiopia most of the emotions, the expression of emotions, is through actions.

Lemlem describes how, in Ethiopian culture, words do not carry feelings—these are expressed through deeds:

Emotional expression, most of the time, is through *doing* something not *saying* something. If he loves you or cares about you, he will do something for you, he won't say it. This is true between couples too; we haven't changed that.

This could be seen as linked to the wax and gold tradition discussed in chapter two: words are not reliable indications of emotions, only actions are. Crying is legitimate, and expected, only at funerals. Emotional pain and discomposure should be kept in the stomach, not expressed openly. Abigail says explicitly that when in pain; 'we do not show our tears'. Rachel described her silent reunion with the mother she had not seen for eight years as devoid of expressed emotions: 'love without words. The body speaks, the eyes'. She says that to this day they have never discussed this time.

Emotional expression through body language, gestures, and actions is deeply embedded in Ethiopian traditional culture (and prevalent in various forms in other cultures, for example Exline, 1974; Payatos, 1983). Parents did not openly express their feelings for their children. When asked how she knew if her parents were pleased with her Ester answered, 'they would not show it', and when they were angry 'they did not talk'. Orna knew her parents were pleased with her because they 'did not comment'. Ethiopian tradition made it common for children to hear their parents' opinions about them via a third party, this was reiterated in the study by Berhanu (2006). Noa explains:

> I know that my mother was proud of me, but she would never say it. I'm different, because I never got that, I can tell my son *I am proud of you*. We did not grow up like that. Not that they didn't want to tell us, in fact they told other people. I would go to the neighbours and hear it from them—*she said you are her eyes...*

Naama learnt from her neighbours that her father was cross with her, and Liora—that her father praised her. Edna spoke of *a look* that expressed love and the feeling of being hugged, without words, and *the look* that expressed anger. Liora and Yafit both referred to the look of disapproval which aroused fear in them as children, and Aberash said she always knew what her mother wanted from her *by her eyes*.

All these examples are from the intermediate, 1.5 generation, who learnt and internalized this form of communication in early childhood as part of a community. In Ethiopia, the intricate language of the body, gestures, *the look* and facial expressions required people to be focused and attentive, to contemplate and understand what was being said without words. The new generation, born in Israel, has not learnt how to read these signs and signals, as Lemlem put it; 'they miss all the cues'. Moreover, their attempts to communicate directly and express their wants, needs, desires, and refusals often arouse the animosity of the adults, who consider them simply rude. But the younger generation are using *dugri* (direct) speech (Katriel, 1986) which the older generation find inexplicable and unacceptable.

7.6 Inter-generational Communication

> Often when adults talk, it takes a long time to understand what exactly they are saying... you must listen to the meaning of what they say and not the words themselves. You need a lot of patience to listen to what the adults have to tell.

Tigist continues to explain that the children born in Israel do not understand this type of communication, including the ones who know Amharic, since a literal translation of the words does not explain the sentence. Thus, they are left without the meaning of what was said—the wax without the gold.

The fact that the second generation has not learnt the ability to solve such sayings from their parents or grandparents seems to suggest that this type of communication requires the existence of a community and is not to be left to individuals. This also provides partial explanation for the impatience of the younger generation towards the adults, as Worknesh says: 'they don't listen. You tell them something and they always have something to answer. They say *what do I care? Here it's not Ethiopia*'!

The inability of the younger generation to listen to their elders is something that came up in all the interviews with the adults, as did the issue of respect. This latter also came up as the core of Ethiopian culture which both the first generation and the intermediate, 1.5 generation would like to pass on to their offspring.

But without a shared language, most of the grandparents and grandchildren are not able to communicate verbally, causing great frustration. Tsehai said that her children

> don't understand. They keep asking me *what is grandma saying? We don't know her language*!

Lemlem describes a similar situation:

> My mother has fluent Hebrew, but with my father or with the other grandmother it's about a sentence and a half. My husband's mother blesses them, they say *Amen, Amen*, and we tell them what she said—*study, be successful, and if someone insults you ignore them.* That is the advice she gives them.

Verbal communication between adults and children in a hierarchical society is aimed at ensuring the obedience of the children, not at increasing their knowledge about each other. Thus, adults say about the children that they 'do not hear' or 'do not listen' when they mean that they *do not obey*. At the same time the children are not being heard either, as Noa explains:

> The way we grew up, children have no voice. Even if you give an opinion, you are told *what do you know? you are a child.*

A child is not considered a partner for conversation, and if one of the sides must make an effort in order to communicate then this is expected of the child. Modesh complains that her children do not know Amharic:

> It hurts. The Russians speak Russian. Their children answer them in Russian. It hurts. This never happens with us.

The comparison with immigrants from Russia arises in several interviews and is always worded to imply that the fault lies with the children, as if they were the ones who decided in what language they should be spoken to. The agency of children in this matter should not be underestimated, as shown by Tuominen's study (1999).

Enye says that her grandchildren 'don't want to talk Amharic' and her husband adds 'we try, but they don't accept it'. Other grandparents have similar experiences:

> Sometimes they say *Grandma what are you babbling?! Say it in our language!* (Almaz)

> It's very hard. They don't understand [me], they ask *Grandma what?* (Worknesh)

In most of the families I interviewed, even the grandchildren looked after by the grandparents did not know Amharic. This is a significant paradox: if the grandparents are looking after the grandchildren on a regular basis, and complaining that they do not know Amharic, why do they not use the opportunity to teach them? The answer is supplied by Eneye, who says that when she talks to her grandchildren in Amharic:

> They tell me *no, no Amharic, we are not Ethiopian, stop it!*

Shani, who lived with her parents for five years while they saved to buy an apartment, says that her children were speaking 'half Hebrew and half Amharic'. Then her parents demanded that she teach them Amharic. Shani reasoned with them, suggesting that they would do a better job because they know the language better, and they could utilize their time together to teach them. But her father replied: 'but you are the parents, they listen to you'.

In other words, the grandchildren do absorb some Amharic words they hear from their grandparents, but the grandparents are not consistent in their use of the language, and do not see themselves as having authority over grandchildren born in Israel. Meanwhile, the grandchildren themselves behave as locals and sometimes object to being spoken to in Amharic, making it harder for their grandparents, who in any case have lost their confidence and traditional status after the transition to Israel. Besides this, it is important to remember that direct verbal communication is not the grandparents preferred form of communication, because in Ethiopia they primarily relied on body language, facial expressions, stories, and proverbs, most of which are not understood by their Israeli-born grandchildren.

It is interesting to note that most of the parents in my study who did consider it important that their children learnt Amharic did not ask the grandparents to teach it. Genet and Miki are teaching their children Amharic via an app on the computer, Aberash sends her children to Amharic lessons at the local community centre, and Yaniv's parents sent him to learn the blessings from a *Kess* (Rabbi) when he was younger. There were some families in which Amharic was taught at home: Abigail said her grandchildren learnt from the other grandmother, Yisrael asked his father to teach him, and Tsehai said that her husband teaches their daughters.

Liora and Shy made a conscious decision to speak Amharic at home, even if the children 'answer in Hebrew, the main thing is that they should understand what is being said to them'. It is important to Shy because 'language is very important'. Even if sometimes it seems artificial, since the youngest has little knowledge of the language, 'he sits there, and we *deliberately* talk in Amharic'.

To Liora it was less clear why the children needed to know Amharic:

> To my husband Shy it was obvious that they needed to know [Amharic] but not to me. Now I see how they bond with other Ethiopians, connect with the culture, listen to music in Amharic, it made it apparent to me that we needed to have Amharic at home.

Nevertheless, Liora also says:

> Most of the explaining, so that they understand really well, I do in Hebrew. But in day-to-day talk at home we speak Amharic, so that they don't forget.

The children answer her in Hebrew, their knowledge of Amharic does not include the subtleties of the language, but they are well able to communicate with their grandparents:

> They don't always know what is hiding behind the word, they simply translate it. I pass on the message, I tell them in my language. Then it's OK, they understand. I see them talking to Grandma and Grandpa in Amharic.

In other words, Liora and Shy's children are not completely competent in Amharic, but they can carry a conversation, which opens a channel of communication with the grandparents. But there is another side to their knowledge of the language: at school their daughter Shira uses Amharic as a secret language with her Ethiopian Israeli friends. Shira said:

> If we have a secret we speak in Amharic. It makes us proud. We have another language. It's special.

Knowing another language gives meaningful content to their dissimilarity as a distinguishable minority in the school. Shira described in her interview how generalizations were made at school towards the Ethiopian Israeli girls; using Amharic as their own secret language gives them added value in their own eyes and provides positive content to the *Ethiopian-ness* forced upon them.

Sometimes language can be used to keep secrets in the family, as Danny describes: 'if I want to tell my wife a secret, I can tell her in Amharic', which his children do not understand. Orna uses the same tactic:

> If I don't want the children to understand I use words in Amharic. Then my daughter says *now you've found a system!*

Language as a source of misunderstandings between parents and children came up frequently in the interviews, often with the qualification that other reasons are also present to complicate things between them. For example, Worknesh tells how the local school recommended sending her son to a boarding school, even though he was doing very well in school. Her daughter Noa reminds her that

> He didn't know Amharic and you didn't know Hebrew. You did not understand each other!

Worknesh nods and confirms this:

> Yes, I spoke Amharic, he spoke Hebrew. I would ask him for my *Natele* [scarf] and he would ask Noa what that was. We had a problem with the language.

Of course, if Israeli society at large and the school in particular had aimed for greater cultural and linguistic inclusion, it would have been easy to think of alternative solutions—less drastic and with hindsight less damaging—which would have enabled the child to stay with his family.

Naama says that her father has no idea what is going on in her life and explains this:

> I don't share, since it's hard for me, his lack of Hebrew, and it's too difficult for me to explain things in Amharic, and to be honest I don't really want to.

In other words, the language is one element of the lack of communication between them, alongside a lack of motivation to share information about her life with her father, which is not exceptional for an independent young woman in her thirties.

Naama was separated from her father for many years, when he arrived in Israel the reunion was fraught with difficulties which included the language. 'We spoke in Hebrew', explains her mother Yafit, and then her husband was suspicious, she recalls:

> *Aah you are cursing me, you are talking about me.* What could I be saying to my daughter about her father? I answered him, she's your daughter! [But Mahari was adamant] *No, you are cursing me, you are not being respectful.*

Lacking fluency in a shared language makes communicating difficult, and yet there are families in which creative methods have been developed to overcome this. For example, Genet describes her mother Almaz as 'very dominant' in her children's lives, and that her daughter

> loves to hear her Grandma, she says that in Ethiopia Grandma was a very big helper of other people.

This grandmother-granddaughter bond has developed largely due to Genet who, aware of the language difficulties, goes to a lot of trouble to encourage communication between them in creative ways:

> we try and have opportunities for cooperation between them. It is something that we build slowly. For example, using weaving or clay, things they can do together. It has to be at her own pace.

7.7 Conclusion

The narratives in this chapter demonstrate the complexity of changing family communication across the generations following immigration. Traditional forms of communication prevalent in Ethiopia—the cultural toolkit containing non-verbal language, honorific morphology, folk stories and proverbs, emotional expression through actions—are all becoming less effective in the new context. The second generation, soaked in local culture and nurtured in Israeli schools and pre-schools, do not understand the intricacies of such means of communication, which to them are confusing and elusive. In many families Amharic itself is taking on new roles: to hold secrets, to call the children to order, even to salvage remnants of the culture. In other families it is a living language serving a lifeline to the grandparents, coupled with creative ways of bridging the gaps when this is lacking (more on this in Chap. 12). Where adults in the family have been unable to master Hebrew and meet the new cultural expectation of more direct, open conversation, a growing gap between the generations is filled with an awkward silence. All these affect and complicate relationships, sometimes in painful and distressing ways. While some adults may be aware of the reasons behind this (and therefore make allowances and cope with this better), children are more likely to succumb to their subjective experiences and simply feel rejected, ignored, or misunderstood.

References

Bennet-Martinez, V., Leu, J., & Lee, F. (2002). Negotiating biculturalism. *Journal of Cross-Cultural Psychology, 33*(5), 492–516.

Bennet-Martinez, V., Leu, J., & Lee, F. (2006). Biculturalism & cognitive complexity: Expertise in cultural representations. *Journal of Cross-Cultural Psychology, 37*(4), 386–407.
Berhanu, G. (2005). Indigenous conceptions of intelligence, ideal child, and ideal parenting among Ethiopian Jews in Israel. *Journal of Cognitive Education and Psychology, 5*(1), 47–71.
Berhanu, G. (2006). Parenting (parental attitude), child development, and modalities of parent-child interactions: Sayings, proverbs, and maxims of Ethiopian Jews in Israel. *Journal of Cognitive Education and Psychology, 5*(3), 266–287.
Blaker, R. M. (1984). quoted in Wynne, L. (1988). An epigenic model of family processes. In C. Falicov (Ed.), *Family transitions: Continuity and change over the life cycle* (p. 90). Guildford Press.
Boer, E. (2006). *Uncertain territories: Boundaries in cultural analysis*. Rodopi.
Burr, V., & Dick, P. (2017). Social constructionism. In *The Palgrave handbook of critical social psychology*. Palgrave Macmillan. ISBN 9781137510174.
Duranti, A. (1997). *Linguistic anthropology*. Cambridge University Press.
Exline, R. (1974). Visual interaction: The glances of power and preferences. In S. Weitz (Ed.), *Non-verbal communication: Readings with commentary* (pp. 65–98). Oxford University Press.
Foucault, M. (1980). *Power/knowledge: Selected interviews and other writings, 1972–1977*. Vintage.
Foucault, M. (1982). *The subject and power. Critical inquiry, 8*(4), 777–795.
Hong, Y., Benet-Martinez, V., Chiu, C., & Morris, M. (2003). Boundaries of cultural influence. *Journal of Cross Cultural Psychology, 34*(4), 453–464.
Katriel, T. (1986). *Talking straight: Dugri speech in Israeli Sabra culture*. Cambridge University Press.
Mok, A., & Morris, M. (2009). Cultural chameleons and iconoclasts: Assimilation and reactance to cultural cues. Bicultural expressed personalities as a function of identity conflict. *Journal of Experimental Social Psychology, 45*, 884–889.
Oyserman, D., & Lee, S. W. (2008). Does culture influence what and how we think? Effects of priming individualism and collectivism. *Psychological Bulletin, 134*(2), 311–342.
Payatos, F. (1983). *New perspectives in non-verbal communication*. Pergamon Press.
Shany, M., & Geva, E. (2012). Cognitive, language, and literacy development in socio-culturally vulnerable school children–the case of Ethiopian Israeli children. In *Current issues in bilingualism* (pp. 77–117). Springer.
Shuster, Y. (2012). *Immigration and multilingualism amongst Ethiopian immigrant children*. Doctoral thesis. Hebrew University, Jerusalem.
Swidler, A. (1986). Culture in action: Symbolism and strategies. *Americal sociological review, 51*(2), 273–286.
Tuominen, A. (1999). Who decides the home language? A look at multilingual families. *International Journal of the Sociology of Language, 140*, 59–76.
Wynne, L. (1988). An epigenic model of family processes. In C. Falicov (Ed.), *Family transitions: Continuity and change over the life cycle* (pp. 81–106). Guildford Press.

Hebrew References

Sever, R. (2001). Absorption or integration? Terms for examining issues of multiculturalism. *Gadis, Z*, 43–53.
Sever, R. (2004). Immigrant absorption in education: Policy and research. *Megamot, 1*, 145–169.
Shany, M. (2006). *Acquiring the written language amongst Ethiopian immigrant children: Cognitive, literacy, linguistic and environmental aspects*. Research paper for the Ministry of Education. Haifa University

Chapter 8
Perceptions of Children According to Their Birthplace

'Children born in Ethiopia think differently, their perspective is different', says Liora. It is a statement I am to hear repeatedly from G1 and G1.5 parents, and it carries an implication that this difference is intrinsic, that Israeli-born children are in some profoundly inherent sense *not the same* as children born in Ethiopia.

Every parent–child relationship involves three specific aspects which are especially pertinent in the context of transition: the inevitable dissonance between affection and rejection which are present in all relationships, the real child and the *ideas* about this child, and the cultural framework in which these first two were formed, which includes *expectations* about childrearing and parenthood. Caring deeply for someone so totally dependent carries simultaneously positive and negative emotions which every parent is familiar with, boundless affection and devotion and at times helplessness and desperation (Diem-Wille, 2014). Every culture mediates emotional ambivalence in its own way, just as each culture carries concepts of the *ideal child* and *parental ethnotheories* (discussed in Chap. 3) which shape ways of nurturing and concepts of child development. These ideas do not change with transition, what changes very rapidly are the *children* born into the new country. Liora's and other parents' similar statements reflect an observation of this change, which introduces new challenges to parenting and is attributed to the change in *location*. But what has really changed is the *effect* of culturally specific parenting suited to the context of the country of origin. In other words, the cultural toolkit used for raising children in one country has different results in another country, which brings us back to Swidler's (1986) paradigm of settled and unsettled lives. In unsettled lives, unfolding at the intersection of two cultures with different (sometimes opposing) value systems and strategies of action, how adults interpret and negotiate the changes they see in their offspring in comparison to the children born in the country of origin, can provide valuable insights into what is happening in immigrant families. Many of the families in my study maintain an invisible perceptual partition between the children—those born in Israel and those born in Ethiopia—although

© The Author(s), under exclusive license to Springer Nature Switzerland AG 2023

N. A. Shmuel, *Children's Wellbeing in Immigrant Families*, Children's Well-Being: Indicators and Research 26,
https://doi.org/10.1007/978-3-031-31917-4_8

generally not openly discussed, the children are painfully aware of this. To illustrate this phenomenon and its results, I will concentrate on one family.

8.1 The Sehalu Family

Eneye and Fentahum have six children: Orna (40) arrived in Israel aged 10, Habtam (32) was just 2 years old, Maayan (30) was born in Sudan and arrived as a baby, Sarah (29) and Shimon (19) were born in Israel. Another brother (36) arrived when he was 6 and did not participate in my study.

A year after her arrival in Israel, Orna was sent to boarding school, as was her brother a few years later. Today the parents regret this bitterly, saying that at the time they were struggling financially, and this was the solution suggested by the authorities. With moist eyes they describe the children as 'coming home like guests'. Habtam became the eldest child at home, and to this day she has a crucial 'parental' position in the family taking responsibility for solving things. She describes this necessity as compulsive:

> I can't explain it, don't know when they [her parents] gave this to me, it's as if they planted something under my skin and they activate it whenever they need something. It's very frustrating. Even more so since this only applies to the three eldest children. The younger ones just don't care, they are immune.

This altruistic sense of total commitment is common in cooperative communities such as existed in Ethiopia, less so in individualistic Western societies. Habtam describes her younger siblings as 'self-centred', their connection to the family loose, less obligating. But Habtam herself, newlywed and living a 2½-h drive away from her parents, functions as an extension of them without thinking twice—when they need her, she is there. Her parent's requirements and desires, often connected to her younger siblings, are constantly at the top of her list of priorities, balanced precariously against her other commitments. The ability to be aware and considerate of her own needs and desires comes with great effort, she describes how it has taken her years to even consider putting herself first.

Her sister Orna, the eldest child, talks eloquently of the chasm which exists between the siblings—the older three G1.5 and the younger three, G2, who:

> are neither here or there, they are stuck in the middle, they don't feel like they belong there [Ethiopia] and they don't feel they belong here [Israel].

She goes on to explain that the younger siblings do not understand what is obvious to the older ones:

> we who were born in Ethiopia still have the value of respect [for our parents], all sorts of values that were inculcated in us as children. I don't see that in them [her younger siblings].

8.2 Impertinence and Lack of Compliance

In most participant families the parents and older siblings described the G2 children as impertinent and lacking compliance. While Ethiopian culture is characterized by the interviewees as respectful, in contrast Israeli culture is considered as impertinent, often rude and inconsiderate of others. Thus, in the Ethiopian community normatively unacceptable behaviour, especially of children to their parents, would include assertiveness, insubordination, talking back, being stubborn, outright refusal, voicing an opinion, interrupting an adult conversation, and raising one's voice. Tigist says that in Ethiopia:

> There is no way children would be impertinent to their parents, to any authority figure.

But in Israel, as many interviewees described, there is 'a lot of disrespect'. Lack of compliance, children saying *no* to a parent, is regarded as parental loss of control. This is a huge challenge to Ethiopian parents, as Edna explains:

> The children asked me how you say *no* in Amharic, I couldn't find the word, so they went to ask other people, they all told them: it does not exist! There is no such word! There are all sorts of ways of refusing, but not the actual word.

In other words, non-compliance in Ethiopia was cunningly formed to evade directly declining, through *wax and gold*[1] terminology. In every household in Israel children are refusing their parents, the common adage is *lo ba li* loosely translated this means 'I don't want to'. G2 children adopt this phrase easily, much to their parent's displeasure. This is how Lemlem describes it:

> This *lo ba li* drives me crazy. It's like [I say] eat, [they say] I don't want to. Forget about asking them to do things, even if you just want them to eat, it's *lo ba li*!

Lemlem says about her three children:

> This saying no, I don't want to, I don't feel like it—these words drive me crazy. Sometimes I just want them to behave the way I behaved [to my parents], but this is impossible. I know I am judging them through my own eyes, as I was as a child. And after I get angry, I think about it for a minute, they don't know that world [Ethiopia], so why am I comparing them to me? This is really a difficult conflict for us.

Non-compliance and outright refusal are behaviours which Ethiopian parents find especially challenging, touching a cultural nerve that stimulates various responses. Lemlem is aware of this, she does not want to judge her children by Ethiopian standards, but inevitably finds herself doing so. Realizing that her children are growing up in a different reality, she nevertheless expects to receive a little of the respect she remembers giving her parents.

> I tell her, I wish you would just obey me! Do you know how I behaved to my mother? And she says: *OK Mum, what do you want from me?* My husband and I are always telling them how we respect our parents. Maybe we'll get a quarter of that!

---

[1] The term is explained in detail in Chap. 2.

The changes accompanying immigration force parents to face their own past, the ability to react to the children in the present moment requires a lot of personal effort and self-awareness. Inevitably parents compare their relationships with their children to their own relationship with their parents, where immigration has introduced a culture clash into the equation, this becomes a painful process of self-reflection.

> I want them to respect me like I respected my parents, they are good children, don't get me wrong, but there is no comparison! (Lemlem).

The *good children* in Israel are far from the polite obedient children of Ethiopia, who did their chores without even being asked. This is the model of the ideal child engrained in parents' minds, even if they are culturally flexible and open-minded it is hard for them to come to terms with the change.

In this case, immigration has produced a culture clash that emphasizes two opposing extremes—respectful obedience and defiant non-compliance—which elevates the power struggle in the family, often resulting in fierce altercations between parents and children. When this happens on a regular basis, the end result can be complete disconnection. Maayan describes a family like this—her cousins, Avi and Addis talk about their friends who have reached this point, where there is little or no contact at all between them and their parents. Once ties are severed, they are difficult to mend, the loss is tremendous—from the children's point of view this means both personal connections and the inter-generational pathway to their cultural heritage. In Ethiopia, growing up in close-knit communities, children always had other relatives to turn to, but in Israel, with the scattering of the community and general breakdown of supportive networks, this does not always apply. Many young people in the study described themselves as 'unprotected' or having an 'unsupportive childhood' involving 'strict authoritarian parenting'. Dana described herself repeatedly as 'submissive, an unprotected child'. Authoritarian parenting leaves no option for negotiation, distancing children from their parents and often leads to submissive or rebellious behaviour, the former involving self-denial and the latter self-destruction. The resultant conflicts—overt or covert—lead to a general breakdown in communication, fixating submissive or rebellious behaviour as the preferable strategy when dealing with people of authority. This can be seen in schools, as student–teacher clashes, and in the army, where often Ethiopian Israeli soldiers excel as officers or end up in military prison. In 2014, for example, they comprised 15.4% of those in military prison, although being only 3% of conscripts (Israeli Channel 2 news 15.5). Obviously, there may be many additional reasons for this, but this is part of the story. This issue has also been discussed by Edelstein (2014).

8.3 Back to the Sehalu Family

Orna fails to understand her younger siblings, she is vehemently against using colour as an excuse for lack of success:

> I cannot say I am disadvantaged. I believe in hard work and making an effort. I won't use my colour as an excuse, I'm used to the fact that I constantly need to prove myself. Once I learnt that, it just became a part of who I am.

As a new immigrant, Orna understood she needed to make an effort to prove her worth in order to belong, she accepts her own and her parents struggles as part and parcel of the process of integration. And like her parents, she expects her younger siblings to do the same. But they did not emigrate, they were born here, and they expect to have equal opportunities as their birth right, without making any special efforts.

Sarah is 11 years younger than Orna, when I asked her what her parents expect from her she sighed heavily and said very quietly:

> That I should manage, be successful in my studies, get ahead at work, make a family…the same expectations all parents have from their children. I think it's the same. I mean standard expectations.

Her face is very sad as she speaks, she knows that so far, she has failed to fulfil these standard expectations. She is not, as Habtam said of her, indifferent to what her parents think of her, she has internalized their disappointment to think less of herself. She then adds that her parents expect

> that if something happens, I won't wait for the last minute to tell them. And that I should succeed all the time.

Nobody succeeds all the time, people learn through failure, an important parental message is that of encouragement—to reflect to the child who fails that they are capable of succeeding, to inspire them to believe in themselves and try again. Habtam knows this, in her interview she recounted an occasion when she failed and her father told her: 'it's all right, you are capable of doing it'! But the G2 children never got such a message or did not internalize it.

Maayan, 30, defines her connection to her parents:

> Complicated. I was often rebellious, often wanted to be different, I don't want to be like my sisters…a lot of the time [as a child] I was depressed.

About her younger sister, Sarah, Maayan says:

> She was more neglected than me. She was much more rebellious and much more problematic. I don't think she sees it like that. But she is the only one who actually managed to change schools. And as soon as she did, she got in with the wrong people and let herself do all sorts of things I never let myself do, like the fact that she smokes.

In her interview, Sarah describes 'many moments' that she finds it very difficult to be with her family:

> I don't get along with any of them. So often I find myself here, at home, sitting by myself, and nobody takes any notice of me. So I just get up and go back to my apartment.

She describes herself as 'a rebel' and tells me how she broke all the rules, insisting on leaving the religious school her parents chose for her, registering herself to a secular school, smoking, going out late, and dressing immodestly. The teenage clashes with her parents have created a rift between them that today is almost insoluble. Habtam says she always knew when her father was pleased with her, but Sarah does not remember any such occasion. The feeling that she was a constant disappointment to them, that they were always more pleased with her siblings, that there is no special quality about her valued by her family, is a feeling that has deeply damaged her self-image. She is sad and tearful as she speaks to me. In Maayan's interview, she groups herself together with her younger sister, Sarah, and says:

> Looking back, I can always see the unfairness. It will always haunt me.

In the Sehalu family the balance of the traditional hierarchy according to age has been broken, the culture clash differentiating the children according to their birthplace has created a painful rift in the family. Maayan has many examples of this, in all of them she is treated unfairly by her parents, which has convinced her they value her older siblings more. Even in Ethiopia, sometimes children found it difficult to accept the hierarchical relations between siblings, but at least they could see the logic behind it. In the Sehalu family the younger children cannot understand the logic of their differential treatment, which combined with the breakdown in communication has distanced them from their parents and left them feeling undervalued.

This is also reflected in the way the various children describe their parents. Orna and Habtam each (separately) described their parents as caring, supportive, and helpful: 'they tried to give us everything'. The three younger children described their family as 'an average Ethiopian family'. Sarah added:

> Father was old fashioned, mother was more modern, more understanding, from the point of view of the language, and also being in control and all, so she was better. My father was very tough, very primitive. He belongs to the *older generation*.

This last she adds emphatically, as if it explains everything—her father is *primitive* and *old*, her mother younger and more modern—the dichotomy is striking, she has defined the chasm which cannot be crossed. Young people in Ethiopia were so respectful of their parents such a thing would never have been said: calling her father both old and primitive in one breath demeans his value, delegitimizes his world view, and differentiates him from the rest of the family. When I asked Sarah what she meant by this she added:

> He understands less, he is less updated, less informed. He doesn't talk to us in Hebrew at all, our mother is much more able to converse in Hebrew, she does talk to us and she's much more open minded.

On the other hand, her sister Habtam said about her father:

> He is stubborn. That is the best word to describe him. He is so stubborn, that it's his way or the highway.

Habtam sees her father as insistent on his way regarding his own and his children's lives, as was common in Ethiopia for the male head of the household. She does not judge him for this and states it as a fact—this is how he behaved in the family. She values and appreciates her father even though he is analphabetic:

> When he sat with me and said—do your homework, it never occurred to me that he had no idea what I was writing. I just understood that I had to do my homework. This really motivated me later on.

Habtam's connection with her father is based on mutual understanding and resides on a shared language and culture:

> There is a very good vibe between us. My younger sisters don't have that, they wouldn't just sit and talk to our parents. They don't do that. But I can just sit with him, and he'll tell me about Ethiopia, what he did, what he thinks, or just talk to me about what was on the news.

For Habtam, just sitting with her parents opens a channel of communication which is not available to her younger sisters. It involves the unfiltered intertwined flow of culture and connection that bonds them and creates continuity across the generations. Her younger sisters have been effectively excluded from this interchange because the cultural rift between the generations has created an invisible barrier between them. Their father, Fentahun, is aware of this in other families, he talks about it with sad eyes, and I wonder if indirectly he is talking about what has happened to some extent in his own home. All his children, at least now as adults, encouraged by their mother, treat him with respect, even if they no longer share information with him or seek his advice. To a passing observer he would appear to have retained his status in the family, but it is empty of content: he does not make the decisions nor is he aware of all that is happening in his children's lives. In contrast, his wife Eneye has not made do with a hollow superficial status in the family, she has made great efforts to learn Hebrew, complete a minimal education, and keep up with what is going on around her so that she can maintain a significant role in her children's lives. Maayan admires her for this:

> She was never like a typical Ethiopian mother, and I say this with great admiration: she always put her children first, which is something most Ethiopian adults don't do. Or for example when there was a big family event, it wasn't like—the parents arrange it all and we just wait to be told—she wanted to hear what we thought.

Maayan says her mother even seeks her advice on what she wears:

> The fact that she would even seek our advice shows that she was not concerned with her own ego—not like *I'm your mother and that's that*—she knows how to listen to us, to be our friend.

Eneye practices authoritative parenting, her parental authority is clear, but it is built on connection, through cooperation. In contrast, her husband, Fentahun, bases his authority on his status, which has been undermined in the new reality.

Maayan explains that this change in her mother is recent, and it was based on

> not wanting to lose us, like in so many families, even in my own cousin's family, where there is no connection between parents and children—they don't talk to each other at all.

8.4 Normative Behaviour in Ethiopia and in Israel

There were other participants in the study, aside from the younger children of the Sehalu family, who described their families as 'typically Ethiopian' or 'the average Ethiopian family'. Shira (13) described herself as 'normal in every way' when she talked about being Israeli, in other words 'normal' is equated with Israeli.[2] The children growing up in Israel have adopted Israeli-Western concepts of normalcy regarding their families, thus Sarah calls her father 'primitive'. Ester (26) talked about her parents as having 'old-fashioned opinions'. The internal concept of cultural normalcy guides behaviour (Kim-Pong, 2015), ways of educating are matched to these concepts, which determine if children's conduct is considered positive and desirable or negative requiring reprimand (Rubin & Boon Chung, 2006). Noam said that his parents raised him 'like they should' and that he raises his daughter 'as he should'—cultural normalcy dictates what 'should' be done in parenting. On the cultural divide of unsettled lives, what this means is no longer clear or necessarily agreed upon.

Conduct considered respectful and polite by one community can be seen as reserved and timid in another. In Ethiopia, as in many African and Asian societies, the normative educational emphasis is less on self-reliance, assertiveness, and self-expression (all normatively valued in Israel) but more on obedience, compliance, and the humble consideration of others. Of course, this is a generalization which must be taken with caution, since there are variations on this in all of these societies. But the tendency to value restraint, prudence and cooperation, communal harmony and respectful behaviour are common components of Ethiopian parental ethnotheories. Thus, Ethiopian traditional education guides the children to internalize humanistic values, also most mentioned by elders of the community in my study when asked what they most wanted the next generation to inherit: a caring attitude, politeness, modesty, and respectfulness. But the second generation have internalized local norms, often leading to a severe culture clash (found also by Berhanu, 2001, 2005).

The Sehalu family has been presented here as an example of this, not as a *typical family*. I did not find such a thing, each family in my study was unique and special, each found their own way of coping with their unsettled lives. When the second-generation participants referred on occasion to their families as typically Ethiopian, I see this as shorthand for describing commonalities associated with Ethiopian culture and immigration. This should not be confused with gross generalizations unhelpful in understanding this community. Although they may often share similar cultural toolkits, personal and family strategies of action interwoven into the very fabric of daily life are particular to each family or individual.

For example, families have varying degrees of emotional expression: Dov described his parents as

> very strongly expressing their love—with hugs, and kisses—these were very common, but when they were angry—wow did they express that too!

---

[2] Which can also have various meanings, as discussed in Chap. 13.

In contrast, Lemlem described her family as very sensitive, quoting her mother as saying 'if anything happened in this family you'll all fall apart'! Yafit repeatedly talked of her family as very special, her mother coming from

> a long line of Rabbis, seven generations back, strung together like a precious necklace.

Families vary in their patterns of communication, for example Dana talked of the differences between her parents' relatives:

> My father's extended family is very different from my mothers. You can see it. In my father's family they are all closed up, less communicative. On my mother's side if you don't communicate, you're not worth anything!

There are differences in the degree of family cohesion or cooperativeness, for example Genet said:

> Personally, I find it hard with my husband, because he comes from such a different family to ours, they were raised in the city, they each only look out for themselves!

Naama spoke of her mother's family:

> My grandmother comes from a charming family, the sisters [her mother and her siblings] are really close, actual soul mates.

Families vary in their attitude to education, as Teruneh said:

> I come from a family where education was top priority, even if it came at the expense of something else. My father preferred to hire paid help for the fields rather than letting us miss school.

Social status also distinguished certain families, for example Liora said about her mother:

> She was very well known in Ethiopia. Everywhere I went, everybody knew who she was. She was a good woman, which gives me strength, and pride to have been born into such a family.

Shy describes his family as

> always economically viable. I remember my father giving clothes to poor people for the festivals.

Families varied in the extent to which the *respectful distance* between adults and children was observed, for example Liora described this as nonexistent in her family, and Habtam remembers her close connection to her grandfather who never worried about 'the respectful distance which was supposed to be'.

Abynesh describes families in Ethiopia who did not punish their children, and adults who would patiently talk to children rather than reprimand them. In other words, in every culture there is the expected norm, and people adjust themselves around it, there will always be those who behave differently. Thus, this mosaic of parental and family conduct presented by the study reflects the diversity of this community, which was apparent in Ethiopia as it is in Israel. It seems that for families who were more verbal, flexible, and attentive to their children in Ethiopia the transition to Israel is easier. For example, Liora said that she could 'sit and talk to her children' because this is the way she herself grew up. Behaviour considered exceptional in Ethiopia paved the way for an easier adjustment to life in Israel, perhaps preventing the full force of the culture clash felt by other, more *traditionally normative* families. Similarly, although less explored by this study, there is also the question of local integration into specific Israeli Jewish sub-cultures with their varying norms and expectations.

References

Berhanu, G. (2001). *Learning-in-context. An ethnographic investigation of mediated learning experiences among Ethiopian Jews in Israel* (pp. 253–261). (Unpublished doctoral dissertation). Gothenburg University, Sweden.

Berhanu, G. (2005). Normality, deviance, identity, cultural tracking and school achievement: The case of Ethiopian Jews in Israel. *Scandinavian Journal of Educational Research, 49*(1), 51–82.

Diem-Wille, G. (2014). *Young children and their parents: Perspectives from psychoanalytic infant observation*. Karnak.

Edelstein, A. (2014). The main causes of anti-social behaviour among former Ethiopian youth in Israel. In E. Witztum & N. Grisaru (Eds.), *Social and clinical aspects of Ethiopian Immigrants in Israel* (pp. 153–184). The Jewish Agency for Israel and Ben Gurion University.

Kim-Pong, T. (2015). Understanding intergenerational cultural transmission through the role of perceived norms. *Journal of Cross-Cultural Psychology, 46*(10), 1260–1266.

Rubin, K., & Boon Chung, O. (2006). *Parenting beliefs, behaviours, and parent-child relations: A cross cultural perspective*. Psychology Press.

Swidler, A. (1986). Culture in action: Symbolism and strategies. *Americal sociological review, 51*(2), 273–286.

Chapter 9
Cultural Flexibility, Hybridity, and Children's Wellbeing

Describing families in general terms as *culturally flexible* or *culturally conservative* refers to long-term patterns of behaviour which shape the reality in which children are raised—with a certain tolerance for change and responsiveness to the current moment or endeavouring to preserve set cultural values and strategies of action. In practice these issues are complex, as all families can sometimes be flexible and sometimes conservative, or flexible about some things and not others, or one parent more flexible than the other. Going back to Swidler's (1986) definition of culture as a toolkit that is formed and renewed constantly in time and place, inevitably containing anomalies and inconsistencies, the issue of cultural flexibility reflects precisely the ability to adapt and match the contents of this tool kit to new contexts. Immigration sharpens perceptions of cultural differences, initiating a process of conscious and subconscious choice and innovation versus strict adherence to the old and familiar. It is this constant covert and sometimes overt dilemma which contributes to the sense of being *unsettled*. This is especially potent between the generations, as families juggle the delicate balance between past and present, personal and collective, daily life precariously balanced on the slippery continuum between conservatism, flexibility, and change.

9.1 The Basis for Parental Authority

> If the father in Ethiopia was forcefully authoritarian, here he is understandingly authoritative (Dov).

Dov goes on to describe how explanations and 'direct talk' are replacing parental commands. 'Here instead of demanding [compliance] one has to ask for it', says Dany, and Shy explains that 'we cannot force conformity'. These fathers are shifting the basis of their parental authority from status to connection, backed by reasoning

© The Author(s), under exclusive license to Springer Nature Switzerland AG 2023

N. A. Shmuel, *Children's Wellbeing in Immigrant Families*, Children's Well-Being: Indicators and Research 26,
https://doi.org/10.1007/978-3-031-31917-4_9

rather than punishment. It is a fundamental change in parental attitudes which applies to mothers as well: Modesh describes how in Israel parental connection is built on words, repeatedly she stresses the importance of talking to children. Her daughter Ester says:

> When I was little my father was very strict, very restrictive, always telling us what to do and not allowing many things. Mother would say—*well, all right*, she always agreed to things. In time they both became more permissive. They still have *outdated opinions*, but compared to how they used to be today they are much more lenient, not completely open-minded but more so…

Ester has distinguished between her parents—her mother was always more flexible than her father, a pattern evident in other families in my study. Ester's parents buried their first two children in Sudan, it is likely that part of her father's protectiveness was an effort to keep his Israeli-born children safe. Ester remembers this as unreasonable restrictiveness, but she recognizes that he has changed over the years and is more flexible with her younger siblings. She calls her parents' opinions 'outdated'—setting them apart from the modern Israeli 'open-minded' mainstream which she encounters through her native Israeli peers.

Other studies (for example, Rosenthal & Roer-Strier, 2001; Roer-Strier, 2001) have shown that after immigration parents tend to preserve traditional parenting attitudes and behaviours, based on cultural perceptions of the ideal child. Thus, in the new context, changes observed in the second generation are still likely to be interpreted by their parents according to traditional logic. G2 children were often described by G1 and G1.5 participants in my study as rude, disobedient, and inattentive, many adults see this as a deterioration of values and lack of sufficient discipline rather than an adaptation to Israeli society. The result is often either an escalated use of coercion and restriction in an attempt to rectify this situation, or parental withdrawal (the present-absent parent).

9.2 A Different Sort of Communication

Dany describes how Ethiopian custom dictates receiving food with outreached hands, and rising when the elders enter a room, both signs of respectful behaviour. And yet in contrast in Israel, he finds himself imploring his children to eat, and on entering the room they remain seated while he stands looking for a place to sit. Dany is smiling when he tells this, he is explaining how he must adjust his parenting to this new situation with patience and understanding, ending by saying

> I am very different from my own father. I need to be their friend, so they tell me things. To get close to them so they feel close to me.

Dany has forsaken the *respectful distance* required by Ethiopian tradition for the sake of connection. He is not offended by his children's behaviour—he recognizes this as cultural adjustment and does not see it as disrespect. This shifting perspective fosters his patience in situations which would otherwise lead to conflict.

Avi appreciates his mother for raising him and his brother by herself in Israel and adapting her parenting to the new reality:

> She understood that the way children were raised in Ethiopia is not the way to raise children born here. I really appreciate that she made this change. She always pushed me to study; she never said you need to go to work. She also understood that if I have a girlfriend, I need to be able to bring her home without being ashamed. In other [Ethiopian] families it is not like that—if you bring a girl home you are expected to marry her.

These parents are initiating a different pattern of communication than was prevalent in Ethiopia—both more verbal and more direct, suited to their children's needs and not adherent to tradition. Their dialogue is aimed at bridging connection rather than teaching children their place in the hierarchy, opening new options of compromise and negotiation aside from obedience or rebellion.

Miki provides another example of this, saying:

> I sit with him [his son] and explain patiently, also by personal example, so that he knows how to behave (Miki).

Miki has denoted two important elements which make this change effective: patience and personal example. In the traditional hierarchy there was one unspoken rule for adults and another for the children. Setting an example in the sense Miki refers to, and holding such an intimate conversation, while both seated rather than the adult standing over the child, are creating a sense of equality which breeds trust and attentiveness. Some adults might reject this as condescending, undermining parental authority. But in the *new context* it does exactly the opposite: this is precisely what builds authority based on connection.

These culturally flexible parents are changing the contents of their toolkit to fit the context in which they live. Some are very aware that their children are no longer surrounded by many other supportive adults, as they were in the villages in Ethiopia. For example, Liora says:

> I talk to them. In Ethiopia there were lots of people around to tell me, to educate me. My children just have us, me and my husband. So we have to talk to them.

These adults no longer expect their children to learn everything of their own volition, simply by vigilant observation, or to decipher an obscure proverb or absorb knowledge from the community. Instead, they are talking directly to their children with simple explanations and instructions. Not only this, but they are skillfully combining elements from their traditional cultural toolkit with new methodologies, as Genet explains:

> My parenting comes from observing my mother and adding to that more verbality, more listening, to give the children space but to be there to direct them.

This new type of parenting is not concerned with relative status or cultural perceptions of respectful distance, it is attentive parenting geared towards the children's current needs, providing them a safe space in which to grow.

What makes some parents able to do this, to be culturally flexible, and others not?

The answer is complex and involves both the abilities of the parents and the nature of the absorbing environment. Immigrant parents are often struggling with their own adjustment to the new society, including their social status, identity, and self-image (for example, Wagaw, 1993; Salamon, 2011). Coping with these is preliminary to any changes in parenting methods, which depend on many factors, such as personal skills of self-awareness and self-reflection, support networks, educational background, and more. In stressful situations, such as facing the uncertainties of life in a new country, while feeling unsettled and possibly dejected, it is difficult to activate self-reflection and open-mindedness, the natural tendency is to rely on automatic cultural reactions and interpretations (Shapiro, 1988). This is where the host society can step in and be supportive and encouraging, but sadly more often tends to be critical and alienating.

9.3 The Experiences of the G2 Children

For many adults, as Dany described, the experience of parenting in Ethiopia was fundamentally different from the experience of parenting in Israel, and often included an intuitive non-verbal almost mystic intimacy, as Edna describes:

> My parents *knew*, without talking to me on the telephone, without calling me ten times a day, they knew exactly what I was doing. My father could look at me and he *knew* if I had gone astray.

In this quote, Edna was talking about her father in Israel, but in most families this deep intuitive connection did not survive immigration: most G2 children do not have an adult capable of such deep perception of them. Thus, the intuitive knowledge Edna was referring to now depends on verbal connection, and where this is lacking, parents are not necessarily conscious of their children going astray. Dany, Shy, Liora, and others are all aware of this, it is one of the reasons they advocate for talking to children. But many G2 children have a different experience. Addis refers to his childhood as 'not very embracing', and including 'very strict discipline'. Dana repeatedly refers to herself as 'an unprotected child', her narrative reflects her disconnection with her parents; she describes her father as 'not a parent' and her mother as totally unaware of her experiences and needs. The breakdown in communication in these families coupled with cultural conservatism has effectively severed amicable inter-generational relations. As Shy explains:

> There are families in which the children refuse to speak Amharic, they see their parents as primitive, nothing interests them, not even Amharic music, they fight over the TV channels [not to watch the Ethiopian channel their parents prefer] like a war…you can see how disconnected these children are from their parents.

Abigail also describes this:

> The parents don't understand the children, don't know how to get close to them. It's not their fault. Then the girl goes partying, stays out late, and to him [the father] this is a catas-

> trophe! There are lots of arguments about this. The mother is more flexible, the father is against it, and war breaks out.

The repeated use of the word *war* to describe family conflict emphasizes the severity of the situation, in which the result is inevitably, as Abigail says with a heavy sigh; 'we lose our dear ones, our children'. Keeping control of the children by traditional methods is a lost battle, waged on two fronts: between the parents and the children and between the parents themselves, when each adopt differing strategies. Naama describes how her brothers 'have developed tactics for persuading our mother', because it is possible to talk to her, while the father's refusal to the children is non-negotiable. She says that:

> If anybody will get hurt by this it is my younger brother, he's very sensitive, he takes it really hard.

Naama is used to the fact that she cannot talk to her father, but her younger brother finds this situation unbearably frustrating.

The upset of power relations within the family, traditionally based on age and gender, has unleashed an overt and covert power struggle between the sexes[1] and between the generations to varying degrees in all families. At best this is negotiated or managed, at worst it turns into outright war, the victims inevitably being primarily the children caught up in the conflict. Disconnection leaves them unprotected and vulnerable, the loss is not only of parental understanding and support, but also of knowledge about and connection to their cultural heritage and roots. Where there are G1.5 siblings, uncles, or cousins who can step up and become their support network the G2 children are not alone, but not all of them have these.

9.4 Educating for Assertiveness

> If they [her children] want to be impertinent let them be impertinent. I don't want them to be trodden on, I want them to stand up for themselves, to be able to argue. (Liora).

Genet proudly describes her daughter as having 'her own opinions' and 'if she says no then it's no'! These parents are changing their expectations, the ideal child is no longer passive and submissive, they recognize that to survive in Israeli society their children need to develop a certain stubborn assertiveness. Liora is willing to let her children practice this at home, she is training them to stand their ground:

> I am proud of them for saying no. In my culture this is not possible. Even if you want to say no, the word reaches your tongue, and you swallow it. I don't want my children to be like this. I want them to be able to say no and explain themselves.

In a separate interview, her husband Shy smiles proudly as he describes his children as having Israeli impertinence. These parents are willing to accept impertinence and refusal as part of preparing their children for the new competitive world

[1] Further discussed in Chap. 11.

they are living in. These parents are changing both their strategies for action, their interpretation of their children's behaviour, and their expectations to match the context in which they live, while maintaining parental authority and involvement in their children's lives. Moreover, the parents' flexibility at home is crucial in enabling the children safe cultural passage between home and school, and in the long run encourages their growing aptitude for hybridity.

9.5 Setting Rules and Boundaries

Matan explains his understanding of how Ethiopian immigrant parents think:

> Their head is still over there [in Ethiopia]. They can react with force, or say something, but they know they cannot use force, they are beginning to accept this.

All forms of corporal punishment have been banned in Israel since the year 2000. But accepting the rules is not necessarily acceptance of the child or his or her behaviour. What the parents are accepting, often, is their own reduced status and helplessness. As Genet said about her mother:

> It is a fact that there [in Ethiopia] she was the educator, she had the authority as a grandmother. Here she cannot educate, she has no authority over the grandchildren.

Physical punishment is ruling by force, causing pain is not part of an educational process. The perception of power relations which gives legitimacy to physical punishment preserves the respectful distance effectively blocking open communication between parent and child.

> If he [her son] is afraid when he is little, then later he won't walk all over us (Shani).

Like Shani, many parents believe that children should be fearful of their parents, punishment in this case is perceived as the means to induce obedience. The idea of reciprocal cooperation induced by an egalitarian relationship is a new and unfamiliar concept in many of these families. It involves relinquishing the hierarchical paradigm and substituting it with an alternative model, in many sub-cultures of Israeli society this has not yet happened. What can change more easily, is the form of punishment:

'If one gives a punishment, it should not be a slap', says Ziv, who goes on to explain that he never hits his children, instead he talks to them. Ziv is basing his parental authority on connection rather than status, he foregoes the rule of force, no longer expecting his children to be obedient as his father expected of him. He might still punish them occasionally, but not using force, his examples include denying them television or pocket money. Like Dany, Shy, and other parents who are changing strategies, Ziv is aware that children who fear their parents do not confide in them but tend to hide things and even lie.

Recollecting her own childhood and referring to herself as an attentive parent, Noa says that her child:

> will receive what I never did… I want him to know that he *does* have someone to turn to, it's very important to me.

Similarly, it is important to Genet to be present in her children's lives 'by my own definitions' which she details as 'to talk to them, to listen to them, to be there'.

Some of these parents are completely deleting the respectful distance between the generations, opening new forms of communication which make them more available to their children. In relationships built on trust, sharing, and learning from mistakes (rather than coercion and punishments) the child becomes partner in their own education. The cultural flexibility which enables this also enhances the potential for cultural transferal across the generations—children in these families are more likely to be interested in hearing stories about Ethiopia or learning Amharic, as described by Liora, Shy, Bossana, Ziv, Genet, Lemlem, Aberash, and Edna.

Shani, her husband Teruneh, and their three children lived for 5 years in her parents' apartment. This is common in Israel while young couples are saving to buy their own apartments. The issue of punishment raised an argument between Shani and her parents which is still unresolved:

> In our culture, if a child misbehaves, then—*kwantut* [a pinch]—this is part of the educational system. Sometimes we do this following my parent's advice because we lose control, but it doesn't really help! It doesn't work! It's just a pity.

Shani is frustrated about 'losing control', she uses this phrase repeatedly during the interview. Without alternative educational methods, she resorts to her parents' solutions, but these are ineffective. Her husband, Teruneh, says that it is hard to teach the children boundaries, that he finds himself repeating the same words 'twenty thousand times' and when he looks after them, they 'recoil'—in other words, his authority is based on persistent threats. Shani and Teruneh are looking for a way to control the children without using force, but parental authority based on connection is not about controlling the children, it is about guiding and influencing them.

> In Ethiopia children are expected to understand [intuitively]. So I want to use that system, but it doesn't work. So then I think, I'll talk to my son, but he—[she covers her ears and sticks out her tongue, indicating that this is what her child does]—it's so hard—neither the Ethiopian nor the Western systems work!

Shani and Teruneh are impulsively mixing strategies of action from both cultures without any persistent system, this is what is not working. They are trying to adopt new methodologies within the restrictive hierarchy, which is hard to relinquish because of the desire to remain in control. But the effect is losing control without establishing any basis for parental authority.

This type of chaos is evident in many families, and mentioned by Ester, Nechemya, and others, where open confrontations and battles of willpower replace the orderly negotiation of everyday living. Ester describes how her father:

> always wanted order at home, like at lunch time or for doing homework, he would always say there is a time for this and a time for that, but we never did it, everything was always just chaotic.

Noam remembers himself as a child falling asleep in the living room in front of the television and finding it difficult to get up in the mornings (consequently he describes having a set bedtime for his daughter as important to him). Contributing to the chaos is lack of communication in the family—the fact that things are not talked about openly and negotiated, and the fact that in many families children and parents live in separate, even opposing, perceptual worlds. This is what growing up on the cultural divide looks like, it is the epitome of unsettled lives. Many children growing up in such families have difficulty adjusting to structured settings such as the expectations at school and in other frameworks.

9.6 Parental Presence, Protection, and Vulnerability

When the family is struggling financially it's very hard. You really feel this. You see frustrated parents, arguments, disagreements, blame, sparse Sabbath meals, and the children don't understand...they complain, why isn't there this food and that food...and there are no books, and they want clothes...and phones...it creates a lot of arguments and frustration because you can't explain it to them properly, they don't understand that not everybody can afford things. There were periods when my parents were managing [financially], these were better periods, calmer. (Naama).

Financial difficulties often accompany immigration and affect the whole family, even if the parents are adapting and adding new strategies of action to their parenting toolbox, their lack of resources is restrictive, as Naama's mother, Yafit, explains:

> I know what children need, how to develop them. But when something is stopping you, you just cannot do it. I encourage them verbally, whether they succeed or not.

She is talking about not being able to give her children the sort of support that might help their success, such as extra lessons or participation in extra-curricular activities. Nevertheless, she is always encouraging, because she knows that however hard her children try, they start off at a disadvantage. Naama's description of her childhood before her father arrived in Israel reflects this:

> my mother worked two jobs, that's how I remember her, I saw very little of her. She came home shattered and exhausted. I remember myself as a latch-key child.

This is a very different reality from the way children grew up in Ethiopia surrounded by community, to be a 'latch-key child' is to be *alone*. This narrative and others illustrate how the financial situation and availability of supporting relatives to share caring for the children while their parents work is crucial for children's wellbeing after immigration.

The need to provide for their families keeps many fathers away from home for long hours, as Dov explains:

> He used to get up at three or four in the morning to go to work, when he came back in the evening he was exhausted and lacking in energy, he just went to sleep and that was that, we never saw him.

Noam describes a similar reality:

> They [his parents] had to work to support us. After school we went to the community centre till four-thirty then we came home alone, one of our parents would arrive about half an hour later. They didn't really have time for us.

Most of the immigrant parents had menial jobs that demanded a lot of energy and long hours. Instead of the safe space of the local village with an abundance of adults to supervise them, many children spent their time in after-school programmes or home alone. Aberash describes the difference:

> In Ethiopia the home and the outside were the same because everybody cared for the children with the same values.

Abynesh describes herself 'not sleeping for six years' after arriving in Israel, because she was so worried about the unknown dangers of her new surroundings. Parents struggling financially were not always able to keep their children safe, Yael talks about this with anger and sadness, saying that in Ethiopia 'nobody ruins your children'. Three of her children are today mentally damaged adults who live in institutions, she blames other people for their situation, believing they were damaged by experiences at boarding school or elsewhere. In the interview it is obviously very hard for her to talk about it, her explanations are fragmented and incoherent:

> I went to work, and the children mixed with all sorts, you don't know who is good and who isn't. It was hard for me. When I brought the three of them here, they were all healthy, and now… the three of them are not well, not well at all. All sorts [of people] come, from different countries, you don't know who you can trust with your children.

Her daughter Dana is very critical of her parents regarding what happened to her older brothers, saying:

> It's not an accomplishment to be a good parent to an easy child. It's the child that challenges you that needs attention. But they didn't give them attention, they sent them to boarding schools.

Dana seems to be implying that her brothers were neglected before they went to boarding school, where they arrived with a certain vulnerability:

> In boarding-school some children are strong and some are weak. They were weak, very weak. They came back damaged.

Dana is inferring that her brothers may have been molested or worse:

> They could not cope, they were really stupid, they did not know how to distinguish between good and bad. So if someone told them to take off their clothes they would just do it.

The tragedy of this family reflects the inadequacy of the system to assist them, to care for these children, support them, and keep them safe.

In many interviews parents referred to luck or God as determining their children's development, failures and successes being attributed to fate or a higher power. 'From their point of view God is responsible for everything', says Tigist about her parents. And Modesh rejects her daughter's praise by saying; 'if you are blessed with good children, it is not difficult to raise them'.

The concept of *iddil* in Amharic—luck or fate—as determining child development relinquishes responsibility from the parents and may lead to passivity (Rosen, 1986). According to Berhanu's study (2006), parents in Israel perceive fate, themselves and the schools in Israel as responsible for child development. He noted that there is no fundamental change in child-rearing practices, for example most parents do not celebrate children's birthdays, something which is practiced in most subcultures in Israel and has the potential for a meaningful emotional interaction with the child. In the families he studied, children were mostly left to play unsupervised, with little active interaction between parents and children. As in Ethiopia, children were not encouraged to ask questions or seek information from their parents, who still rely on them learning from their surroundings of their own volition. This attitude is counterproductive, as my study reflects, since it results in children who know very little if anything of their parents' language and culture. For example, Modesh's daughters do not know Amharic or how to cook *engera*, she attributes this to their unwillingness to learn, while they say she never taught them. In other words, neither generation has taken responsibility for the transferal of cultural knowledge between them.

Berhanu's research (2005, 2006) also found that most parents do not play with their children and were mostly passive in their interactions with them. In contrast, I found great variety in parental behaviour between the families in my study, with parents who are adding to their cultural toolkit methodologies suited to local contexts, including actively teaching their children Ethiopian cultural heritage as illustrated in the forthcoming examples. The differences between parental strategies might be attributed to levels of education, parental awareness, and willingness to learn new things—through active participation in parent meetings at school and parenting groups. Abynesh said she never missed even one meeting of the parenting group at school, even while she was pregnant and after she gave birth. Both she and Rachel (separately) described such meetings as very helpful, enabling self-reflection and sharing. Rachel talked about herself before she went to these meetings as 'always angry' with her children, feeling that they were ungrateful for everything she did for them. She completely changed her attitude:

> I was just giving and giving all the time and I felt my children owed me. I wanted them to thank me, to appreciate me. Even if they did something good, I never praised them. Now I do. *Thank you for doing that, thank you for taking your sister and bringing her back, thank you for enabling me to get to work on time*.

Recognizing her children's efforts to help her encourages them to shoulder some of her responsibilities and reduces arguments at home, her new attitude creates a partnership of action—they are all on the same side rather than pitted against one another.

9.7 Merging Cultures

Mulu describes how in all areas of life—music, food, language, and cultural codes—she is combining the foundations of both cultures to create 'the best of both worlds'—a suitable cultural mix in which to raise her daughter:

> I base her nutrition on healthy foods from the Ethiopian kitchen—so our traditional food and also Western food. The same with music, and language, we speak both, and all sorts of cultural codes, so it's a mix.

Included in this mixing of cultures is the internal acceptance of their joint value, and the effort to match the appropriate mix to the specific context. Aberash says the same about mixing educational methods she uses to raise her children:

> I try to merge what there is here with what there was in Ethiopia. There we were told not to raise our gaze, not to look adults in the eye when they talk to us. If they tell you to do something you have to do it, you don't have an opinion about it, whether it suits you or not, you do it. But here it isn't like that, so I consult my children and give them choices about what they can do, this helps both them and me. I don't tell them *you have to do that*, I let them choose.

Aberash does not give her children orders they must obey, as was customary in Ethiopia, she gives them choices to enable them to take responsibility and share household chores out of their own preference. Thus, she is avoiding power struggles and encouraging an atmosphere of cooperation and shared responsibility at home.

Aberash's home is also a place where stories 'bond between us to this day', as she says. Most parents can remember stories they were told as children, these are easier to pass between the generations, even in a different language, than proverbs—which often use local imagery and allegories, carrying messages in the *wax and gold* tradition.

Here is a wonderful example of stories acting as bridges between the generations:

> Every situation I found myself in, if I argued with my father or was rude to my mother, if I was punished in the army or whatever happened, I always told my grandfather, and he had a story, like a metaphor about what had happened to me and how I get out of it.

Yisrael, a soldier, comes to seek solace from his grandfather Gebre when he is troubled, and Gebre skillfully uses stories to reach across the generations and cultures to have meaningful conversations helpful to his grandson. Yisrael admires and appreciates his grandfather and his stories from the past, which have a powerful presence in his life and give him the strength to cope with current dilemmas and difficulties. Stories told out of context, in a different time and place, transport cultural meaning across the generations (Bauman, 2004). This interchange is made possible because Yisrael understands Amharic, even if his ability to speak it is limited.

Stories are a universal tool for building inter-generational connection and transferring cultural values, as illustrated by a study on Oromo-speaking children (Tadesse, 2018) whose folkloric performance of storytelling serves as a way by which they learn survival skills and grow connected to values of their society. This process of communication across the generations is based on sharing both a language and perceptions of reality, both of which do not inevitably apply to immigrant families experiencing unsettled lives, as demonstrated by the Sehalu family in the previous chapter. In fact, most of the second generation in my study did not know their family's immigration story and have little or no knowledge about Ethiopia at all, or their parents' childhood. The merging of cultures can only take place where there is sufficient connection to enable it, where closeness to a parent or grandparent inspires the desire to know them and even to emulate them—as Edna said about her father 'I want to be like him, but differently'.

9.8 Hybridity and Wellbeing

'In Israel I need to be both Ethiopian and Israeli, I try to combine the two', says Aberash, who has described her home as 'an Ethiopian home in Israel'. Combining two cultural systems as her internal reference mode and the basis of her parenting has made Aberash and others hybrid or bicultural, meaning that they have full competency in both cultures (Benet-Martinez et al. 2002, 2006). Thus, Genet describes herself as reserved and modest when in the Ethiopian community, using indirect communication—'talking in circles', while

> outside [the community] anybody who sees me says *you're not Ethiopian!* It starts with the language, it's important to me to speak correctly, so I have adjusted to both cultures. And I can be very Israeli, the jokes, the verbal jiving…

Spontaneously, without thinking about it, Genet matches herself to her surroundings, this is the essence of hybridity: culture-specific strategies of action are triggered by context, as are thought processes—accessing culture-specific knowledge to understand reality. Hybridity is especially common amongst the G1.5, but also applies to some of the G2 and even G1, for instance, Shy (G1):

> If I think about commenting on the news I heard, I think in Hebrew, not Amharic. I don't translate myself. Since I am here, I manage very well with Israelis, from the point of view of self-expression, at work, I know the culture. If you know the language, you know the culture. If I have a problem in this country, I know it might take me time, but I can solve it.

Shy is involved in Israeli society, thinks in both languages, and is confident of his ability to manage. Just as his wife, Liora (G1.5):

> I am Ethiopian by my colour, behaviour, culture, stuff like that. But I give to my country [Israel], my son is in the army, I want him to be a good soldier, I give what I can to help, visit him on base, come to parent's day, keep updated, especially now, I want to know what is happening, to take part in decision making, this is my country, my place.

Hybrid parents are better able to understand the world their children live in, to be involved in what is going on around them and help their children bridge harmoniously between the two cultures. Lemlem says that when she visits Ethiopia she 'knows the language, enjoys the food, and knows how to behave'. As a school counsellor in Israel she uses 'this knowledge with the Ethiopian parents I work with'. But she also says:

> I work with everybody, especially Israeli parents. That is where my own Israeliness expresses itself, through the advice I give parents in the schools, the board meetings, in the municipality. I teach in the college, there are no Ethiopians there.

Lemlem is confident in her abilities in both cultures, and it is this confidence which enables her to function calmly and efficiently both professionally and as a parent. Thus, she can navigate the refusal of her own children to obey (discussed in the previous chapter).

When Shira talks about her parents, she refers to refusal as something which 'brings out their Ethiopian side'. Refusal is the epitome of disrespect in Ethiopian culture, hybridity acts as a buffer mediating responses to this. Hybrid people have more than one frame of reference, Bennet-Martinez et al. (2002, 2006) refer to this as 'cultural frame switching' activated by cultural cues which may be actual (such as food, language, clothes) or implicit (such as expectations and social or family roles). Refusal is a cultural cue that elicits a severe sense of disrespect, but hybrid people can also re-interpret this as something else, such as assertive independence, enabling an amicable response to the current moment rather than conflict.

What enables or enhances hybridity? The answer is cultural knowledge, a clear sense of personal identity as both complex and dynamic, sensitivity to cultural processes, bilingualism, and cultural competence—meaning knowledge of cultural codes and expected behaviours in both cultures (LaFromboise et al., 1993; Chen et al., 2008). All these are fostered by an environment that appreciates and encourages diversity and are hindered when there is pressure on new immigrants to assimilate. The more parents maintain their involvement in both cultural communities, the more hybrid they become. Immigrants may have varying degrees of cultural knowledge, may be more culturally competent in some areas than in others, in other words this is a constantly changing continuum rather than a dichotomy. Local culture is also varied, especially in Israel, and so immigrants may experience varying degrees of hybridity in different contexts (as reflected in other studies, for example, Bar-Yosef, 2001; Sharabany & Israeli, 2008).

Every culture has preconceived notions of how people should behave, how lives should be lived, what it means to be a man, a woman, a child. At least to some extent, hybridity frees parents from these preconceptions, since it opens awareness to the fact that there are many ways of being, and every situation can be interpreted by differing perspectives. Hybridity itself invites the natural dissolution of all assumptions, a readiness to watch and listen before responding, as cultural knowledge is triggered by context. This often breeds in hybrid parents the unique ability to accept the slow discovery of each child, rather than the rigid determination to mould the children in a certain way.

Thus, children who grow up steeped in more than one culture often develop an inbuilt acceptance of complexity and the legitimacy of being more than one thing. Where diversity—between and within people—is acceptable and valued—children can develop multiple identities and yet feel whole. They may gain not only a better relationship with their parents but also learn to be more accepting of the diversity within themselves and others.

Similar to the use of different languages, the more cultural frame switching is practiced, the easier it becomes, and the more it develops complex thinking processes (Hong et al., 2003; Benet-Martinez et al. 2002). Thus, many G1.5 who are both bilingual and familiar with traditional body language can bridge between the other two generations (G1 and G2). Mostly they do so willingly, shouldering some of the responsibility for the children of the second generation. But not in all families is there somebody like this, thus Sarah says 'there is nobody who advises or supports me', and Dana constantly refers to herself as an 'unprotected child' and describes herself coping alone with many difficult situations as a young child. Lack of support and outright conflict are all part of the experiences of such G2 children at home. While the basis is cultural, as described by Dana, Sarah, and others, their subjective experience may often be one of personal disapproval and rejection. Not only this but going out into Israeli society they often experience a similar type of rejection based on their categorization by colour as Ethiopian. Depending on its potency and consistency, this *double rejection* can be a very harsh and damaging experience for children, leaving them both vulnerable and marginalized (to be discussed further in the next chapter).

Hybridity makes people adept at switching frames of reference; this flexibility enables them to adjust to changing social situations. Many of the intermediate, 1.5 generation, are skillful at this, like a swimmer changing naturally between breaststroke and crawl. To continue the analogy, in contrast, many of the second generation have not learnt to swim properly in either style, often previous experiences serving to undermine their confidence in swimming at all. Without clear intergenerational guidance, many of the G2 are drowning in the complex intercultural milieux, unless rescued by concerned G1.5 relatives. This is not to say that G2 are incapable of coping on their own, after all there are those who became leaders in their families after their elder siblings left for boarding schools (such as Habtam and Ester), and others who have built self-efficacy through challenging army service (such as Addis, Avi, Yisrael, and Yaniv), or have educated themselves in the Amharic language and culture (Miki, Dana, and Maayan). To go back to the above analogy, they are competent self-taught swimmers. Their search for meaning cannot be answered by the traditional knowledge of their elders, such as family genealogy. They are searching for knowledge which will combat the prejudices of Israeli society and expect to find this in books and not through their grandparents. As Naama explains:

> I buy every book that has connection to Ethiopian identity. I feel like I must fill this void inside me, because my parents didn't want to give me this information or thought it was not relevant for me. As an academic I must know… I wasn't born here, I came when I was five, I need to read about the country I came from.

Naama implies that her parents missed their chance to provide her with this information, now she is searching for it herself. Dana said something similar when she refers to the need:

> to have something that is mine, from my ancestors, not from here, because that belongs to them [the Israelis]. That's how they have defined it.

Dana is searching for identity as a right, not a privilege, she was born in Israel and all her life has tried to fit in, now she is looking for content to the Ethiopian identity which has been forced upon her.

Hybridity is not entirely a conscious choice, but dependent on many factors, both personal (language acquisition, cultural flexibility, support networks, etc.) and social (national and local policies encouraging or discouraging diversity). The Israeli tradition of assimilating immigrants, with the ethos of building one nation out of multiple cultures arriving from the Diaspora, has faded but not disappeared. Recent immigration coupled with President Rivlin's Four Tribes initiative[2] has paved the way towards a new dialogue on multiculturalism in Israel which is beyond the scope of this book. What is important to realize is that as our understanding of hybridity broadens, it is possible to see culture as a mosaic of customs, beliefs, and perceptions, representing values and strategies of action, thereby changing our concept of differentiated ethnic cultures to a complex view of reality in which all cultures are varied and their different combinations still create even more variations and differences. It is only through perceiving this complexity that we can begin to understand the lives, challenges, and strengths of the new generation born into immigrant families.

References

Bar-Yosef, R. W. (2001). Children of two cultures: Immigrant children from Ethiopia in Israel. *Journal of Comparative Family Studies, 32*(2), 231–246.

Bauman, R. (2004). *A world of others words: Cross-cultural perspectives on intertextuality* (pp. 1–11, 128–158). Blackwell Publishing.

Bennet-Martinez, V., Leu, J., & Lee, F. (2006). Biculturalism & cognitive complexity: Expertise in cultural representations. *Journal of Cross-Cultural Psychology, 37*(4), 386–407.

Benet-Martínez, V., Leu, J., Lee, F., & Morris, M. (2002). Negotiating biculturalism: Cultural frame switching in biculturals with oppositional versus compatible cultural identities. *Journal of Cross-cultural psychology, 33*(5), 492–516.

Berhanu, G. (2006). Parenting (parental attitude), child development, and modalities of parent-child interactions: Sayings, proverbs, and maxims of Ethiopian Jews in Israel. *Journal of Cognitive Education and Psychology, 5*(3), 266–287.

Berhanu, G. (2005). Indigenous conceptions of intelligence, ideal child, and ideal parenting among Ethiopian Jews in Israel. *Journal of Cognitive Education and Psychology, 5*(1), 47–71.

[2] https://www.runi.ac.il/en/research-institutes/government/ips/activities/4tribes

Chen, S., Benet-Martinez, V., & Harris, M. (2008). Bicultural identity, bilingualism and psychological adjustment in multicultural societies: Immigration based and globalization based acculturation. *Journal of Personality, 76*(4), 803–837.

Hong, Y., Benet-Martinez, V., Chiu, C., & Morris, M. (2003). Boundaries of cultural influence. *Journal of Cross Cultural Psychology, 34*(4), 453–464.

LaFromboise, T., Coleman, H., & Gerton, J. (1993). Psychological impact of biculturalism: Evidence and theory. *Psychological Bulletin, 114*(3), 395–412.

Roer-Strier, D. (2001). Socialization in changing cultural contexts: A search for images of the 'Adaptive Adult'. *Social Work, 46*(3), 215–228.

Rosenthal, M., & Roer-Strier, D. (2001). Cultural differences in mothers' developmental goals and ethnotheories. *International Journal of Psychology, 36*(1), 20–31.

Salamon, H. (2011). The floor falling away: Dislocated space and body in humour of Ethiopian immigrants in Israel. *Folklore, 122*(1), 16–34.

Shapiro, E. (1988). Individual change and family development: Individuation as a family process. In C. Falicov (Ed.), *Family transitions: Continuity & change over the life cycle* (pp. 159–180). Guildford Press.

Sharabany, R., & Israeli, E. (2008). The dual process of adolescent immigration and relocation: From country to country and from childhood to adolescence – reflection in psychodynamic psychotherapy. *The Psychoanalytic Study of the Child, 63*(1), 137–162.

Swidler, A. (1986). Culture in action: Symbolism and strategies. *American Sociological Review, 51*(2), 273–286.

Tadess, J. (2018). Folktales reality and childhood in Ethiopia: How children construct social values through performance of folktales. *Folklore, 129*, 237–253. https://doi.org/10.1080/0015587X.2018.1449457

Wagaw, T. (1993). *For our souls: Ethiopian Jews in Israel*. Wayne State University Press.

Hebrew Reference

Rosen, H. (1986). *Questions and answers about the behaviour of Ethiopian Jews*. Published by the Hadassah Women's Organization and the Ministry of Absorption.

Chapter 10
Education and Schooling

When my eldest son Daniel was 4 years old, I was horrified to hear him chanting a rhyme he had picked up in pre-school calling his own father 'stupid and brown'. Some days before Emmanuel had casually suggested that I should be the one to take him to pre-school, apparently, he had heard the children taunting Daniel and thought this could be avoided if he didn't show up. Following a conversation with the pre-school teacher about all this, I wrote a book explaining where Daniel's father came from, she used it to talk to the children about being different and equal. When the book was published (Shmuel, 1991) I discovered it was the first children's book in Hebrew with a brown-skinned protagonist. The book changed Daniel's reality in pre-school and is used today by educators to talk about colour.[1] This was 30 years ago, and yet this subject came up in all my interviews with parents and young people as they described their experiences with school or pre-school. Obviously, this is not the only thing happening in these institutions, but for many children of the second generation these formative encounters frame all the rest.

This chapter will address this issue, and the relationship between immigrant families and the state education system through the experiences of the participants in my study, including their educational background and attitudes towards education and ways of learning. I will also discuss the significance of the celebration of the Sigd festival in Israeli schools (since 2008) and the effect of school experiences on inter-generational relations. Finally, I propose a hypothesis of *double rejection* experienced by the second generation, who are often perceived as *the other* both at home and at school.

The narratives of participants in my study are arbitrary accounts of personal encounters, not necessarily representative of immigrant experiences in the Israeli educational system. It is important to remember that Jewish parents in Israel can

[1] Following this book, I wrote another seven books for children, four for teenagers and three for adults, they can all be seen on my website: http://en.naomis-books.com

© The Author(s), under exclusive license to Springer Nature Switzerland AG 2023

N. A. Shmuel, *Children's Wellbeing in Immigrant Families*, Children's Well-Being: Indicators and Research 26,
https://doi.org/10.1007/978-3-031-31917-4_10

choose schools based on geographic location and religious or other preferences, but also that immigrant parents are not usually equipped with the information necessary to make such choices. Most teenagers arriving in Israel were automatically sent by the authorities to boarding schools, younger children were generally referred to national religious schools.

People in settled lives experiencing life's challenges rely on their cultural conceptual framework, past experiences, and the presence of some form of support network to help them cope. But people in unsettled lives, in-between conceptual frameworks, where past experiences were linked to a very different context and a support network is often not available, may be overwhelmed by the challenges facing them. As demonstrated in the interviews, many of the adults in these children's lives were not necessarily equipped to assist them, or even aware of what the children were coping with. Another factor to consider is that children in settled lives are negotiating inherent conflicts between their world and the world of adults, while the children of immigrant families are faced with the formidable reality of negotiating inconsistencies between *two* adult worlds: that of their parents and that of their teachers and other adults in the host society (Zhou, 2009). When these two worlds are acutely different in cultural expression, expectations, and practices, the harder it is for the children to bridge between them.

10.1 Education and Immigration

Most of the 19 first-generation participants did not have any formal education, two studied a little in Ethiopia (Dany in high school without graduation and Tareke was one of Yonna Bogale's students[2]), Shy completed 1 year of university studies in Israel, three completed courses with certification in Israel; Abraham as a crane operator, Yafit as a child-minder and Abigail to run local workshops for elderly people. Almaz was a midwife and mohel[3] in Ethiopia, she had no formal education. In their own community, most of these people are considered knowledgeable, their wisdom based on life-experiences and ancestral knowledge passed on verbally from previous generations.

Of the 15 G1.5 participants 8 were academic (Genet and Mulu are social workers, Tigist is a nurse, Edna and Dov are teachers, Teruneh and Lemlem are graduates of master's degrees, Orna just completed her undergraduate degree). Three G1.5 participants began university and dropped out (Tsehai, Lee, and Noa), four never studied higher education (Matan works for the prison authority, Rachel, Aberash, and Liora have all taken various in-job training courses working with the Ethiopian immigrant community).

---

[2] Manager of the chain of Ort schools created for the Beta Yisrael community in Ethiopia.

[3] A Mohel (usually a man) circumcises male babies 8 days after their birth in Jewish communities.

Six out of 16 G2 participants were first-generation academics in their families; Shani and Miki completed undergraduate degrees, Naama and Habtam completed master's degrees, at the time of my research Dana and Ester were in their final year of undergraduate degrees (both today work as teachers). Two G2 participants were soldiers (Avi and Yisrael), two were recently discharged soldiers (Yaniv and Yisrael). Shimon was awaiting civilian national service, Shira was still in high school, and Noam had dropped out of school when he was 16. The rest had all completed high school, some with graduation and some without, Maayan started university but dropped out.

Western culture tends to value science and provable knowledge, which is usually taught through formal education using trained teachers and books. Genet asked her mother

> how she became a midwife and mohel, she said *I observed*. I asked her what she meant, and she said she saw her uncle performing circumcision and thought *there is no reason I can't do that if I train my mind, I can do it.*

Genet was so impressed by this, she decided to adopt this attitude:

> I want to be creative, I have intelligence, emotional intelligence which is not always appreciated.

Genet went on to explain how studying at university to be a social worker utilized another, more analytical type of intelligence, while she was referring to something more intuitive:

> I think I can *look* at something and understand it. To look and really *observe*.

She repeats this insight when she talks about teaching her own children:

> At home we *look*, we *see*, and we *observe*. I actually say those words, it's like a game—to look, see and observe—they already adopted this way of thinking and I love that.

Genet is describing the learning process in Ethiopia based on intuitive understanding through observation, to which she has now added verbal instruction and explanations. Thus, Genet is fusing two different cultural learning methods, thereby equipping her children's innate hybrid toolkit with both. This is the eminent embodiment of hybridity.

Children's informal education in the Jewish villages in Ethiopia was based on learning through observation, children spent a lot of time with the adults and were motivated to take part in what was going on around them, they wanted to learn to fit into adult society. In contrast in Israel, as in most Western countries, children often cannot perceive the relevance of what is taught in schools to their daily lives. At the same time, issues of identity and belonging are becoming powerful factors in the school and pre-school experiences of the second generation.

10.2 Colour

Aberash says that when her eldest son was 5 years old,

> he started to tell me he didn't want to be Ethiopian, that he didn't like his skin colour. Once when we were brushing his teeth, he asked me to cover his skin with toothpaste. I asked him why, and he said *in pre-school they call me cushi*[4] *I don't like my colour.* Until he was five, he never spoke to *Ferungim* [white people]. He thought brown [people] don't talk to *Ferungim*.

This child's experiences have created a dichotomy in his mind between brown and white people, shaping his self-image with negative connotations. The feeling has been enhanced as he grew older, at the time of the interview he was 11:

> My eldest son is really Ethiopian. His colour bothers him a lot and he talks about it. Anything unpleasant that happens [he says] *it's because I am Ethiopian*. He was born here. I don't see that he is really an Israeli child who can fit in with the *Ferungim*. Something will always bother him.

After the incident with the toothpaste, she bought him the book *Chocolate Child* (Cohen, 1998) and asked the teacher to read it in pre-school, she says that it helped him. Aberash is concerned about her son and says that she is determined to 'work on it', by trying to strengthen his self-image through teaching him Amharic and Ethiopian customs. Similarly, Orna recalls how her daughter wanted to change her colour:

> More than once she asked me when her colour would change, she said *I've had enough, lets change my colour…*

In response Orna told her about Ethiopia and says, 'I always tell them that they are judged by their actions not their colour'.

Pre-school age (4–5) is the time young children become aware of physical differences between people, skin colour is one of these. Their subsequent reaction is very much dependent on how the adults around them respond to their observations—encouraging a positive attitude to human diversity or (inadvertently or deliberately) promoting preference for similarity and fear of differences. Children pick up on both overt and covert messages, which exist in books, pictures, films, and the environment in which they play. Diversity can be celebrated through all of these or eliminated by default, the message is quickly internalized by brown-skinned children as inclusive or alienating of *themselves*. The children of most other immigrant groups are not visibly different, they blend into the crowd indistinguishably, brown-skinned children do not. Thus, the second generation of Ethiopian descent struggle with issues of identity and belonging which begin in pre-school and are often painfully enhanced in school.

> I was always reminded [that I am Ethiopian]. They always made a point of telling me who I am, what I am, where I came from. Whenever there was a school play, we had to be the

[4] Negro. Although cush is a term used in the bible to denote people of African descent, the word today is commonly regarded as derogatory and not to be used.

> Ethiopians. In school they always looked at us as.... *you the Ethiopians*. But I wanted to be Cinderella, why didn't they let me be Cinderella?

Maayan recalls this with tears in her eyes, she was the only child in the class in a drama group, and yet when children were cast for the annual school play marking the end of their elementary education, she was not even considered for the main role. Her teacher could not conceive of the idea that Cinderella could be black. This became the painful epitome of Maayan's experiences in school: she was always above all else *the Ethiopian*.

Many of the G2 participants recalled similar formative experiences during their childhood which distinguished them from the 'normative' white Israeli children and marked them as different by skin colour.

Shira studies in class with three other Ethiopian Israeli G2 girls, during her interview she refers to herself as Israeli, but when talking about school she calls herself 'Ethiopian' and says that the teacher always groups the four girls together and generalizes about them. It is the only time in the interview when she stops smiling and looks angry, then she says passionately 'I hate generalizations, I always have to respond'. Her responses often get her into trouble with her teachers, although she is an excellent student.

Racism and stereotyping in schools were the subject of Mula's study (2010), her dissertation begins with a moving personal account of her own experiences on arrival in Israel and later as a teacher. Sagiv (2014) studied second-generation Israelis of mixed Ashkenazi and Sephardic ethnicity and found that their initial awareness of ethnic identities and the expectation that they define themselves according to one or other ethnicity was associated with their experiences at school. The prevalent social hierarchy of identities, both overt and covert, coupled with disproportionate attention given to ethnic identities in Israeli society, serves to fixate attitudes towards the various groups and enhance stereotyping and prejudice. Without an extensive national investment in anti-bias education, the common terminology of *them* and *us* in which the specific groups this applies to change according to context, creates a constant dichotomy of identities, damaging to both individuals and society. Comparing Israeli reality to other countries (especially America) and importing various theories regarding race and racism distorts the complex experiences of Ethiopian Israelis and presents a simplified and often misleading story in terms of *black* and *white*. This has particularly detrimental results for the Ethiopian community in Israel.

Firstly, the common misdirected assumption that guided many absorption initiatives, especially in relation to schooling, was that G2 children needed assistance in overcoming *cultural deficits* to fit in and get ahead. Rooted in prejudice and an Israeli tradition of assimilation and paternalism, this attitude was also prevalent when dealing with immigrant groups from other African and Islamic countries in the 1950s. The alternative, to base the adjustment of new immigrants on their abilities, strengths, and intelligence inherent in their cultural tradition, is a relatively new concept which has not yet completely taken over the Israeli absorption-acculturation narrative and practice. An example of this is the underrepresentation of Ethiopian

Israeli children in programmes for the gifted and talented, discussed by Lifshitz and Katz (2015).

The second detrimental result is that many Ethiopian Israeli children and youth are adopting the *disadvantaged narrative* based on colour, paving the way to marginalization and lack of motivation to even try and fit in (socially, academically, in school or in the job market).

Yaniv and Habtam (both G2) described many examples of feeling 'pushed out' (Habtam's words) by discriminatory remarks. Yaniv recounted long stories of not being let into clubs when home on leave from the army where he served as a combat soldier (his white friends were all let in). But both these young people can balance these stories with positive experiences in Israeli society—Yaniv describes the 4 years he spent as the only Ethiopian Israeli in his military boarding school as the best time of his life, Habtam has succeeded tremendously both academically and in her government job. They may be critical of Israeli society but have not rejected it completely, their strategy in life has been to overcome prejudice and prove themselves, something Addis talks about repeatedly in his interview (more on this in Chaps. 13 and 14). But where the 'disadvantaged narrative' takes over personal initiative diminishes, and it is a slippery slope to marginality.

The third detrimental result, is that the *black-white* narrative pits the entire community against the Israeli white majority, preventing any real introspection in the Ethiopian immigrant community. This narrow perspective blocks any attempts for personal or community improvement, since all the problems are attributed to the black-white dichotomy. A more accurate perception of the complexity of both internal and external processes occurring following immigration would enable personal, familial and community self-examination, awareness, and initiatives for improvement dependent only on themselves.

10.3 School Experiences

During the interviews participants were asked in general terms about their school experiences, there was no specific question relating to prejudice or discrimination. Of the 16 G2 participants 4 recalled being discriminated against at school (Dana, Naama, Shira, and Maayan), 4 recounted positive school experiences and said they were never discriminated against (Miki, Yisrael, Shimon, and Leah), and the other 8 did not relate to this subject in the school context (though 4 of them related to this issue in other contexts; Yaniv, Habtam, Avi and Addis, discussed in Chaps. 13 and 14).

Like Aberash's son, for many G2 children pre-school or school attendance involves a formative first experience of *being different*, shaping both their attitude to society and to themselves. Dana has many examples of overt discrimination she experienced in elementary school, for example the time when another girl refused to sit next to her:

> I was sitting here, like a leper, and she sat over there, she even moved away from the table, so my germs wouldn't be able to get to her.

She remembers being offended, but also not understanding why, and says 'I did not understand it as racism'. In this instance and others, the teacher did not intervene on her behalf. On another occasion the teacher asked all the children to bring lice combs to class, but only checked the heads of the Ethiopian Israelis. Once Dana was accused of hitting another child and the teacher pulled her by the hair. Dana had no-one to share these experiences with, she says:

> I was such an unprotected child…I knew that if I told my mother she would say *you must have annoyed the teacher* or something like that. There were occasions when I tried to tell her, and she just said *you must have deserved it.* She had complete faith in the educational system, to the extent that even being hit, or having my hair pulled, was acceptable.

Dana is angry when she speaks about this, saying that she learnt not to tell her parents what was going on and felt 'unprotected'. When I asked her if she could understand their attitude as new immigrants, she shakes her head and says:

> No. you would always protect your child. So you came from an underdeveloped country, so what? So your child can't tell you anything? It's an appalling lack of protection. Like talking to a brick wall.

In Dana's narrative, she was left to cope alone with a teacher who did not understand her and even hurt her, while her parents offered her no support. Her elder brothers were, apparently, severely damaged by things that happened to them in boarding school. Her parent's inability to protect their children is something that makes Dana determined to act differently, she says she is 'preparing for all sorts of things'. When I ask her what she means she explains:

> To work on my own identity, the identity in the mirror, to see that you are black, to know where you came from.

In other words, she sees her own self-acceptance and knowledge about her culture of origin, as a source of strength. In fact, she goes on to say; 'knowledge is power, I have nothing else'. Dana has accepted as unavoidable that her skin colour distinguishes her but has decided to give her identity content that goes beyond this. This is a conclusion that Mekonen (2010) also arrived at when examining the effect of a programme enhancing the cultural legacy of youth from Ethiopian immigrant families in boarding schools. This is the reason why the public attention given to Ethiopian customs and heritage 30 years after their arrival is important, and not a wasted effort as Jaffe-Schagen (2016) seems to suggest, since it will not undo all the mistakes made by the establishment in their absorption or counteract discrimination. But what it can do, is give the second-generation cultural knowledge they can be proud of, and a sense of belonging to a thriving resilient community with a rich cultural heritage (more on this in Chap. 14).

As a child, Naama accepted her position in class as 'the good girl with low grades'. She describes herself as 'quiet and polite', saying 'I was the best-behaved girl in class, I used to sit like this', she folds her hands and sits upright, then laughs. 'I was very respectful', she continues:

> all the teachers used to tell the class *we want you to learn from Naama.* I used to draw too, so I made all the classroom decorations. They had this image of me as a good, quiet respectful girl and I fitted myself into this. I had no ambition. I never complained. It never occurred to me that nobody noticed me, that nobody expected more of me, nobody expected good grades. They were all please with 70% and so was I.

Naama fitted in perfectly with the stereotype of the quiet polite Ethiopian child, and her teachers had no expectations of her, nobody noticed that

> a lot of the time I didn't understand what they were teaching. It was very hard for me.

But one day a new teacher arrived in the school, and she expected more of Naama:

> This teacher really paid attention to me. At first, I found it very embarrassing, because I never even paid attention to myself. I couldn't understand why she did. She kept asking me questions about myself, nobody had ever asked me questions about myself, and I was not interested in answering. It embarrassed me. But she didn't do it like a teacher, she was really something more than that. I think I only really started studying properly because she encouraged me.

Since then, Naama has successfully complete both an undergraduate and a master's degree and is today studying for her doctorate. Her ability to see herself as capable of achieving more than average started when one attentive teacher noticed her and encouraged her, believing that she could do better.

The issue of prejudice, its effect on children and ways of preventing it, has been extensively studied in other countries (for example, Aboud, 2003; Doyle & Aboud, 1995; Creaser & Dau, 1996; Igoa, 1995; Reddy, 1996). And yet it seems from this study and others, for example Anaki (2017) that many teachers in Israel lack appropriate professional training on this issue, or even basic awareness. The educators interviewed by Anaki expressed the opinion that parents and children of Ethiopian origin were influenced by 'baseless and wrong' misconceptions about living in a racist society, detrimentally influencing their attitude towards the school. Anaki also found most educators thought immigrants from different countries should assimilate, and any parent who does not actively encourage their child to do so is putting the child at risk. In fact, many educators saw the Ethiopian parents as 'risk factors' to their children, as 'weak, with no parenting skills, lacking in knowledge and ability to deal with Israeli reality'. These educators also considered Ethiopian culture itself as a risk factor, being 'primitive' and 'holding them back'.

Berhanu (2001, 2005) who studied the issue of underachievement of Ethiopian Israeli youth in schools came to some interesting conclusions. Berhanu categorized three parameters of educational gaps: personal (the students themselves), as a group (compared to other groups in the school), and institutional (the school compared to other schools). According to Berhanu, these three parameters shape the learning process, which occurs in these three contexts: institutional, social, and cultural. To understand how educational gaps are created, it is necessary to look at the interaction between these three contexts. The assumption that underachievement of Ethiopian youth is the result of low motivation, lack of parental support and cultural gaps creates a situation whereby the school effort to assist these students is focused on extra lessons (mostly in Hebrew) and ignores the wider contextual conditions of learning and the institutional attitude to diversity. Thus, the focus is on helping them 'catch up', while the real problem is lack of understanding of and consideration towards their cultural background (findings reiterated by other researchers, for example: Sever, 2004; Shmuel, 2015; Shemer, 2009). In short, students are unlikely to achieve well when their parents and culture are undervalued by the teachers and the system.

Even teachers apparently empathic to the Ethiopian students in Anaki's study (2017) were ignorant of their perspectives and experiences, lacking knowledge about their culture of which they tended to be critical. All these educators (teachers and headmasters alike) voiced the need for further training in cultural competence. Entering a system that lacks cultural knowledge, in which educators have no idea what the students and their parents feel or think on issues of identity, belonging, and school discipline, has a strong influence on student motivation to succeed (Berhanu, 2005). Discipline in school is an important concern for immigrants in transition from a hierarchical society basing authority on power relations to a democratic society basing authority on dialogue and connection; the whole teacher–student relationship is forged differently in these two systems. According to Berhanu, the inter-generational rift caused in Ethiopian families by immigration creates children who find it difficult to cope with authority figures. Lack of understanding on this issue coupled with lack of appreciation for their culture of origin and for diversity in general undermines students' motivation and ability to learn, thus enhancing rather than diminishing differences in the level of school achievement (Berhanu, 2001, 2005).

For the past 30 years, I have been visiting schools throughout Israel as guest author, over the last 15 years I have also been training teachers in cultural competence and context awareness (Shmuel, 2020; Shmuel & Shimon, 2012). The vast differences between the schools I encounter is striking, while some are very aware of the significance of celebrating diversity and understanding the cultural background of their students, many are not. This seems to depend on personal initiatives of dedicated enlightened headmasters and staff rather than national policy. Education takes place in context; it is not just an individual process. Underachievement of Ethiopian Israeli students is a failure of the system detrimental to all. Berhanu's research (2005, 2006) grapples the complexity of this issue by considering both the school and the home environment of these children. While the former is not sufficiently invested in diversity education and understanding their students' cultural backgrounds, the latter are also not preparing children for coping with their new reality. But this is not a 'cultural deficit' or lack of parenting skills, rather it is an emphasis on humanistic cultural values which served them well in Ethiopia but do not equip the children with skills necessary in Israeli schools such as speed, initiative, self-expression, curiosity, and problem-solving (Berhanu, 2005, also discussed in Dotan, 1987). In other words, the parental cultural toolkit suited to a totally different context is ineffective in preparing the second generation for what they meet in Israeli schools. While the schools themselves are unequipped and unprepared to cope with issues of bias and stereotyping and tend to attribute student failure to the children themselves or their cultural background rather than the system that is failing them.

Children struggling with two totally different and opposing cultural systems and their own sense of isolation are unlikely to manage devoting themselves to the learning process (Berhanu, 2001). As Orna stated, it seems that many of the second generation 'are not here and not there'—lost in the invisible space between the two cultures, struggling with issues of identity which thwart their efforts to fit in. Effectively, they are trapped in the grey area, often feeling increasingly excluded from both cultural communities (more on this in a moment).

Both Orna and Tigist talk about younger siblings who have dropped out of school, Tigist says that 'the young people of today give in far too easily', remembering her own immigrant childhood and the efforts she made to study and succeed.

Tigist arrived in Israel when she was 8. After her first year, during which she fitted in very well in a regular class in a good local school, her family moved to more permanent housing in another town. This time she was assigned to an immigrant's class in which 'we were told we were not capable of joining in', and she 'spent most of my time outside'. Being a very industrious child, by the time she was 12 Tigist started looking for an alternative school, she found herself a religious boarding school for girls. She says at the time her mother could not understand why she wanted to go, and took a lot of convincing, but Tigist managed to persuade her and today says it was a good choice.

Tigist was obviously a resourceful child, able to communicant with her mother well enough to convince her, and Abynesh attentive enough to listen to her. I have come across other examples like this, reflecting the agency of immigrant children in determining their future. But more often the children just remain stuck in schools that do not suit them. Orna describes accompanying her mother to her sisters' parent meetings, and being told 'they have so much potential, but don't apply themselves' (possibly the most common comment heard by Israeli parents in parent meetings). It is convenient to blame the students or the parents rather than examine the system.

I feel it important to give credit to the many diligent educational staff who are aware of these issues and make great efforts to improve the situation. Thus, in one school I visited some years ago, after my meeting with the students one of them (an Ethiopian Israeli child in the fourth grade) came up to his teacher (who was standing next to me) and said, 'I am proud of my school'. She smiled at him and asked him why, and he said; 'because you are not afraid to talk about colour'. In such a school this child can feel like any other, can value himself as a human being with multiple identities, and can participate in all activities in the school as an equal.

10.4 The Boarding Schools

The common policy of sending immigrant youth to boarding schools came up in many of the interviews as having far-reaching consequences for both the children and their families. Nine of the G1.5 participants (Mulu, Tigist, Edna, Dov, Orna,

Teruneh, Lee, Rachel, and Matan) and three of the G2 participants (Yaniv, Miki, and Yisrael) attended boarding schools. Mulu describes this as:

> A traumatic experience, this separation without agreement, without discussion. You are not consulted, they do with you what they want, like an object. It was hard for me and even harder for my parents.

Often this was initiated by the absorption authorities soon after arrival in Israel, after the hardships of the journey and sometimes prolonged separations, many G1 parents found this very stressful and felt that they were not given any other choice. 'Nobody asked us', says Abynesh, and recalls how the children were taken to see the boarding school without their parents' knowledge.

Abigail and her son Dov were separated on the way to Israel. Soon after their reunion, 5 years later, Dov was sent to boarding school. Abigail becomes very emotional when talking about this and insists it was not her choice, that they were told it was the only option for her son to study. Dov recalls how his parents cried, and he felt severed from the family, especially his grandparents who had raised him. And yet he talks fondly of the boarding school, where he had good experiences and says, 'they gave us things our home could not'. In the long run, from Dov's current perspective, it was the right choice for him, but he is painfully aware of the price paid in disrupted family relationships.

Habtam talks about the rift in her family caused by her sister Orna going to boarding school, and how hard this was for her. She says:

> Only later I realized that my mother thought there was no other option. It was presented as a fact, they were not told to choose, like other people.

When I spoke to her parents they presented it as a financial decision, they could not pay for school and so agreed to have the two eldest children sent away. A decision they regret to this day, saying that it left 'scars'—a term Habtam also used in her interview. There is a sense of helplessness in these narratives, parents who had only just arrived and with hindsight feel they made bad choices or were coerced into allowing their children to be sent away. Their children are ambivalent about it, for some of them it was a good experience, others describe it as more damaging than beneficial. For Aberash it was her first separation from her mother, and she 'cried a lot', but she also says that her adjustment strengthened her so that today there is no difficulty she cannot overcome.

After the eldest children left, their younger siblings took their place. Sarah describes the siblings who went to boarding school as 'no longer a part' of what was going on at home. Her sister Orna says she felt alienated from her siblings when she visited home, she talks about 'not knowing them at all'. Maayan says it took them years to reconnect.[5]

---

[5] My research only touched on this issue, a much more extensive study is necessary to determine the effect of sibling separation and the differences between the experiences of girls and boys in boarding schools.

Orna describes the experience as difficult, but in order not to make it harder for her parents she never told them this. She also recalls traumatic moments, for example getting her first period away from home and missing her mother. Today she says she would never send her child to a boarding school and finds it difficult to recommend this to other parents, something that her job on occasion requires of her.

Habtam, who effectively became the eldest at home, feels guilty for 'having all the opportunities' which her sister Orna did not have. She also says that if it was done to enable Orna to study then what was the point, since Orna never graduated high school but was streamed to a vocation as a secretary. Obviously under the right circumstances she was capable of more: Orna recently completed her undergraduate degree. Her return home at the age of 18 was equally traumatic, Maayan remembers her sister losing weight because she was not used to her mother's cooking.

Habtam thinks the boarding school was good for her brother, there are others who have good things to say about the boarding schools; Matan, Teruneh, Miki, Tigist, and Yaniv. But for all these participants aside from Miki the move was their choice, the decision was made together with their parents. Miki was left alone in Israel with his younger brother, when he was only 10 years old. He has only praise for the people who looked after him:

> They helped us, they made us who we are, they gave us everything, a good education, love, they were really like parents.

It seems that going to boarding school was not necessarily a bad thing if it was done with consent and to good institutions.

Edna describes her father's decision to send her away as 'cruel', and says that at first, she was angry with him. With hindsight she says that the boarding school gave her a lot, enabled her to graduate and to fit in socially, so 'they made the right decision'. Nevertheless, she also says she would never send her own child to a boarding school.

Lee arrived before her parents, her experiences in boarding school were 'really hard'. The local children did not accept the newcomers, whom they cursed and quarrelled with. Since her parents had not yet arrived, they had nowhere to go for holidays. And yet when her parents did arrive coming home permanently was not even an option, and Lee felt 'disconnected' from her family, she says 'I felt I was not their daughter'.

> Our roots were strong, but the children who were born here and went to boarding schools, they had no backbone. Their parents were not available to give them a backbone, nor a strong identity, they were just lost. These are the people who are broken, unable to create a normal life, a family, a career, addicted to all sorts of substances. (Mulu)

The ability of 11- and 12-year-old children to cope with their experiences in boarding schools was dependent on their own resilience as well as the type and quality of the institution they arrived in and the degree of support they received there. Mulu is making an important distinction between the resilience of the 1.5 and G2 children, saying that the latter are much more vulnerable. As a social worker she has met many such children in a professional capacity:

> Two or three more children were born into such families and they can't survive either in such a home, with no guidance.

Her words echo the story of the Demse family (further discussed in Chap. 12) and suggest that the damage done by the policy of sending immigrant youth to boarding schools likely had far-reaching consequences on many families, including the younger children who stayed at home. Some of the institutions were run by poorly qualified staff and the only native Israeli children who were sent there came from problematic backgrounds. Mulu talks passionately about this, she feels that a great deal of damage was done to many children, who not only did not study but suffered breakdowns, some of them ending up in prison or committing suicide. She was very much involved in helping her brother Yaniv choose his boarding school, which she says was a completely different experience because it was a good institution of his own choice. Yaniv's school was not far from home and they visited him frequently, with his instructor in constant contact with their mother—none of which applied when Mulu was in boarding school.

The quality of the institution to which children were sent was crucial, there were also very good schools. For example, in 1979, Chaim Peri came to manage the Yemin Orde Youth Village and founded the idea of what has become known as 'the village way',[6] inspired by the African proverb 'it takes a whole village to raise a child'. The 'village way' recognizes and enhances cultural identity through personal narratives, as well as teaching valuable life skills alongside knowledge in a welcoming home environment where the participants feel valued and are encouraged to contribute. It is a totally different concept from a boarding school, based on the idea of providing teenagers a community in which to thrive rather than simply a school where they also sleep. In Chaim Peri's vision young people's formative years present an opportunity to turn their life story around by creating an environment changing their focus from survival to leadership. Chaim Peri has been widely renowned for his educational work, in 2012 he received Israel's Presidential Medal of Honour for his lifework. The 'village way' has since been adopted in dozens of institutions throughout Israel, including in the Arab sector. These initiatives have taken many children classified as 'at risk', including immigrants and refugees, and literally change their life course opening up new opportunities and choices. Many of the graduates from Yemin Orde have impressive accomplishments, notable amongst them is Shimon Solomon, who became a member of the Knesset (Israeli Parliament) in 2013. Preceding this he successfully used the *village way* methodology to establish a youth village in Rwanda for survivors of the genocide. Since then he was manager of the Kfar Silver agricultural youth village near Ashkelon, and, from March 2022, Israel Ambassador to Angola.

None of the participants in my study went to Yemin Orde, but all the G2 participants who attended boarding schools had very positive experiences. Yaniv says this was 'the best time of my life'. Both Yaniv and Yisrael were the only Ethiopian Israelis in their boarding schools, both said they never experienced any kind of

[6] https://www.derechkfar.org.il/

discrimination. They were also both very much involved in choosing their own boarding schools, in both cases an elder sibling was instrumental in helping them persuade the parents that this was a good choice. These were, apparently, good institutions with an awareness for diversity education and sensitive staff.

Even children relatively settled in local schools were eventually at some point encouraged to move to boarding schools. This was the case for Worknesh's son, and it was not a good experience. When I interviewed the family, Worknesh recalled that it was his school that had suggested the move, and Noa reminded her that it was because there were behaviour problems and they could not understand each other. Eventually the boy returned home to complete his high school graduation, but recounting the story raises emotions and causes arguments during the interview. This narrative and others suggest that more attention should be given to the specifics of the institutions chosen to send new immigrant children and ensure their safety, as well as providing other alternative choices for parents to consider.

10.5 Parental Involvement

Rachel's son tested as gifted at school, when she called to register him for the exceptionally gifted programme, she recalls the secretary making sneering remarks '*you too? Who told you* [to register]'? Rachel is angry when talking about this, she adds that her son told her:

> An Israeli parent would make a fuss about it, but you're always like that, you parents, that's why we're treated differently.

By 'like that' he meant too quiet and polite, not assertive like native Israeli parents, not standing up for their children but rather trusting the system. Mahari went to parents evening once and told the teacher to be strict with his son Yisrael, not to hold back on punishing him. The next day Yisrael came back from school and told his mother, Yafit, that the teacher was picking on him and he didn't want his father going to parents evening again. Thus, parents are often struggling to negotiate differing cultural expectations, seeing their role as enhancing teacher authority rather than representing their children's interests.

Dov teaches in an elementary school where he tries to keep the parents involved in their children's progress. But often when he asks the parents to come to school their response is that the teacher should deal with whatever problems there are, and not bother the parents. In Ethiopia this is how it was, parents were not invited to parent–teacher meetings, it was expected of the school to deal with the students as they saw fit, including punishing them if necessary (Poluha, 2007; Shmuel, 2010).

Maayan works in a boarding school for children who have been expelled from other institutions, this is their last framework available for rehabilitation. Most of the youth in this school are of Ethiopian origin. Maayan is very critical of their parents, saying that they expect somebody else to deal with their children and won't even come to the school when invited. The reasons for these parents relinquishing their responsibility may be complex, including past negative experiences with other schools and dependency on the Israeli authorities inadvertently fostered by absorption policies. Mayan says:

> They see the boarding school as replacing the parents. That we should take responsibility, cope with them, be there for them, and they should just be updated about what is happening. They have taken themselves out of the equation, as if it's not their place.

But there are parents who act differently, taking responsibility, always struggling to keep involved even without knowing the language or being familiar with the system. Thus, Genet remembers her mother 'coming to all the parents' evenings at school:

> We used to tell her she didn't need to come because everything was all right, and she would say *I'll go, and I'll hear, and I'll decide if everything is all right.*

Abynesh set out to bring her son home from boarding school after she realized he was not happy there. The authorities tried to dissuade her, telling her that in the local school he would not study, he would deteriorate, but she insisted. When her daughter (Tigist) went to boarding school, Abynesh travelled for a whole day on three buses with a small baby on her back to see where her daughter was sleeping and make sure she was all right. She says:

> I am her mother, how can I send her alone? I need to see who her teacher is, who the headmaster is. Three times I went, by myself, to her parent meetings.

Abigail also insisted on visiting her children at boarding school and getting the phone numbers of their counsellors so she could keep in touch. She says:

> It's always important to visit the children, it's so hard for them to be away from home.

Abynesh and Abigail might have been passive when they arrived in Israel, traumatized by their difficult journey via Sudan, and so their eldest children were taken to boarding schools. But once they had adjusted to the new country, they initiated contact and took back their responsibility for their children.

It is interesting to note that none of the fathers participating spoke about such things, in fact only one interviewee (Edna) mentioned a father in this context at all. It seems to have been the initiative of the mothers to be involved in their children's education.[7] Parental ability to be involved and supportive to children after immigration depends on several factors, including knowledge and understanding of the system, cultural flexibility, and attentiveness to the children. As is apparent from the interviews, immigrant families are also susceptible to absorption policies determining where children go to school, and their ability to make decisions about this is dependent on the information they are given and their own confidence to take the initiative.

---

[7] The gender division at home is further discussed in the next chapter.

10.6 Celebrating the Sigd Holiday in Israeli Schools

The Sigd is a traditional celebration unique to Ethiopian Jews celebrated 50 days after the Day of Atonement. The Sigd is described by Rabbi Dr. Shalom Sharon (2016) as creating a bridge between the personal introspection which the Day of Atonement requires, and a collective community reflection on the historical devastation caused to the people of Israel by improper human conduct. The assumption is that to be worthy of the ascent to Jerusalem, repentance and fasting on the Day of Atonement are insufficient. What is necessary is a *collective* atonement, bridging between the personal and the social. The Sigd simultaneously reminds the people of their covenant with God forged on Mount Sini when receiving the bible and reaffirms that covenant through the aspiration to return to Jerusalem. Climbing the mountain while fasting and praying was a reminder of the affinity of all Jews, their commitment to God and to each other.

Up until now, I have framed this book around the themes prevalent in the narratives from my interviews, but the Sigd festival was hardly mentioned by them. Nevertheless, I feel it important to relate to this festival for two reasons: firstly, it has become a prominent national festival (since 2008) commonly celebrated in schools and therefore having significance in contributing to the heightened presence of Ethiopian culture in the schools. Secondly, the prevalence of this festival as well as other significant landmarks enhancing the Ethiopian immigrant's narrative and giving it a prominent and legitimate place in Israeli society, was largely instigated by leading figures from the Ethiopian community itself (to be discussed further in Chap. 14).

Only Tsehai mentioned the Sigd festival, as a way of celebrating Ethiopian culture with her Israeli-born children. Why others never mentioned it is a point for speculation, my guess is that it probably slipped their mind or is not terribly important to them. From my own experiences visiting schools throughout the country, I would like to suggest the significance of the festival and what it does and does not do for Ethiopian Israeli children.

Firstly, the celebration of the Sigd in schools gives the Jewish Ethiopian narrative visibility and makes their story part of the school curriculum. This in itself is important, because it is both *inclusive* and *distinctive*, giving the children both a sense of their uniqueness and their entitlement to belong. Secondly, the celebrations often initiate events where parents are invited to tell their stories and there is a general celebration of elements of Ethiopian culture, creating significant bridges for the G2 children between home and school. Thirdly, generally the new narratives describing their Aliyah today give prominence to the Ethiopian initiative, they are no longer the poor Ethiopians who were rescued by Israelis but heroes in their own right who initiated and implemented the journey. Finally, these events sometimes encourage more open discussions around issues concerning the community, in which children and young people might find opportunities to make their voices heard.

What the Sigd celebrations in school do not do is undo or delete existing problems, reduce bias and discrimination, or magically make everybody suddenly cohesively united (Jaffe-Schagen, 2016). Worse still, sometimes celebrating the Sigd is the *only* reference to the children's cultural heritage, and beyond this they remain isolated, ignored, or misunderstood.

10.7 Noam's Truancy

Rosenblum et al. (2008) studied the hidden dropout phenomenon amongst Ethiopian immigrant youth (aged 14–18), meaning students registered in school and therefore not listed as dropouts, but with poor attendance. They found that the dropouts had more of a social support network and experienced less stress than students who remained in school. They suggest several explanations for this, including the importance of the peer group as a support network after immigration, especially if youth feel alienated from the mainstream, and are struggling with issues of identity and belonging. Interestingly this study was carried out in boarding schools and did not relate to school variables. In another study, Mengistu (2014) found a connection between perceived discrimination and truancy (both overt and covert) amongst Ethiopian immigrant dropouts. In fact, any reactions to discrimination can be seen as a manifestation of resilience, even if the result is socially maladaptive behaviour such as truancy (Ungar, 2008).

When he was 16 Noam stopped attending school, he was not officially documented as having dropped out till a year later. He says:

> I blame myself. Because I left. It wasn't that I was expelled, or they didn't want me there.

But it also seems from his narrative that nobody took a genuine interest in what was going on in his life:

> I felt that I just couldn't sit and learn. There were times when I told the teacher *I'm going to the bathroom* and just never came back.

Indicating that there were warning signs that Noam was about to drop out, but nobody picked up on these.

When he was a teenager Noam was quick to get into trouble, but today he has changed his ways:

> A person can call me *cushi* and it's not a problem. You can curse me, it won't kill me. Maybe it will hurt me a little, but I'll say, so it hurt, so what? Did it damage me? But when I was sixteen and someone cursed me or whatever I would immediately act with violence. Today I say, where will that lead me?

This narrative seems to suggest that issues of social rejection and racism experienced with peers may have been a contributary factor in his truancy, though he did not elaborate on this.

Noam was just 1 year old when he arrived in Israel with his parents. He had three brothers, the eldest was recently killed in a car accident, the other two are younger than him. When he was growing up the family lived in a poor neighbourhood in one of the large cities, his parents have always been struggling financially. Noam recalls hardly seeing his father at all as a child, saying about his parents ‘they didn’t really have time for us’.

There are probably many reasons for Noam dropping out of school, including the multiple contexts influencing his life. Noam was labelled as ‘youth at risk’ after an altercation with the police, whatever assistance he was offered did not prevent his dropping out of school.

Today, Noam’s youngest brother Yaniv admires him especially because he made some big changes in the last few years:

> He was always kind of unstable in his life, I remember him always getting into trouble. Like the black sheep of the family. But look at him today, he’s happy, he has a woman who loves him, they just had a child. He’s really changed for the better. He’s a family man, he does stuff, he worries, he’s a big brother.

Settling down and having a family, being responsible and caring, apparently contented in his life, are indicators for Yaniv that his brother has overcome the stormy period of his life and changed his ways. His reference to Noam’s position in the family seems to suggest that these stormy periods were forged both at home and at school, that Noam may have experienced *double rejection* (detailed below). Today Noam lives on a kibbutz where he works regularly and takes care of his new family, at the same time he keeps regular contact with a daughter from a first marriage and finds the time to be a significant big brother to his younger siblings.

Obviously, the whole issue of truancy, causes and consequences, requires further research, but Noam’s story points to the multitude of issues facing immigrant youth alongside the aftereffects of growing up in a family in cultural transition. These include belonging to low-income families, in poor neighbourhoods, often without a supportive community network, and attending low-level schools in which there is insufficient understanding or concern for their complex and challenging reality.

10.8 Double Rejection

The idea of double rejection is not a value judgement on Ethiopian immigrant families or Israeli society, nor is it the norm for second-generation children, most of whom seem to have *back-up caregivers* who take the place of their parents at times when that relationship is stressful or ineffectual. Nearly all the second-generation participants in my study mentioned somebody whom they could talk to and would help them when they felt low and were encountering problems: Addis and Avi had Genet and her brother, Yisrael had his grandfather, Noam and Yaniv had their sister Mulu, Maayan had her sister Habtam. These relatives, mostly of the one and a half generation, buffered the effects of whatever else was happening at home and helped these young people pull through and forge themselves a precarious cultural pathway. Miki talks of the staff at his boarding school as being ‘like parents’ to him. But there are others who explicitly said they had no-one: Dana talked about herself as an ‘unprotected child’, Sarah said she had nobody to turn to and often felt ignored by her family. Sometimes extenuating circumstances mellowed the effect of the intergenerational rift, for example Dana was instrumental in caring for her damaged brothers, Ester and Habtam inherited the privileges of the first-born since their siblings were in boarding school. For these young people their roles at home gave them significance in the family which bolstered their self-esteem and softened the culture clash. But in the absence of back-up caregivers or special family roles, lack of support and outright conflict at home based on cultural and linguistic misunderstandings and failing communication can leave youth of the second generation dangerously isolated. This is not a sudden breakdown during adolescence, it is a consistently increasing lack of synchronization between children and the adults caring for them built into the very fabric of their childhood in ever repeated negative experiences of not being listened to or not being understood. As Adler (Dreikus, 1994) postulated, children inevitably feel inferior to the adults around them, but when belittled or rejected, persistently disapproved of and criticized, this inferiority can become an intrinsic part of their self-perception. Children do not rationalize their situation as being the result of cultural transition and misunderstandings based on the culture clash and growing up in unsettled times; the fact that their parents have expectations of them forged in another context, that they are using a parental toolkit suited to another culture. The children simply feel *personally* rejected and unworthy of affection. They go out into the world without that invisible protective shield of having family support and encouragement and knowing their own worth. Thus, intrinsically vulnerable, they enter pre-school and school where they often encounter the second devastating rejection by being labelled, overtly or covertly, as the *other,* often categorized by colour as *the Ethiopians*. This second rejection matches the first in the sense that it re-confirms their inferiority to others, internalizing a self-image of inadequacy that is like a self-fulfilling prophesy. Again, as Adler suggests, nobody can feel they belong if they feel inferior. These children, held captive at the far end of the continuum between settled and unsettled lives by this double rejection, despite being born in the host country, are effectively desolately lost. In other words, they are rejected at home for not being Ethiopian enough and rejected at school for not being Israeli enough. They are essentially in between the two cultures without having appropriated either as their own, and their overall experience is one of being excluded, with all the dire consequences of this. Of course, all this may apply to varying degrees, depending on individual, family, and school circumstances, and may lead to various bumpy pathways through which people attempt to compensate for feelings of inferiority: by excelling, by disrupting, or by passivity. To bring these youth back into the fold and give them hope is to create nurturing environments in which they can feel wanted and worthy, which is exactly what the 'village way' does, and what acutely aware members of the intermediate 1.5 generation sometimes manage to do. It is also important to remember, that families are complicated and can contain simultaneously positive and negative processes and interactions. Thus, experiencing rejection paradoxically may be combined with experiencing loving care, as demonstrated by Dana in her narratives (detailed in the next chapters).

References

Aboud, F. E. (2003). The formation of in-group favouritism and out-group prejudice in young children: Are they distinct attitudes? *Developmental psychology, 39*(1), 48.

Berhanu, G. (2001). *Learning-in-context. An ethnographic investigation of mediated learning experiences among Ethiopian Jews in Israel.* Doctoral dissertation. Gothenburg University, Sweden.

Berhanu, G. (2005). Normality, deviance, identity, cultural tracking and school achievement: The case of Ethiopian Jews in Israel. *Scandinavian Journal of Educational Research, 49*(1), 51–82.

Berhanu, G. (2006). Parenting (parental attitude), child development, and modalities of parent-child interactions: Sayings, proverbs, and maxims of Ethiopian Jews in Israel. *Journal of Cognitive Education and Psychology, 5*(3), 266–287.

Creaser, B., & Dau, E. (1996). *The anti-bias approach in early childhood education.* Harper Educational Publishers.

Dothan, T. (1987). Jewish children from Ethiopia in Israel: Some observations on their adaptation patterns. In M. Ashkenazi & A. Weingrod (Eds.), *Ethiopian Jews and Israel.* Transaction Publishers.

Doyle, A., & Aboud, F. E. (1995). A longitudinal study of White children's racial prejudice as a social-cognitive development. *Merrill-Palmer Quarterly, 1982*, 209–228.

Igoa, C. (1995). *The inner world of the immigrant child.* Laurence Erlbaum Associates Publishers.

Jaffe-Schagen, J. (2016). Creating space. The construction of Ethiopian heritage and memory in Israel. *Annales d'Éthiopie, 31*(1), 81–105.

Lifshitz, C., & Katz, C. (2015). Underrepresentation of Ethiopian–Israeli minority students in programmes for the gifted and talented: A policy discourse analysis. *Journal of Education Policy, 30*(1), 101–131.

Poluha, E. (Ed.). (2007). *The world of girls and boys in rural and urban Ethiopia. (pp. 69–90, 134–197).* Forum for Social Studies.

Reddy, M. (1996). *Crossing the colour line: Race, parenting, and culture.* Rutgers University Press.

Rosenblum, S., Goldblatt, H., & Moin, V. (2008). The hidden dropout phenomenon among immigrant high-school students: The case of Ethiopian adolescents in Israel – A pilot study. *School Psychology International, 29*(1), 105–127.

Shalom, S. (2016). *From Sinai to Ethiopia: The Halachic and conceptual world of Ethiopian Jewry.* Gefen.

Ungar, M. (2008). Resilience across cultures. *British Journal of Social Work, 2008*(38), 218–235.

Zhou, M. (2009). Conflict, coping and reconciliation: Intergenerational relations in Chinese immigrant families. In N. Foner (Ed.), *Across generations immigrant families in America* (pp. 21–46). NYU.

Hebrew References

Anaki, M. (2017). *Perceptions of risk and protection amongst educators working with children of Ethiopian descent.* Thesis for master's in social work. Hebrew University Jerusalem.

Cohen, H. (1998). *Chocolate child.* Hapoalim.

Dreikus, R. (1994). *Fundamentals of Adlerian psychology.* Alfred Adler Institute.

Mekonen, B. (2010). *The influence of the Ethiopian Jewish Legacy program on strengthening ethnic identity and social and school acculturation amongst youth of Ethiopian origin in boarding schools.* Masters thesis. Bar Ilan University.

Mengistu, W. (2014). *Youth of Ethiopian origin in cultural transition: Connecting ethnicity and perceived discrimination with covert and overt truancy and risk behaviour.* Doctoral thesis in social science. Hebrew University.

Mula, S. (2010). *The struggle to be normal: Ethiopian students meet racism in religious schools*. Masters thesis. Hebrew University.

Sagiv, T. (2014). *On the fault line: Israelis of mixed ethnicity*. Hakibbutz Hameuchad.

Sever, R. (2004). Immigrant absorption in education, policy and research. *Megamot, 1*, 145–168.

Shemer, O. (2009). From many cultures to multiculturalism: Professional challenges in culturally sensitive work with children and their parents. *Et Hasadeh*. Ashelim. 3. 4–10.

Shmuel, N. (2020). *Exploring diversity: Six-modules for academic courses and professional training*. Erasmus+ Program of the European Union, NEVET Greenhouse of Context-Informed Research and Training for Children in Need, the school of Social Work and Social Welfare, Hebrew University of Jerusalem. Exploring diversity | Demo erasmus+ (erasmus-il.org)

Shmuel, N. (2015). Transitions not gaps: Absorption of Ethiopian immigrants in schools. *Gilui Daat, 8*, 137–146.

Shmuel, N. (2010). *Educational traditions of Ethiopian Jewry: The dynamics of continuity and change* (pp. 71–73). Masters thesis. Hebrew University.

Shmuel, N. (1991). *Aba Hum*. Modan.

Shmuel, N., & Shimon, M. (2012). *Shades of Belonging. Educational pack aimed at providing primary school teachers with practical easy-to-use methods for improving the social and learning environments in the heterogeneous classroom*. Funded by the Merchavim Institute for the Advancement of Shared Citizenship in Israel and Israel-Germany Future Foundation. The complete booklet can be found on my website: www.naomis-books.com

Chapter 11
Gender Perceptions and Roles Following Immigration

Some of the most significant and complex changes following immigration from Ethiopia involve the issue of gender—expectations and roles. These changes are closely linked to the disintegrating traditional hierarchy, which was based on age and gender. As the balance of power in the family shifts, men and women experience these changes differently, mostly without open discussion on these issues, creating volatile situations that affect the whole family. These changes are simultaneous to all the other shifts in the family following immigration and interact with the social stratification of the receiving society. In the mosaic of sub-cultures which make up Israeli society, a range of attitudes and practices regarding gender expectations and roles can be encountered.

Stratification in Israeli society is convoluted, being based on race, gender, ethnicity, socioeconomic status, and geographical location, creating differential distribution of resources, privileges, rights and obligations (Abdo, 2011; Shafir & Peled, 2002). Thus, women's status in Israel varies according to their other identities, detailed by researchers when discussing the feminist movement and Israeli citizenship (Abdo, 2011; Shafir & Peled, 2002; Dahan-Kalev, 2001). The hierarchy is generally considered to be Ashkenazi men, Ashkenazi women, Mizrachi men, Mizrachi women, other immigrant groups, and then Palestinian men and women. But the intersectionality of privilege and oppression complicates this, as both men and women may be privileged or oppressed in different ways, as their social positions and multiple identities may give them agency in some spheres and present barriers in others (Chow et al., 2011). Patriarchy can be seen in public social structures in the division of labour and relative salaries, politics, law, and the military, as well as in family roles and expectations specific to different cultural and religious groups. These systems interlock and overlap, complicated further by the effects of globalization and intermingling of Israeli's various sub-cultures, creating interconnected contexts of differential access to society's resources and opportunities (Chow et al., 2011).

© The Author(s), under exclusive license to Springer Nature Switzerland AG 2023

N. A. Shmuel, *Children's Wellbeing in Immigrant Families*, Children's Well-Being: Indicators and Research 26,
https://doi.org/10.1007/978-3-031-31917-4_11

Negotiating the transition in the overwhelming obscurity of the grey area between the immigrant's culture (also not homogenous) and local variations while struggling to establish an economically viable and nurturing family home, can be a formidable and lengthy task. This issue has been addressed in studies on immigrants elsewhere, for example Espiritu (2009) demonstrates how social structures of power relations affect the lives of Filipino immigrants in America. Incorporating in the analysis the context of adjustment to a highly stratified society reflects family conflicts on money and sexuality not just as cultural clashes but as the manifestation of intersectionality, expressing the interaction of both gender and ethnic inequality in people's lives. Undoubtedly this paradigm is also relevant when discussing Ethiopian immigrants in Israel, as the intersection of gender, ethnicity, and socioeconomic considerations form the context for personal, familial, and community negotiation of the roles, obligations, and expectations of men as fathers and husbands and of women as mothers and wives.

11.1 Changes in Daily Existence in Israel

In Israel, girls are expected to study, thus they marry later, when they are much older, to men of their own choice and not by arranged marriages as was customary in Ethiopia. Couples make joint decisions about where to live and may choose to live near the woman's parents (Simuchin & Shefu-Tsenkel, 2005). There is no special hut for women to go to during menstruation or after childbirth, changing the customary behaviour of women in relation to these events (Anteby, 2000). Women bare fewer children, many work and are financially independent (Wiel, 2005). The clear division of roles in the family prevalent in Ethiopia changes and becomes open to negotiation (Bodovsky, 1989). Men are no longer at the head of extended families as sole decision-makers, as the traditional hierarchy disintegrates, and family units become smaller. Infants enter day care, children go to school, teenagers go to boarding school, thus there is a distinct separation between the world of adults and children, who spend less time together. All these practical changes undermine the traditional balance of power between the sexes, coupled with the inevitable culture clash, this is akin to a social earthquake rocking every household.

11.2 Changes in Perceptions Regarding Gender

> Amongst Ethiopians there is always a gap between men and women. Women are quicker to mingle socially in their new environment. They learn the language more quickly; they look after the children so are inevitably more involved in what is happening around them. (Naama)

Practical changes occur faster than perceptual changes, thus there is a lack of correlation between expectations in the family, inevitably leading to confrontation. When Ester's mother was ill, her father would clean the house and even cook *engera*, but he never expected his sons to do housework. Ester was 'annoyed that they were exempt'. She tried to confront her father on this and he said 'they wouldn't do it well', which Ester saw as an excuse, saying

> they can do it! I don't understand why they are not expected to do anything!

The dissonance between her father's behaviour and his attitude towards his sons pinpoints the paradox: he has changed his own behaviour to help at home but still perceives this as women's work, which he does not expect of his sons. His value system and perception of male and female roles has not changed, but he is flexible in his own behaviour for the sake of his family.

In many families changes in behaviour are evident to prevent open conflict, but the underlying value system has not changed. Thus, Maayan's father wanted to prevent his girls from staying out late, so he threatened to lock the door at ten, but in fact left it open and did not wait up. Dany, who is religious, says that when his sons borrow the car on Shabbat he 'pretends not to notice'. These men are refraining from outright conflict with their children by forfeiting their control over them. They are saving face by not condoning openly behaviour which is against their principles. Peace at home is maintained by a code of silence.

In contrast, many young participants noted that it was possible to talk freely to their mothers, as Addis describes:

> I can talk to my mother without being worried. I used to believe that if I had problems, I was the one who should solve them. I wouldn't share [what was bothering me]....My mother said *don't close yourself up*. Actually, it's easier to talk to my mother.

Liora, Noa, Edna, and Lemlem all stated that they want their children to be able to talk to them freely. These mothers are opening a dialogue with their children in which traditional assumptions can be questioned, open communication with their children is more important to them than saving face.

11.3 Actually or Effectively Absent Fathers

Out of 16 second-generation participants, only 4 talked about their father as having a positive presence in their lives (Yisrael, Shira, Habtam, and Shimon). The interviews with Yafit, Naama, and Mahari indicate that Yisrael's younger siblings find it much harder to communicate with their father (Mahari) and experience less support from him. Three G2 participants talked about their father in relation to family conflicts, describing him as authoritarian (Ester, Sarah, and Maayan).

Six G2 participants described their father as completely dysfunctional (Dana, Yaniv, Addis, Noam, Sarah, Maayan). These present-absent fathers are at home but do not function as fathers, not by Ethiopian traditional standards or Israeli standards. Yaniv said about his father that he 'does not really feeling him' and that 'he's there, in the living room, in front of the TV'. He describes himself as 'giving up on him'. Addis talked about his father as 'in his own world' and said that 'he wouldn't give me five shekels'. Dana said about her father that he 'was never there, was not functional', and that 'he was never a parent'.

Three G2 participants describe themselves as growing up without a father: Miki, whose father left him alone in Israel with his younger brother when he was 10; Avi, whose father did not live with them and died when he was 13; and Naama who was separated from her father as a toddler when he was taken to the army in Ethiopia and he arrived in Israel when she was 16.

Of the 15 G1.5 participants, 7 described their father as a positive presence in their lives (Liora, Noa, Noam, Matan, Edna, Lemlem, Teruneh). Five of the six G1.5 participants who attended boarding school hardly mentioned their fathers at all (Lee, Mulu, Tigist, Dov, Orna). The other three G1.5 participants all grew up without a father; Genet says her father was not a part of her life and she called her grandfather Dad. Rachel and Tsehai's fathers died when they were children.

Some of the fathers were absent because they were working to support their families, as Dov, Noam, Dana, and Lemlem mentioned. Ester's father was an only provider, his wife never worked. Tigist remembers her father as 'always at work', and Orna says of her husband that he comes home after the children have gone to bed. Rachel describes her husband as always either asleep or at work, with the aim of 'giving them [the children] what he never had'. Naama also talked about her father 'working very hard' and how Ethiopian men work so hard 'they miss opportunities with the children, including understanding things'.

It seems that most fathers are actually or effectively absent from their children's lives either because of the need to work and support their families or as a result of personal conduct.

> Usually, I read the children stories. He [her husband] does try sometimes, but mostly he prefers the technical side, doing their laundry or tidying up their room, organizing them. This business of reading to them or fooling around with them on the carpet or watching television with them, that's for me… He doesn't fool around with them; he likes to keep up the façade…' (Shani).

In all Israel's sub-cultures young couples mostly maintain the traditional division between the parents to varying degrees: the father tending to be more authoritarian (stressing obedience and discipline) and the mother more permissive and communicative. The façade Shani was talking about upholds the 'respectful distance' which was expected in Ethiopia, but it also creates a barrier to personal connection and deep involvement in the children's lives.

In Israel, new challenges are added to parenting, like choosing and being involved in pre-school and school education. Fathers who leave this to their wives are missing out, as Nama explains:

> My father has nothing to do with their [her siblings] education—buying books, going to parent meetings. Even if my mother can't do this, the children won't agree that he [father] will get involved because he doesn't understand anything… so the division is very clear. Well, they can see that it's possible to laugh and to argue with our mother, to tell her secrets… because she won't use them against you. In the same way they know that it's not possible to talk about everything with my father, because he is inflexible and doesn't under-

> stand, or misinterprets things... you can't ask him for things over which there is disagreement. These characteristics are common amongst Ethiopian fathers.

These inflexible and inaccessible fathers are preserving their traditional status, which in Ethiopia came with authority, but in Israel has become void of content. At best it maintains the children's polite, respectful behaviour, while leaving the fathers uninvolved in their lives. Most of the young participants in the study referred to their father as distant and silent. The bond with the fathers that has been severed or diminished leaves an abyss between the generations, which makes not only communication impossible, but also cultural transferal. This seems to be the collateral damage accompanying this community's immigration.

11.4 Involved Fathers

Genet's grandfather Berihun and her uncle Mamu described in detail how tradition, practical farming knowledge and family genealogy were passed from one generation to the next through daily living in the Jewish villages in Ethiopia. Shy's father often travelled away from home in Ethiopia, but his son felt very connected to him:

> I loved my father very very much. I used to sleep with him. When he went away to some event in a distant village for three days I used to take his clothes and sleep with them. There was no electricity in the village, but I used to sit opposite the door [waiting for him]. Because of me it was difficult for him to go out.

Shy's father had a presence in his life even in his absence, he was his protector and the anchor of his cultural identity.

Adults of the intermediate (1.5) generation, such as Matan, Dov, and Tigist, still recall shepherding or working the fields with their fathers, who obviously had a very significant presence in their lives. Children need to see their parents as people they can aspire to be like, this is made possible through a deep connection that breaches the narrow confines of culturally defined duty to reveal the multi-dimensional person within. Edna recalls listening to her grandfather pray as a young child, she still remembers all the words for these prayers and says that he is the one who planted faith in her heart. In Israel, this natural process of inter-generational transferal is almost non-existent, any transferal at all depends on the fathers' abilities to adapt themselves to changing circumstances and through this flexibility become accessible to their children (like Dany, Shy, and Tareke).

Lemlem speaks about her mother as 'the minister of finance, education and social security', what seems to suggest the mother took all the responsibilities in the family. And yet Lemlem talks about her father as her inspiration to study, saying:

> He always told us to study, that studying was the way to self-discovery. He used to say *knowledge is power*. Even in Ethiopia, he never said *get married and have children, bring me grandchildren*, like others, no, he always said *you will go to Israel, and you will study.*

Fathers guide their children, setting their sights for the future, they can be both the source of change and continuity by encouraging children to adapt to a changing world while keeping their heritage and traditions. This is the leadership of competent, culturally flexible fathers at the crucial time of living unsettled lives after immigration.

Miki arrived in Israel when he was only 9, his father left him and his younger brother in a boarding school and went back to Ethiopia. As an adult he understands that 'it is up to me to search for my roots', he did so recently by seeking out his father and making the effort to know him as a person, saying 'he can tell me many things'. Miki was cared for very well in a good boarding school, he grew up sufficiently rooted in local culture to be able to set out to seek knowledge about his Ethiopian roots from the primordial source: his father in Ethiopia.

Edna's parents divorced in Ethiopia because her mother insisted on taking her children to Israel via Sudan. Aware of the dangers of such a journey, her grandfather caught up with her before she crossed the border and managed to take Edna back with him. Later her father, who thought walking to Sudan with the children irresponsible and reckless, followed them:

> My father came to Sudan with the connections he had, gave her [mother] food and took back with him whoever he could. She was after birth, so the baby stayed with my mother, and my two-year-old sister who refused to be separated from her. She died in Sudan.

Despite the divorce, the father encouraged Edna to keep in touch with her mother during their 7-year-long separation by writing letters, he also made a point of taking her to visit her mother's relatives. In Israel, when she was in boarding school, he visited her regularly and made sure to make her the centre of his attention on the weekends that she came home:

> When we [she and her sister] came home for Shabbat, they [father and stepmother] made sure not to have too many guests. They had the big family gatherings on the Shabbat when we were not home, so that [when we came] they could give us their utmost attention.

Edna's father was an exceptional father in Ethiopia, where he 'always put his children first' and even gave them best pieces of meat much to the amazement of his guests. In Israel, he continued to be a devoted father and make his children's needs his priority.

Similarly, Noa's father was devoted to his children:

> My father raised us. He sang to us and told us stories. He took us out for ice cream. He rented us movies. He bought us bicycles. He did things that other [Ethiopian] fathers didn't do. Other immigrant fathers thought it was shameful to be seen with the children, to run along with the bicycle. My father wasn't like that. He was with us, talked to us, sang to us.

These fathers were responsive to their children's needs in their new environment without being restricted by the narrow confines of cultural tradition. In the parent groups I facilitated in the Ethiopian community men often voiced the fear of being seen as ruled by women, for example if observed hanging out the laundry or pushing a baby in a pram. In other words, social expectations limit behaviour, but there are fathers who do not care about appearances.

Dov is very much aware of the changes he is making in his own version of parenting:

> In Ethiopia there are clear rules—father says something, it needs to be done. Of course, I have a tendency to educate my child in this fashion, but here it doesn't work. I tried! And truthfully, the fact that we enter a new life, gives us the opportunity to let go of past ideas. Naturally I might think, what would my father do in such a situation? It would most probably be something completely different from what I do with my children. In Ethiopia the father was authoritarian, children had to do what they were told and that was that. I'm not like that. I have changed a lot. My parents used to use extreme measures; they would hit me. I don't do that.

Dov is aware of the tendency of every parent to educate their children using the methods familiar to them from their own childhood. But he has made a choice to do things differently, has concluded that in the new context these methods are ineffective and even detrimental. Dov also makes an important observation about the nature of transition as an opportunity to 'let go of past ideas' not in the sense of relinquishing cultural heritage, but in negotiating new cultural pathways more suited to the new environment. Dov's parental toolkit is different from his father's because in his negotiation with transition, he is deliberately changing his parenting methods to suit the new context.

Noam also states:

> My father educated me with methods that belong over there [Ethiopia]. I educate using both methods—from there and from here.

Noam has two children from different relationships, he makes great efforts to be significant in the lives of them both, even if this involves a certain amount of confrontation with his former partner. Since he sees this child only once a week, he is determined to make their meetings meaningful.

These fathers are aware of the necessity to invest time and effort in building a connection with their children, as well as adapting their parenting styles to the new reality. Children are responsive to this investment; it inspires them to try and understand their parents even when communication with them is compounded by language and culture. Thus, Yisrael says:

> To my father it is very important that I should be serious, use the head on my shoulders, be organised and plan ahead. Every time he comes into my room and there is a sock on the floor, he'll say *how do you expect to get anywhere if you have a sock on the floor? Do you think it is logical that so and so…* he wants me to be in control of my life and be practical.

Yisrael is aware that his father's comment about the sock is not trivial, that it is part of a world view containing implications for his own future. His ability to understand this is based on the effort he is making to follow his father's logic, despite Mahari's poor Hebrew and unclear imagery, because they have a deep connection. Yisrael is Mahari's first son born after the reunion with his family following an absence of about 10 years, these special circumstances seem to compensate for the linguistic and cultural obstacles between father and son that make communication so difficult.

It is connection which motivates learning from one's parents, as Dana describes:

> My Amharic is good because of my father. My father was enthusiastic when I showed an interest in his books, so I started to read with him. Then I did five units in Amharic [for matriculation] and he was very pleased with this. Now I can read fluently, and this is our warm connection. Me and my father, we really got close.

This is the same Dana who was so critical of her parents in the interview, saying that her father was not a parent at all. And yet reading Amharic together sparked a 'warm connection' between them. This example illustrates what Foner (2009) has noted, that relations between the generations in immigrant families contain inconsistencies and contradictions, that conflict can exist alongside cooperation and caring.

11.5 Mothers

Genet explains how she understood her culturally perceived role in life from a very young age:

> At home I was educated towards something very specific: *family*—to marry and have children and that was it.

When Bosana cried because the other children went to school and her parents forbade her to join them, her father sat beside her and said:

> Why are you so sad? If it is possible you will study, if not—what does it matter? You will have a home like your mother, you will get married and bear children like your mother.

In Israel new choices are available for girls; to choose who and when they marry, and how many children to have and when. As Orna explains:

> I have been given an opportunity. The fact that I came here and I can choose my husband, that I can choose how many children to bear…

Women in Israel also have the choice of studying and/or working, unlike their mothers in Ethiopia who, as Lemlem says about her own mother, was 'completely focused on raising her children'. Lemlem says 'there is no comparison' between her mother—who gave her undivided attention to the children, and her own reality—as she juggles work, studies, and childrearing. Mulu feels the same way:

> In Ethiopia it was much easier to raise children because life was tribal, everybody grew up together, everybody helped. Mothers didn't go anywhere, were much more attentive to their children, gave them love and warmth, that emotional safe haven which sadly is missing today. The modern woman is trapped in a snare; she has to be a mother, a wife, a housewife, and have a career. This damages the quality of education, of parenting, and the children as well as the women pay the price.

Mulu is talking about the heavy load of motivated, career-oriented women, struggling to be attentive mothers at the same time as working or studying, something Lemlem, Orna, and Genet all spoke about as well. Other studies have shown that this can come with a price, for example Dion and Dion (2001) found that amongst Korean immigrants in Canada women tended to suffer more from depression than men. This was especially so amongst working women of high socioeconomic status, in other words a better financial situation and being educated did not necessarily improve women's mental health. Their conclusion was that amongst immigrant groups, factors that improve their financial situation do not necessarily contribute to the wellbeing of women—who are expected to fulfil both new and traditional roles. This *double burden* of responsibilities, both at home and at work, is what led to depression. Sometimes it can also lead to illness; Abigail gave birth soon after arrival to Israel, she missed most of the *ulpan* (Hebrew classes) and insisted on immediately going out to work despite her husband's objection. With six children at home and an uncooperative husband, her health deteriorated resulting in several hospitalizations. Many working mothers, such as Tsehai, Liora, and Orna, were assisted by their own mothers taking care of their children after they gave birth. Yafit says that she only managed to survive because of her parents, and that 'an Ethiopian woman who lives near her parents is sure to flourish'.

Other studies have demonstrated the determination of immigrant women to be significant mothers, for example Unger and Sever (2012) studied Ethiopian immigrant women in Israel and their relations with pre-school institutions their children attended. Contrary to common opinion, they found the mothers assertive and involved, determined to maintain maternal responsibility. In another study on successful Ethiopian immigrant women in Israel, by Walsh and Unus (2012) the women described their parents as supportive and involved in their lives, despite struggling with the language and financial difficulties. All the interviewees ascribed their own success to being stubborn, relentless, and optimistic. Perhaps it is the personal narrative attributing themselves agency and ability which enables these women to get ahead (Plunkett, 2001).

When talking to the women participants of my study, I got the impression that in searching for the middle road between the cultures they live in, and coping with personal and family struggles where important life decisions must be made, they often lack close confidants who could share in their deliberations. Neither the men in their lives nor the women in their community seem to take on this role. Wilfully pursuing one's dreams is not necessarily encouraged by a society based on collectivism, neither is developing self-reflection, which can be seen as questioning traditional roles. Thus, often women are not only coping with multiple conflicting tasks in and outside the home, but they are doing so in relative isolation. Their struggles have no legitimacy either in their home communities or in their wider local social networks, each supportive of contradictory norms. Of course, this very much depends on which particular sub-culture of Israeli society they live in, and the attitudes and sensitivities of close relatives. But it seems that often negotiating the intersection of gender and culture with family and social expectations can be a lonely business.

In conversations with women of the older generation (G1) they often attributed events in their lives to fate or a higher power, frequently mentioning God in reverence as responsible for everything. They did not seem to see themselves as responsible for how their children turned out. Their daughters of the intermediate generation (G1.5) are more inclined to talk about personal effort, they appreciate and look up to their own mothers and grandmothers, seeing them as role models, even if their own lives are very different. Many aspire to be like the older generation, and many often act as bridges between their mothers and their younger Israeli-born siblings (G2).

11.6 Gender Socialization

Mulu wants her daughter to 'be whoever she wants to be', a statement releasing her child from the narrow confines of cultural expectations. But these expectations are still existent in people's minds after immigration. Thus, Modesh describes herself as a young girl in Ethiopia retreating to an inner room when guests arrived, as was expected of her, saying 'we were taught to be ashamed'. This feeling still haunts her; 'I have something in my stomach that I want to say, but I am ashamed'. Being 'ashamed' has been internalized by Modesh and other women as an inhibition which prevents them from standing up for themselves in public or even voicing an opinion. As girls they were socialized not only to modesty but also to silence. Poluha (2007) describes boys in Ethiopia as taking up more physical space than girls, who cower their bodies and lower their gaze in the presence of men. She also describes the expectation, internalized by young girls, not to play on the street, to remain at home, available to their parents and siblings to assist with household chores, and to hide themselves when guests arrive.

Shira (13) was born to Liora and Shy after two boys. She says that she 'is expected' to help at home, she sees this as logical. While I interviewed her father in my home she cleaned their apartment of her own initiative. Her mother Liora says:

> The girls are at home more, closer to their mother, less outside, therefore daughters need to be socialized, so they can teach their own children.

She is talking about girls in Israel, and of her own daughter she expects 'to be more open, patient and forgiving'. Then she thinks for a moment and adds:

> Boys should be like that too, but boys are more outside, more at work... even though now it's more similar [for boys and girls] but I expect the girl *to be a woman*.

Traditional concepts of qualities attributed appropriate for girls persist after immigration even amongst parents who show high levels of hybridity. To Liora girls are inherently more domestic than boys, they mature earlier and are generally more open and helpful of their own volition. Since the boys' primary domain is external to the home, they are more adept outside, she continues to explain that at home they are only likely to help if told what to do.

Shira knows intuitively what her mother expects of her, it is what her grandmother expected of Liora; to be 'a good woman' who knows how to cook and behave as anticipated.

Gender-specific expectations in Ethiopia were embedded in the language, thus a girl who behaves like a boy was called boyish—wondawend—and a boy who behaves like a girl girlish—*setaset* (Poluha, 2007). There was more tolerance for the latter—a boy was expected to argue sometimes and do things his own way, while a girl was likely to be severely punished for not fulfilling her gender role and labelled 'bad' (Poluha). Similarly, in Israel, gender-specific expectations may lead to fierce conflicts, with repercussions especially for girls. Shani (G1.5) provides an example of this. Shani lived with her parents after she married. Even though her husband had a good job in which he received cooked meals, her parents expected her to cook for him before he came home. She says that she became angry and told them:

'*Are you trying to make me the little woman?! We are not in Ethiopia*!'

At the same time, she would dress up to go out and sense her parents looking at her disapprovingly:

> I was constantly in conflict with them. [I felt/said] let me flourish, let me succeed! But I would get dressed and their body language said: *is that what you're wearing? What is that? What is that short revealing thing? Is it a shirt?*

Shani got this message from their gaze, it made her feel that while she was struggling for independence, they were shackling her to tradition:

> Their attitude defined my identity in narrow terms as a woman, *the woman in the kitchen*. I was trying to define myself according to what is acceptable in the modern era.

Shani was struggling to distinguish herself from the narrow confines of the traditional female role as her parents defined it and allow herself to be a free emancipated woman. Her own daughter she describes as 'much too fragile' and seems to be reflecting her own vulnerability. As she struggles to explain to me what she wants for her daughter, she mixes between the terms assertiveness and aggressiveness. She belongs to two cultures with opposing expectations of women, it is not by mistake that she cannot explain herself. Perhaps, in Israel, both men and women are searching for a new equilibrium between assertiveness and aggressiveness, between coercive manliness and attentive sharing, between self-fulfilment and endless collective generosity, between self-definition and conformity to social expectations. Therefore, Shani is confusing assertiveness and aggressiveness; in Ethiopia, a blatantly assertive woman would be considered offensive and disrespectful, it would be appropriate to treat her with aggression. Shani is balancing herself and her daughter on the fine divide between the two cultures, in the confusion the two terms become synonymous to her. She sees her young daughter as fragile—at the intersection of her identities as Ethiopian and a woman—then describes herself as 'not tough enough' to be able to help her.

Gender-related values often clash after immigration, when tradition demands modesty as girls seek newfound freedom (Tummala-Narra, 2004). Cultural pathways are colliding, the result includes garbled and confusing messages passed from mothers to their daughters. Thus, Lee cannot understand why her mother complains about her clothes—saying she is dressed immodestly. Lee is wearing jeans, her arms and legs are covered, but to her mother Worknesh this is not good enough, good Jewish girls in Ethiopia wore skirts not jeans. Young female immigrants, especially from traditional patriarchal societies, are often restricted by their parents more than boys to shield them from the influences of what is regarded as a promiscuous society (Dion & Dion, 2001). These struggles are prevalent not only in the immigrant community but also in some sub-cultures of native Israelis. In negotiating the spaces between settled and unsettled lives, between the older and the younger generations, between change and conservatism, between religiosity and secularism, young immigrants can always find local partners for rebellion in the diversity of Israeli society. But while experimenting with boundaries and challenging authority are recognized stages of teenage development in Israel, to the elders of the new immigrant community such behaviour, especially from girls, is considered so abhorrent it can lead to harsh responses, even ostracism. As Worknesh explains:

> Trying to be boyfriend and girlfriend, to see if they match, this is not good. What does it mean to *try*? This is not acceptable! God does not like it.

There is a big difference between arranged marriages for girls aged 8–13, and young women of 20 or 30 choosing their own partners. Worknesh goes on to say that young people no longer respect their parents and don't listen to them. Her daughter Lee arrived in Israel at 15 before her parents, and even after their arrival a year later remained in boarding school. She says:

> My parents expected… that we study, only study. Here girls study and also have boyfriends. [They said] *No, no boyfriend, just study!* If I talked on the telephone [they said] *who are you talking to?* Like that. It was really hard. I just studied and look what happened.

What happened is that Lee married very late and never bore children. At 45 she is inferring that her parents are at least partly to blame, saying:

> They had unrealistic expectations, *don't talk to boys*. It was extreme.

Lee's parents expected her to avoid having relationships with men until she was ready to marry, out of respect and obedience she complied and feels she paid a heavy price. In contrast, Tigist at 32 lives with her boyfriend, and says her parents know 'not to confront' her on this. When 30-year-old Maayan told her mother she had adopted a dog, her reaction astounded her: her mother said, 'better you should have adopted a child'!

Maayan was horrified by this remark and cites it as an example of how much her parents do not understand her and her life. The cultural gap which has been added to the generational gap in these relationships seems too wide to be bridged. According to 35-year-old Naama, it is a conceptual gap that exists also between men and women in the Ethiopian community:

> Sometimes it is really hard for me to understand the way Ethiopian men I have dated think, and these are *young* men. Then I think to myself, maybe I have *disconnected myself too much*. That is my feeling. I am disconnected from the source. I can't understand them anymore.

Naama has come so far from the traditional way of thinking about gender and relationships, that she cannot understand the men she dates from the Ethiopian community. When such gaps in perceptions occur within the family, where one might expect to be most understood, the resultant misunderstandings may lead to fierce emotions.

It seems that to some extent, the baby is being thrown out with the bathwater—in the sense that these young women rejecting the traditional roles assigned to them by their community, are severing the ties that link them to their cultural identity as a whole. Naama refers to herself as 'disconnected from the source' implying an unmendable rift which not only distances her from a set cultural pathway but effectively severs her ability to even understand this pathway. Naama says about her sister that she 'shouts at my father in a loud voice', something which would be unheard of in Ethiopia. Naama's teenage sister is not only refusing to heed her father, but she is also actually telling him what to do. Naama calls her 'super-feminist'. In face of such mutiny, there will be little or no cultural transferal between this teenager and her father Mahari, and the increasing volatile clashes are undoubtedly detrimental to them both.

Edna is well aware that most girls in Ethiopia were not encouraged to study, she says:

> My father was told, *you are educating your daughter you are ruining her*. He put me on his knees and taught me how to count. I counted using stones. Slowly he took them away from me and said *think for yourself*. He taught me the times table while bouncing me on his lap, and when I knew it he sent me to school.

When she notified her father in Israel that she was planning to marry a white man, he completely amazed her by saying:

> *Of course you are, I always pushed you to study.* There he was telling me that most Ethiopian men would be put off by my education.

Her father admitted to her that this had worried him, that she might never get married, but it never stopped him from encouraging her to study. Edna's fathers' attitude was the exception, more often even after immigration telling girls to study is lip service, seldom backed by changing expectations of them at home creating suitable conditions for them to be able to do so.

11.7 The Marital Relationship After Immigration

> At home with my partner I am much more Ethiopian, I am much less expressive, less demanding. Much quieter. Yes, there is the Genet you can see, but at home I restrain her.

Genet is an assertive, strong-willed educated woman, who consciously restrains herself in the presence of her Ethiopian husband, whom she describes as active and responsible at home, taking care of their children when she studies and supportive of her decisions. Genet wisely combines elements from both cultures in managing her life with her partner, she has re-created the delicate balance of power between the sexes which existed in Ethiopia on her own terms—her respectful behaviour enables him to be an active supportive partner.

My interviews did not include direct questions about spouses, but in describing their daily lives in detail and their ways of educating their children, one might expect the partners to be mentioned. And yet only 8 of the 20 married women and two of the divorced women had something positive to say about their partners, in the context of shared parenting or sharing or seeking advice, all of these belonged to the intermediate generation (G1.5). Ten women never once mentioned their partners during the interview (three G1.5, two without children, and all the others G1). Four women mentioned their partners in a negative manner, as absent parents or in conflict with them (two G1.5 and two G1). Only 4 of the 11 married men interviewed mentioned their wives in a positive way, all G1. The other seven married men did not mention their wives at all.

My sense is that these findings are not arbitrary but reflect the fact that most G1.5 women have created relationships based on partnership, joint responsibilities, and shared parenting. While most G1 women have coped with parenting in the new country on their own, as Tummala-Narra (2004) found often happens after immigration for financial, cultural, and personal reasons. Other studies, for example Hondagneu-Sotelo (1992) found that amongst Mexican immigrants to the USA, coming from a patriarchal society, the balance of power between the sexes changed after immigration. In any case, patriarchal constraints are not uniform, women in the same culture can have differing experiences. For example, there are women who worked in Ethiopia, and there are also women (such as Abigail) whose husbands tried to prevent them from working in Israel.

When Yafit and her husband quarrelled, she recalls a friend telling her

> You must bow down a little, Yafit, otherwise Ethiopian men have no space. Where is your respect for your husband?

Rachel also talked about the ‘respect for the husband’ that must be preserved as part of the culture:

> I promise you, in every family, first of all there is the respect. The respect between husband and wife must be maintained, meaning whatever the man says, she has to do it. This is sacred till this day! Nobody can deny it, there is something about the men—*I decide, I determine, I come home and am served food!*—it’s all right, this is our culture, you cannot sever from it completely.

She said this with great conviction, but a minute later contradicted herself vehemently:

> The respect? Gone! It has not been kept! Today, women my age and older, they are getting divorced. You never saw that [in Ethiopia]. Every Monday and Thursday—divorce!

When I asked her if it was because the women are not obedient to the men she says:

> Yes! Yes! they all want to be Israeli! They forget where they came from!

The contradiction in her statements reflects the unresolved dilemma of this immigration; on the one hand, tradition demands respecting and obeying the husband. On the other hand, in their new environment there are opportunity for women to make decisions without asking for permission from or even considering their husbands. Without a system of open dialogue and correlating expectations, as soon as traditionally structured relations disintegrate after immigration, outright power struggles and one-sided decisions ensue. Thus, equality clashes with conservatism, and definitions of national identity are confused with gender conceptions. Rachel says they all want to be 'Israeli' but there are also a lot of versions of Israeli women. She ends up by saying women should 'remember where they came from'—as if this must call them to order, but in the same breath also says of herself that she does not accept her traditional role. The fact that this volatile situation causes many divorces indicates the extent to which men and women are pulling in opposite directions while negotiating the grey area between the two cultures where gender perceptions and expectations are blurred, re-considered and inevitably clash.

In Ethiopia, equality meant something different than what it means in Israel. Couples joined in arranged marriages learnt to adapt to one another, their affection visibly expressed in small respectful acts such as a woman washing her husbands' feet when he returned from the field. Rosen (2009, unpublished) compared this to a woman giving her husband a massage after a long day's work. The act in itself is not necessarily humiliating, since it was part and parcel of a delicately balanced system, in which, for example in public events a woman would give her husband a plate of food and he would offer her a handful of *engera* before eating himself, as a gesture of affection, not status. Behaviour needs to be understood in context, strategies of action are suited to preconceived ideas about what is appropriate for men and for women. When the context changes there is a dislocation between expectations, intentions, actions, and outcomes.

11.8 Three Major Changes

I would like to focus upon three major changes affecting gender relations in the Ethiopian immigrant community in Israel: communication, expectations, and relative status.

Firstly, changes in communication: women of the intermediate and second generations (G1.5 and G2) are not silent like their mothers, they stand up for themselves. As Liora says:

> I can argue. I don't let him [her husband] off the hook like my mother [Emebet] did, she always shielded my father.

Emebet was restrained, she was respectful towards her husband by not arguing with him. Women in Ethiopia used *wax and gold* communication[1] and covert means to get what they wanted. They avoided direct confrontation, maintaining the traditional *respectful distance* between the sexes. In Israel, the communication strategy has changed to being much more direct, women are saying what is on their mind

[1] Discussed in Chap. 7.

unhindered. Rachel says her mother was never angry but describes herself as able not only to get angry but sometimes even to 'bark'.

Mulu says of herself as a child:

> I have a rebellious personality, I always did what I wanted, but not to the extreme... I was always quiet and polite; I was a *good girl*.

Mulu's rebelliousness in Ethiopia was moderated by her respectful behaviour, she never broke the rules. In contrast, Naama's younger sister in Israel shouts at her father. In Ethiopia, open antagonism between the generations or between the sexes was avoided—the respectful distance buffered all conflict. The *good girl* was obedient and respectful (Poluha, 2007). The cultural transition has eroded these barriers to self-expression and direct, sometimes volatile conflict enters almost every home.

Secondly, the change in expectations: G1.5 and G2 women are no longer satisfied with the traditional Ethiopian version of equality between the sexes, which contained gradual adaptation to unknown partners of arranged marriages and covert symbolic gestures of affection. They have *chosen* their partners and expect mutual reciprocity in every sense. Liora explains that her mother showed her father respect no matter what, but she herself: 'I respect him if he respects me, it has to be mutual'. Young women perceive their relationships with Western values of equality, it is not enough for them that their partners should be loyal, hardworking, and non-violent. They want partners who will share equal responsibility for their relationship, their home, and their children. Naama talks of Ethiopian men as '*chauvinistic*', Mayan says that 'Ethiopia is not exactly a feminist state'. In this context, it is worth noting that in 2018, Ethiopia was the first state in Africa to choose a woman president. Sahale Work-Zawde was chosen unanimously by the Ethiopian parliament only days after the new cabinet was formed, one of the most gender-balanced parliaments in the world—containing 50% women. But equality is not just about being given a seat at the table, equality is about relinquishing the power struggle and sharing responsibilities.

Which brings us to the third major change: a change in relative status. Women are quick to let go of the hierarchy that defined them as inferior to men, most of the women in my study have also relinquished the respectful distance between themselves and their children to build closer more intimate parental relationships. But many men sense a loss of status in the public sphere after immigration, often coupled with experiences of prejudice, causing them to cling to the remnants of respect they can maintain at home. The women are aware of this, thus Rachel, despite being unable to demonstrate the respectful behaviour customary in Ethiopia, repeatedly urges all Ethiopian women 'not to forget where we came from'—as if this itself will preserve the fragile crumbling hierarchy between the sexes. To build another form of interaction between partners requires joint effort, beginning with letting go of this hierarchical power-play which results in a constant covert (and sometimes overt) struggle between couples on who has the upper hand. As long as relationships are thus perceived, tending towards a pattern of dominance and subservience, there is no chance of creating the genuine equality that young women yearn for. That is not to say that such genuine equality exists in all sub-cultures of Israeli society, where one can also find chauvinism and violence against women, but that the hegemonic model is more egalitarian, and people live on a wide spectrum between equality and disparity.

11.9 The Language of Power

When talking about their relationships at home, the language used by participants in the interviews is tainted with words denoting the ever-present power struggle between the sexes. Thus, Naama describes her parents as 'both very stubborn' and says that her mother 'will not give in', and 'insists on things she believes in'. Habtam described her father as stubborn to the extent that 'it's his way or the highway'. Dana says her father insisted on speaking Amharic to the children but her mother 'cancelled that for him'. In another context, she described her mother as 'pushing' her father to tell them stories. When talking specifically about her parents' relationship Dana says that her father 'lost' in his marriage, implying that her mother 'won'. Modesh could not understand my question when I asked her who she sought after for advice, eventually she answered in terms of getting permission from her husband. Orna said that in matters concerning the children she might ask her husband his opinion but that she is the one who makes the decisions.

All these examples point to the fact that hierarchical relationships do not encourage open discussion, amicable compromise, and making shared decisions—rather they lead to subservience, permission seeking, or rebellious behaviour. Stubbornness as described above is a symptom of the power struggle and denotes a constant tussle between family members based on age and gender. Yaniv described his mother as the dominant one at home using the expression: 'she has the last word; she wears the pants at home'. Abigail called the conflict between herself and her husband after they arrived in Israel 'war'. So did Yafit, saying:

> There is a problem with education. I want them [their children] to be educated like the modern Israelis… I fight for discipline… there is a war between my husband and me on this. He wants to educate the children with his discipline, like in Ethiopia, not with violence, but with obedience. Not with sitting and talking to them, which could empower them. I want us to listen to each other, like I listen to my child, and he listens to me. Most Ethiopian [men] who didn't study don't understand this. Here in Israel women talk to each other, so they adapt. Men take longer. Meanwhile the children miss out…

Naama was 5 when reunited with her mother Yafit on arrival in Israel with her grandparents. She was a teenager when her father, Mahari, who had been conscripted in Ethiopia when she was still a toddler, arrived. Yisrael and two other children were born during the following years. The long separation between the parents was compounded by the cultural transition. Yafit says that in many Ethiopian immigrant families in Israel, there is 'lack of cooperation between husband and wife', combining lack of communication with a constant power struggle. Describing the situation as 'war' expresses the severity of the conflict, in which the traditional hierarchy and modern democratic concepts of equality between the sexes are in head-on collision.[2] Each family handles this differently, from outright conflict to various forms of negotiation. Perhaps the most common strategy, as reflected by these narratives, is avoidance—of the issue or of each other. Children in such families are living in a warzone, this is how Naama describes it:

> A child needs order, and a coherent view of family function. Well on the one hand they [her younger siblings] see a very chauvinistic father who works very hard to support his family and will clean the house and hang the washing and give them showers… a very involved father. But there are certain things that he will never do, like cooking. And they see a mother who functions like a mother, always cooking, even if she's sick she'll cook. And she never gets any help with that.

Both Mahari and Yafit are involved parents, each according to their own perceptions without any discussion between them. What the children experience, according to Naama, is the covert power struggle between her parents, and the inability to discuss things which she sees as detrimental to family life. Culture and gender intersect to create this volatile situation, head on collision being prevented by inhibition. Balancing childcare on a pinpoint of silence, hardly ever able to discuss in detail important (or unimportant) matters, creates a precarious base for joint childrearing.

In contrast, Edna says about her parents, that even after getting divorced they:

> always spoke the same language, despite not being together, they always gave me the same message—that I must study, it was not a matter of choice.

Edna's parents gave her a sense of security by coordinating their efforts in raising her even though they were divorced and did not agree on many things. The ability to talk through disagreements and share expectations gives children consistency, security, and constructive strategies of action for future relationships. This issue came up also in the interview with Lemlem, who says:

> In our home we are very open. I think it is very important. Children exploit conflict [between parents], keeping secrets with mother or with father. We make every effort to make it clear that in our family there are no secrets.

Families can pull together to create new viable pathways forward when faced with changing situations, or they can disintegrate into a group of separately struggling individuals unable to support each other. This latter scenario can be a temporary bump in the road as they adjust to unsettled lives or become a long-term situation. Ethiopian immigrant families in Israel are coping with a multitude of simultaneous changes, while struggling to adjust to a new country, support their families, and raise their children. Underlying these changes are the shifting power relations between the generations and the sexes, negotiated by each family in their own way. This negotiation includes differing degrees of interaction with local Israeli sub-cultures, each with their own versions of the delicate balance between the sexes alongside other variables of stratification such as ethnicity, age, and socioeconomic status. Paradoxically it seems that the ability to incorporate gradual change, to

[2] A discussion on the use of the term 'war' to denote family conflicts appears also in Chap. 9.

enhance and adjust the cultural toolkit to fit the new context, can soften the effects of the disintegrating hierarchy, while rigidly attempting to resurrect it elevates the crisis to breaking point.

References

Abdo, N. (2011). *Women in Israel: Race, gender and citizenship*. Zed Books.

Anteby, L. (2000). There's blood in the house. In R. Wasserfall (Ed.), *Women and water* (pp. 166–186). Brandeis University Press.

Chow, E. N. L., Segal, M. T., & Lin, T. (Eds.). (2011). *Analysing gender, intersectionality, and multiple inequalities: Global-transnational and local contexts*. Emerald Group Publishing.

Dahan-Kalev, H. (2001). Tensions in Israeli feminism: the Mizrachi Ashkenazi rift. *Women's Studies International Forum, 24* (6), 669–684

Dion, K., & Dion, K. (2001). Gender and cultural adaptation in immigrant families. *Journal of Social Issues, 57*(3), 511–521.

Espiritu, Y. (2009). Emotions, sex and money: The lives of Filipino children of immigrants. In N. Foner (Ed.), *Across Generations Immigrant Families in America* (pp. 47–71). NYU.

Foner, N. (Ed.). (2009). *Across generations immigrant families in America*. NYU.

Hondagneu-Sotelo, P. (1992). Overcoming patriarchal constraints: The reconstruction of gender relations among Mexican immigrant women and men. *Gender and Society, 6*(3), 393–415.

Plunkett, M. (2001). Serendipity and agency in narratives of transition: Young adult women and their careers. In D. P. McAdams, R. E. Josselson, & A. E. Lieblich (Eds.), *Turns in the road: Narrative studies of lives in transition* (pp. 151–175). American Psychological Association.

Poluha, E. (Ed.). (2007). *The world of girls and boys in rural and urban Ethiopia.* (pp. 69–90, 134–197). Forum for Social Studies.

Shafir, G., & Peled, Y. (2002). *Being Israeli: The dynamics of multiple citizenship* (Vol. 16). Cambridge University Press.

Tummala-Narra, P. (2004). Mothering in a foreign land. *American Journal of Psychoanalysis, 64*(2), 82–167.

Hebrew References

Bodovsky, D. (1989). Customs and culture: Implications for professional development. In M. Shavtai & L. Kasan (Eds.), *Mulualem: Women and adolescent girls from Ethiopia in spaces, worlds and the voyage between cultures* (pp. 78–107). Lashon Tsacha.

Simuchin, L., & Shefu-Tsenkel, A. (2005). Merging, change and conserving amongst mothers of Ethiopian origin. In M. Shavtai & L. Kasan (Eds.), *Mulualem: Women and adolescent girls from Ethiopia in spaces, worlds and the voyage between cultures* (pp. 78–107). Lashon Tsacha.

Unger, L., & Sever, R. (2012). I educate them! Ethiopian immigrant mothers and Israeli pre-school. *Cultural Issues in Israel, 14*, 118.

Walsh, S., & Unus, A. (2012). Attached and continuing…keeping the balance. Successful Ethiopian women in Israel. *Society and Welfare*. LG.G. 317–345.

Wiel, S. (2005). Jewish Ethiopian women in transition. In M. Shavtai & L. Kasan (Eds.), *Mulualem: Women and adolescent girls from Ethiopia in spaces, worlds and the voyage between cultures* (pp. 24–29). Lashon Tsacha.

Chapter 12
Family Connection and Wellbeing After Immigration

Connection, culture, and tradition bind the generations—perhaps the extent to which this is so depends on the delicate balance between the forces of change and continuance present in all families (Keith & Whitaker, 1988). In relatively settled lives values and strategies of action are synchronized with cultural pathways, the strains and stresses between the generations contained within available channels of communication. Change is moderated by time, gradually seeped into the fabric of family life, clashes based on age and gender moderated by a shared frame of reference. After immigration, people renegotiate their relationship with the outside world, with family members, with themselves. This process itself, an inevitable part of their new unsettled lives, puts a new strain on family togetherness. Family members adjust at different paces, in different ways, experience varying degrees of stress, optimism, confidence in the future, firmly anchored in set ways or flexibly feeling their way into the new reality.

Relationships produce the glue of family cohesion, supportive and encouraging or stressful and undermining. These are not dichotomies, sometimes they can be both to varying degrees. Connections are forged in context, inclusive of past and present, as well as dreams and aspirations of an unknown future. All this comprises the invisible baggage with which families arrive at their new destination, including more distant remnants from the past—adult memories of childhood, family ancestry, the history of their community. Some of this baggage will be useful in helping the family adapt to new circumstances and environments, some might encumber their adjustment. The conscious and subconscious process of sorting between them might take years. In this chapter, I will use the narratives from my study to understand how these immigrants and their children are negotiating this task, what cultural elements do they choose as beneficial to family connection and wellbeing and how are new cultural pathways forged on the intersection between cultures.

> Our children live in two or three different worlds… here at home is one world, some Ethiopian culture, some Israeli culture, mixed up. And then when they go outside—it's

© The Author(s), under exclusive license to Springer Nature Switzerland AG 2023

N. A. Shmuel, *Children's Wellbeing in Immigrant Families*, Children's Well-Being: Indicators and Research 26,
https://doi.org/10.1007/978-3-031-31917-4_12

> totally to another culture, other behaviours. It is really challenging to raise children to be capable of coping with what is at home and what is outside. (Liora)

Parents' narratives describing their family lives open a window onto their experiences and interpretations of these experiences, in which the merging of cultures is being negotiated. This process is dynamic and continuous, it shakes the family tree both vertically and horizontally—between the generations and between siblings, cousins, and other relatives. As shall be illustrated in this chapter, personal interactions are intertwined with an overt and covert dialogue challenging power relations and cultural paradigms. Each family deals with this in their own way, to be experienced subjectively by its members as personal and cultural construction or destruction.

It is worth remembering that most people live on a continuum between settled and unsettled lives, constantly negotiating the bumps in the road. While immigration is more like an earthquake in the road, there is still a continuum between coping well and total disaster. In other words, as Foner (2009) has noted, relations between the generations in immigrant families contain inconsistencies and contradictions, conflict can exist alongside cooperation and caring. This is probably true in all families, but in immigrant families these processes are enhanced, the unsettled base makes everything more acutely felt.

'I want to be like him, but differently', Edna said about her father, whom she greatly admires. Her desire for continuance coupled with change is a common sentiment of the G1.5 generation, the implementation of which is complex. This is a generation strongly connected to their roots through meaningful childhood relationships with the older generation, often the grandparents.

12.1 Grandparents

Mulu says about her grandfather:

> He inspired me and gave me strength. This strength I remember. He taught me to love Israel, to love people, to love God... so Zionism and belief... including belief in myself, in who I am... these are things I learnt from him.

The older generation in Ethiopia was mentioned frequently as a source of knowledge *about* and connection *to* Jewish culture and traditions, they were instrumental in the lives of many participants in forging their Jewish identity and sense of self-worth.

> I am very connected to my paternal grandfather. I learnt all my prayers from him. If a child cries, I will repeat the words from Grandfathers' prayers. He didn't say them to crying babies [she smiles] he just prayed, and I listened to him. I used to come and see him at sunrise and sunset, those were the times he prayed. I often missed him in the mornings, but I saw him in the evenings. Everybody else was sent away, but I stayed and listened to him, I used to copy his movements. (Edna).

When Edna as a child observed her grandfather in prayer she was internalizing almost by osmosis the essence of his faith, embedded in mind and body by imitation. Her memory of this lights up her face, she adds wistfully 'I am religious for my grandfather, *because of* my Grandfather'. She may well also be alive because of him, he was the one who caught up with her mother before she crossed to Sudan and brought her back, her 2-year-old sister did not survive the journey.

There were other grandparents who took an active role in ensuring the safety of their grandchildren, for example Gebre insisted on keeping 5-year-old Naama with him when her mother Yafit left for Sudan with her peers, telling her that the journey was too dangerous for a child.

> My grandfather told her to go and he would take care of me, so my mother left me with him. As soon as she was gone, he gave me preferential treatment, like a princess! My cousins were jealous, and it didn't really compensate for my need of parents, but I remember him as very protective. It was a very hard time—a year and a half in the village, and then the difficult journey. (Naama).

In his interview Gebre recalled with moist eyes how Naama fell ill in Sudan and nearly died:

> Naama was very sick in Sudan. I thought she was going to die. I lit a lamp and sat next to her all night. I prayed, I told God *I got this child for safekeeping, I promised her mother I would bring her to Israel, please don't take her from me, take one of my own children, just not this one*. God be blessed he let us keep all the children, we all arrived healthy and whole.

Gebre continued to be a very special grandfather in Israel, as Yisrael explained:

> I feel very close to my grandfather, he makes me feel I am special to him, from all the grandchildren I spent most time with him. I used to spend all my weekends with my grandparents since I was small.

Abigail described how her grandmother taught her to respect human diversity and always think positively and have empathy for others. To indicate the concept of equality the grandmother used a simple scale filled with stones and told her stories illustrating the difference between right and wrong, 'she told me never to laugh at people who are crippled'.

These grandparents and others instilled humanistic values, connected their grandchildren to tradition, and in so doing planted within them the seeds of faith, giving them confidence in themselves and their Jewish identity. Their stories conceptually threaded the grandchildren onto the long genealogical necklace (a metaphor used by Yafit) imbuing within them a sense of belonging and purpose (also discussed by Newman, 2007).

Habtam's grandfather was revered by his community, she described him as:

> the source of all education in the family. Every time I said I was his granddaughter; I could see how people respected him. Gradually I understood that he wasn't just my grandfather, he was a very important man.

The community elevated the elderly to a special status as bearers of knowledge and tradition, the special attention given to the grandchildren offset their age-related position at the bottom of the social hierarchy. As this hierarchy disintegrates in

Israel, the role of the grandparents in the family changes. This was very eminent in my conversation with two elderly brothers Berihun and Mamu, facilitated by Genet (Berihun's granddaughter).

> As I was raised and married off in Ethiopia, so I raised and married off my children. But in Israel, I just send them to other people, that they should learn and replicate or take the lead. (Berihun).

Berihun is explaining the change in status of the older generation following immigration. In Israel they are no longer the primary source of knowledge, as Berihun says of himself; 'here I am lacking in knowledge and voiceless'. The older generation have internalized this self-image to such an extent that Berihun and Mamu initially refused to talk to me, convinced that it did not matter to anybody what they had to say. They only conceded after Genet's impassioned plea in Amharic, later translated for me by Bossana:

> Until I finished the army, I wanted to be Israeli, not to be ashamed in front of people, to be with self-confidence. But after my discharge from the army, I wanted to know who I was, who my grandfather was, what he did, who my mother was… when I am with Israelis, they talk about who they are, who their parents are, now I can say what my parents did and where we came from. The next generation will ask us who we are, we need to be able to give them answers.

Genet was describing her own experience as a young woman in the army, believing that her self-confidence and ability to fit in were dependent on becoming like everybody else. In time it became clear to her that what everybody else seemed to have that she didn't was knowledge *about* and connection *with* their family history. It was a turning point in her development, which made her actively seek answers from her mother, thereby remodelling their severed relationship following the clashes of a turbulent adolescence. Today, Genet and her mother Almaz run mother and daughter workshops within the community to encourage inter-generational connection. Genet is passionate about the need for the older generation to break their silence, she knows from experience that the younger generation desperately need their guidance.

But when they did consent to speak, Mamu and Berihun expressed with anger and sadness what seems to them like an insoluble rift:

> Our children are deleting their culture to fit in to Israeli society, and this breaks my heart. Everything learnt in Ethiopia is lost, not just theirs but mine too. I am losing my knowledge as well (Berihun).

The rich culture Berihun grew up on in Ethiopia and wanted to pass on to his grandchildren seems to him to be rapidly disappearing, even he cannot hold on to it, let alone pass it on. The cultural pathways which gave ample opportunity for intergenerational transferal—a cohesive community with a common language and strategies for viable connection—have been effectively eroded or severed. For example, Dov's parents were

> the young pioneers who left the village to walk to Sudan. I stayed with my grandparents because there was no-one else to help them. My father left me with them.

But soon after his arrival in Israel, Dov was separated from them:

> I was very close to my grandfather, but then life changed so much. I went to boarding school, I didn't have any time to travel to visit them, the connection was severed. I wish I had managed to visit them once a month.

Public policy aimed at aiding the assimilation of the children overlooked any consequences to the family, it is impossible to gage the effect of this loss on these children, to whom such relationships were an anchor of self-worth, family roots, and cultural identity.

In Israel many grandparents become babysitters to the second generation while their parents work or study, but these occasions create limited opportunities for meaningful connection, as Liora describes:

> Not everybody has such patience, it is not easy to look after a bunch of children at the age of 75. [...] She [her mother] raised my children, my sister's children, and the children of my two brothers, all since they were babies. So, there are nine or ten unruly children, with no common language, it takes a lot of patience.

The strategies of action for connection between the generations are culturally formed, and in Ethiopia were not based on direct informal engagement with children through toys and games, as Mulu explains:

> My mother cannot relate to any of this [her hand indicates the toys lying on the carpet]. Since I grew up here, this has become an integral part of my parenting, to sit and play with her [the daughter] and soon to read to her, but my mother can't do these things even if she wanted to.

Almaz, the grandmother of Genet's children, admits that connecting to the next generation is challenging, when she tries to play with them, they chastise her; '*Grandma, your confused*!'

The channels of connection familiar to the elder generation from Ethiopia, such as apprenticeship, body language, proverbs, and stories in Amharic, are mostly ineffective in forging bonds with the Israeli grandchildren. Playing games requires adapting oneself to the perspective of the child, learning new skills and rules that are unfamiliar to them, even trying to do so may be a humiliating experience further eroding their already fragile status.

And yet there are grandparents who are forging new pathways of connection to the younger generation, usually at the instigation of the intermediate, 1.5 generation. Thus, Genet buys clay and other craft materials to encourage her mother to make things with her daughters, Tsehai's mother gardens with the grandchildren, Emebet cooks with hers, and sometimes they play cards or *gebeta*.[1] These connections are significant and important, but it is questionable if they are likely to equip the younger generation with a cultural toolkit from their ancestral inheritance. Interestingly many grandparents seem to be aware of this and talk of 'worrying about' the second generation more than they worry about the others in their families. Perhaps these grandparents are aware of the vulnerability of the second

[1] A traditional game: mancala.

generation, mostly growing up without a protective community shield. Several parents of the intermediate, 1.5 generation recalled being told by their parents to be considerate and patient with their Israeli-born children. For example, Shy said:

> If we get angry with the children, they [the grandparents] tell us *not like that. If you are angry with them, they will grow away from you, you need to explain yourself.*

Emebet tells her adult children not to curse their offspring or hit them, to be patient and encouraging. Rachel recalls how her mother rebuked her for leaving her children with a babysitter so she could work two jobs, telling her they would be better off if she spent more time with them. Worknesh told Noa to be patient with her son. The fear of losing connection seems to be eminent, as Abigail said sadly:

> Today there are many families that have lost their children, the parents just don't understand them.

The fear of losing connection is a powerful driving force to instigate change. Nevertheless, sometimes culturally based expectations and misunderstandings manage to thwart efforts to bridge the inter-generational gap. For example, Habtam describes her grandfather's differential attitude to his grandchildren:

> He used to come and visit us, and we always greeted him in the right way, mother said he loved us because we respected him. [When he visited] the other grandchildren they hid in their rooms and didn't come out until he left. We were not raised like that. Because we respected him, he appreciated us.

For many grandparents, connection with the grandchildren is contingent upon their adherence to appropriate traditional codes of behaviour, especially showing respect. This is more important to them even than language, since without respect between the generations there is no basis for a relationship at all. The cultural expectation is that the child should be the one to make the effort, most Ethiopian grandparents will not invest in enticing a small child who is reticent and uncooperative, or worse still rude by their cultural standards, this would only further erode their already fragile social status and self-esteem.

12.2 Three Sisters

The three sisters from the Metiku family, Rachel, Aberash and Tsehai, will illustrate the diverse attitudes and coping strategies available for dealing with the cultural mix formed by the transition from Ethiopia to Israel. The three sisters share a mother, Aberash and Tsehai also share a father and seven brothers. All three sisters are married to members of the Ethiopian immigrant community, but their partners are barely mentioned in the interviews.

Rachel's uncle took her to Israel as an 8-year-old child, after her father died and her mother re-married. She grew up in an orphanage and foster homes until her grandmother arrived. Today she is married with five children and works two jobs to provide them with the home she never had. Once a week she also studies. She sighs often during the interview and looks tired, she does not seem to have any significant support networks, her husband is mentioned only as being either at work or asleep. She introduced herself using her Hebrew name, Rachel, and does not speak Amharic with her children, who also refuse to eat *engera*—she says they get up and leave if she eats this next to them. She also says they object strongly to music in Amharic and tell her to 'switch off that noise', they prefer songs in Hebrew or English. Her expression is sad as she says that her children have 'taken nothing from Ethiopian culture'.

Her sister Aberash arrived in Israel with her parents when she was 12, she was soon sent to a boarding school. Aberash proudly calls her home 'Ethiopian', she makes an active effort to make it so by cooking traditional dishes her children enjoy and telling them traditional stories she remembers from her childhood. Their bookshelves contain many children's book on Ethiopian heritage, including several of my books. Aberash is determined to pass on to her children everything she can of the rich culture she grew up in, including teaching them to respect their elders, be polite, and say the traditional Jewish blessings in Amharic, which they learn regularly at the local community centre. She says emphatically that there is a continuation between the generations and gives many examples of combining the two cultures, saying:

> We were educated well over there [Ethiopia], we understood what was expected of us from my mother's *eyes*, nobody talked very much, we understood the signs. Here you have to say everything twenty times, sometimes even raise your voice.

Aberash smiles as she says this, she is nostalgic about her own childhood but has come to accept that here things are different, there is no bitterness in her voice.

Tsehai was nine when she arrived, she also went to a boarding school as a teenager. Today she is a young working mother of three daughters, busy managing her life, preserving Ethiopian culture is not something which especially concerns her. She says:

> I have many Israeli friends, and I never felt discriminated against or that I don't belong.

But qualifies this with a comment that: 'At some point I am always reminded that I am Ethiopian'.

Her husband makes a point of talking to the girls in Amharic, Tsehai talks to them in Hebrew and cannot remember any of the stories she was told as a child. But she does make *engera* and *buna* at home, and for the *Sigd* festival she will take her girls to a play at the community centre. She described all this in a matter-of-fact way, it appears that her mixed identity is interwoven into her daily life naturally, without a great deal of effort. Her daughters are close to their maternal grandmother with whom they do not share a language, mostly they garden with her or make things together.

Each one of these sisters has found her own way of coping with the cultural mix in her family's life. They may have arrived in Israel with the same cultural baggage, but their experiences and personal choices (conscious or not) in coping with unsettled lives have shaped their strategies for action and the cultural pathways they have forged for their children. All three sisters are strong capable women, working and raising a family through personal agency and hardiness. Agency involves a sense of control, either to change situations or to reframe perceptions about them. Hardiness breeds self-efficacy through feeling influential rather than helpless, involved rather than detached and perceiving change as normative and desirable (Gezentsvey & Ward, 2008). These qualities enhance adjustment through a sense of wellbeing and reduce the element of stress, they can apply to varying degrees and are strongly affected by context, as can be seen clearly in comparing the three sisters. All three sisters belong to the 1.5 generation, but Rachel was only eight when she arrived in Israel without her family, her subjective sense of rejection from both family and society seem intermingled and unprocessed. Her unsettled life has been a struggle in every respect, including financially, and yet she is very much a resourceful survivor. As will be discussed in the next chapter on identity, Rachel feels she has sacrificed everything to become Israeli but has never felt accepted, while her children seem to reject everything Ethiopian. She is angry and frustrated that her children have taken nothing of her culture, which she herself struggles to reconcile with Israeli reality as demonstrated by the discussion on gender relations in the previous chapter. In negotiating strategies for action in the narrow space between two conflicting cultural paradigms, convoluted by a general sense of rejection, Rachel bravely attempts to forge a viable pathway for her children. But losing Ethiopian culture is perceived by her as an inevitable result of the transition.

In contrast, Aberash arrived in Israel with her family and her experiences in Israeli society were more amicable and accepting, she feels comfortable in her new hybrid identity. Aberash has made a conscious choice to ensure her children are educated in Ethiopian tradition, she sees this as important for their ability to cope in Israeli society which labels them as 'Ethiopian'. Her children are fond of stories about Ethiopia, willingly visit the community centre to learn Amharic and enjoy *engera* as well as music in Amharic. The cultural mix in Aberash's home is palpable and harmonious.

While Tsehai does not worry about all this, she is busy living her life in a culturally mixed community where she and her family feel comfortable. She is open to opportunities which present themselves to introduce Ethiopian culture to her children, such as taking them to a play on the Sigd, but she sees them primarily as Israeli, fitting in to the mosaic of Israeli society like their peers of various backgrounds. It seems that in this case a favourable context and an easy-going attitude are paving the way for a mildly hybrid pathway.

This example of three sisters and their differing experiences and coping methods demonstrates some of the various possible scenarios for families after immigration. The interplay of context, encounters, personal agency and hardiness combine to shape the reality of the new generation. Thus, various cultural elements can be harmoniously interwoven into their childhood to encourage various forms of hybridity, or frequent clashes within the family and between family members and their surroundings can serve to form a no-man's land between perceptibly opposing cultures. In this last scenario, the second generation are missing out on cultural elements which could contribute to their own sense of self-efficacy and resilience. Effectively they are unable to appropriate the content of their parents' cultural baggage as their own, without viable access to local cultural capital.

12.3 Rocking the Family Boat: Culture Clash Within the Family

Cultural clashes are often discussed in terms of clashing values, as if actions are inevitably motivated by logic reducible to ideas about how people should live (Swidler, 1986). But people's actions are largely a product of habit, even in parenting an awareness of end-goal motivations is often absent. In other words, we often behave as we did before, or as our parents behaved, unless we are actively in the process of trying to change or improve ourselves as parents or individuals. We also act out of shared assumptions about the world we live in, through a familiarity and knowledge about context in a particular time and place. When that time and place change, such as after immigration, our whole frame of reference is out of sync with our surroundings, this is what forms unsettled lives (Swidler). It is at this point that immigrants begin the subtle often subconscious process of weeding out of the cultural toolbox those elements no longer relevant in the new environment and appropriating new cultural tools. There is no time pause for this, it happens simultaneously to daily life, and it rocks the family boat. The themes that repeated themselves in the interviews in my study expressed the ripple effect of these clashing cultural systems as personal struggles. Expectations and important decisions effecting the family rest on personal and collective perceptions of both strategies of action and ideally desirable outcomes. For example, what is the appropriate cultural mix that will ensure a viable future for the children? Where are the conceptual and spatial boundaries for children's behaviour in the new surroundings? What are appropriate adult responses to misbehaviour or lack of reverence? How should children be reprimanded or encouraged? In most families these questions are not openly discussed, their resolution is negotiated in live time with varying degrees of cooperation and conflict. Instinctive habitual reactions exist alongside differing levels of self-reflection, trial and error, stubbornness, and remorse. Powerful opposing undercurrents of perpetuation and change swing the boat in differing directions, under such conditions it can be very challenging to create steady, viable, and consistent pathways for the next generation.

I have identified five main axes of contention:

1. Between Liberalism and Conservativism

In settled lives cultures are not static or uniform, they include both contradictions, anomalies and diversity all embedded in daily living (Swidler, 1986). But the mixing of cultures that occurs after immigration accentuate set formats of cultural action crystalized in comparison with other, less familiar local strategies. At this intersection between cultures in immigrant families relationships and strategies of action are renegotiated, challenging power relations based on age and gender. Daily conflicts accompany this sticky process as the older generation attempts to control the younger generation or patriarchal patterns are evoked. Both may be instinctive or protective, but the result is conflict, which can be prevented by avoidance, negotiation, or denial. Thus, Maayan's father threatened to lock her out of the house for staying out late, but always left the door open. Dany, a religious man, 'pretended not to see' that his children were borrowing his car on the Sabbath, and always left the keys where they could find them. These men have not changed their value systems, but they refrain from enforcing them, preferring to adopt new strategies of action which keep them in touch with their children.[2]

For many educated Ethiopian women liberalism is an essential quality they look for when choosing a partner, its absence amongst her Ethiopian male peers makes Naama say:

> Today I am incapable of dating Ethiopian men. I hear them talk, and I see black. How dare they say such a thing! My perspective is too liberal, I cannot tolerate even a little conservatism.

In the name of liberalism—a tolerance of a variety of perspectives—Naama is closed to conservatism to such an extent that she rejects all black men, symbolically connecting their culture to a darkness that is opposite to modern enlightenment. Her attitude fosters a blanket rejection of her own traditions; 'I have grown *too far away*, I don't visit [the community], or go to their events'. Her expression changes from one of adamant defiance, when talking about the men she dated and rejected, to a deep sadness as she adds softly, 'suddenly it seems I have exaggerated'.

The dichotomy of Israeli reality does not enable her to restructure definitions; to be a free woman, she must reject her traditional culture as one closed package—gender roles intertwined with all else her rich cultural heritage has to offer. Naama, like Tigist and Maayan, have long passed the age that Ethiopian women are expected to marry, being constantly reminded of this at family gatherings emphasizes the price they are paying for the new cultural pathways they have forged.

2. The Self-image of the Child

The traditional hierarchy created social order, but it also taught children and women their place. Breaking free from these internalized expectations is an uphill struggle described by Shani:

> There are a lot of things that fit Ethiopian culture. For example, as someone who grew up in a big family, when a small child says something, whether it is funny or not, everybody laughs at him. This damages the child's self-image.

When she talks about this, she lowers her voice, even though we are alone in her home. It is an issue she has struggled with for a long time, her determination to protect her child has given her courage to confront her parents about it:

> My middle son gets very upset. He feels humiliated. He says *why are they laughing at me? I'm not funny!* I asked them to treat him like an adult, not to laugh at him. It damages his self-image.

[2] also discussed in the previous chapter.

Traditionally, Ethiopian elders are not concerned with a child's self-image, it is their prerogative to teach the child his place in the hierarchy, amongst the means they use to do so are jovial mockery, ridicule, and teasing. The elders in Shani's family are following tradition, but Shani is worried about her child's self-image, she does not want him to internalize his inferiority in the social order. Herself the tenth child, she is painfully aware of how this has undermined her own self-confidence, and dares ask the elders to treat her son as an adult. Still speaking softly as if afraid of being overheard she refers to her relatives as 'interfering' in her efforts to educate her children, undermining her son's self-confidence. Gaining her own confidence back she says in a regular tone:

> I am trying to find the balance, between our traditional values and values more appropriate to the Western world.

Shani would like her children to feel equal, but in the extended family they are expected to inherently *know* their place in the hierarchy. She is caught between her concern for her son's self-image and her obligation to show respect for her elders. In many families this delicate balance between traditionally expected behaviour and personal wellbeing based on a sense of equal self-worth is constantly being challenged daily. Often it is the intermediate, 1.5 generation who are balancing the needs of the generations above and below them with great audacity, as for example Genet invests in facilitating the bond between her daughters and her mother through creative interaction while carefully maintaining reverence for the grandmother.

3. Between Protection and Restriction

'My parents always like to talk, to express themselves', says Shani, differentiating her parents from the mainstream of silent restraint. She continues:

> They have this mission to protect, to warn us about bad unpredictable things. I appreciate their efforts, but sometimes it is very restrictive. Now I find myself talking to my daughter, trying to warn her about things. Like not taking sweets from strangers. I want to pass on the message without scaring her. I hope I manage to do so without damaging her self-image.

Shani appreciates her parents but rejects their efforts to restrict her with rules and regulations on humility and modesty, which she feels limit her to being 'a little woman' or to remember that she is 'tenth in line'. She wishes to protect her own children from these cultural restrictions, to empower them regardless of age, gender, and colour. At the same time, she wishes to prepare them for the dangers ahead without inhibiting their every step. She herself, caught between the two cultures, hesitates between over protection and temerity, freedom of choice and her obligation as a parent to guide them without encumbering them with cultural limitations. This hesitation often paralyses her parental instincts, making her feel inadequate as a mother. She says, as if it were a good thing; 'we were *afraid* of our father'. The protector's ultimate powers enabled him to also embody the threat, this was his prerogative—the power that kept family order. Shani adds:

> They say that if a child is afraid of you when he is young, afterwards he won't sit on your head.[3]

Like many young parents of Ethiopian origin in Israel, Shani longs for the respectful order of the hierarchy, while simultaneously determined to raise an egalitarian family without internal ranking. She is concerned with her children's self-image and would like them to have free choice, but simultaneously she is afraid of losing control and unable to establish set rules and regulations. The values she inherited from her own parents as the pillars of her childhood have crumbled into a sticky cultural mix of daily living in which her children are experiencing primarily her hesitation and lack of consistency.

4. Obedience versus Consultation

For the elders of the Ethiopian community, to listen is to obey; therefore, children and teenagers cannot ask for advice—this would obligate them to follow it. Thus, sharing information becomes a tricky business, and communication between parents and children is fraught with pitfalls and misunderstandings. Instead of sharing information and discussing possible courses of action, many families live in a web of silence, protecting them from confrontation while hindering any possibility of constructive involvement. Important life decisions are no longer in the hands of the elders, young people choose their own life partners and goals. A sense of insignificance silences the older generation, while the younger generations' search for answers or need of guidance remains unfulfilled. And so, when Maayan asked her parents about Ethiopia they refused to answer her, instead they snapped back '*why do you ask*? *What happened? What woke you up*?'

Tareke has an important message to the parents, to whom he says:

> Stop saying no all the time, buy them clothes, buy them food, help them with their teachers, talk to them. If you don't, you will lose them.

Tareke is convinced that the strategy of coercion, using anger and denial as a means for control, is simply distancing the youth from their parents. Intergenerational clashes are escalating to the point of no return, the elder generation are watching the deterioration of their offspring helplessly, as Gebre explains:

> In Ethiopia we looked after the children together. Since we arrived here everything is upside down, the children don't listen to us anymore, they want to be Israeli—they drink beer, whisky… In Ethiopia the children conformed, their behaviour needed parental approval.

Many parents and grandparents are anxious about the younger generation, feeling that their fate is out of their hands, and the only influence they have left is through prayer. Instead of talking to the children they are now talking to God.

5. Faithful to Tradition or Ambition

The complexity of Israeli reality makes it almost impossible to fulfil traditional expectations of attendance at family celebrations and an immediate response to life

[3] A common idiom in Hebrew indicating overbearing behaviour.

crises regardless of study commitments and work schedules. Inter-generational clashes on this dilemma between family responsibilities and personal obligations are common, as Abraham describes:

> In Ethiopia everybody came to help if something happened. They were self-sufficient, so they could just drop everything and come back to it another day. Here one has to get permission from work, if there is a family event or somebody got sick or died, you have to ask your boss, it creates problems. This is a cultural clash.

This situation reflects the collision of cultural systems—oriented towards social commitment and conserving extended family relations or oriented towards free choice, self-fulfilment, and ambition. What people consider ethical and appropriate in different situations is culturally constructed (Oyserman & Lee, 2008). In an individualistic society personal logic and ambition may be enough to overcome external barriers such as prejudice and racism. But in a collectivistic society, where self-worth is measured by the greater good, such external barriers are sufficient to disable the best intentions. In other words, people who act out of self-motivation are less susceptible to external challenges, while people whose self-perception is embedded in society find it much harder to continue in their efforts when society rejects them. Thus Addis (G2) tells his mother to 'learn to move past' overt and covert racism, but she (G1) cannot be placid about it since it rattles her very being.

Shira at 13 has already decided that this part of Ethiopian culture—obligatory attendance at extended family celebrations—is something she wants no part in:

> All the events, I don't want to be a part of that, absolutely not. I won't go, or be listed, it's nothing to do with me.

The lists she is referring to document arrivals at weddings and Bar Mitzvahs so that guests can be repaid when they host their own events. Shira understands that while these occasions provide unique opportunities for family reunions, they also create their own set of problems, primarily the financial strain on low-income families and the results of an abundance of unsupervised alcohol. Her father, Shy, is very critical of all this:

> We have turned drinking into our culture, we are experts on beer. Once a week maybe this is all right, but every day? Where was there such a culture in Ethiopia? This has been invented here.

This behaviour, which is regarded as cultural, represents the post-immigration crisis of this community, and not its traditions. The traditions include hospitality, which was extended to all guests via the traditional *buna* (coffee) and *tele* (a home-made beer from cereal, water, and yeast). The alcoholic element of this latter traditional drink was minimal, often enhanced during celebrations. Since *tele* also has nutritional value, in Ethiopia it was offered to children as well. In Israel this traditional drink has been replaced by shop-bought beer, which has higher levels of alcohol and no nutritional value, without sufficient awareness of its potential addictiveness and long-term negative results (discussed in Shmuel & Rosen, 2007; Budowsky et al., 2012).

12.4 Cultural and Religious Compromises

Edna admires her parents for having adjusted to Israeli society, saying 'their world was shattered, and they embraced change'. This change enters the essence of what brought them to Israel: The Jewish faith and how to practice it. Edna admits that she does not know how she would react if her son 'came home one day and said *I cannot eat the food you cook*'. But in many families this is what happened, for example when Dov came home from his religious boarding school. He recalls this sadly, saying 'there is a great rift with tradition', going on to describe how difficult this issue is even today for both himself and his mother. His mother Abigail also spoke about this in her interview, describing her original dismay, but her face softens as she remembers how respectfully polite he was at the time.

Edna recalls telling her father she was vegetarian, but he did not believe her. Acutely aware of what was going on between the community and the Israeli religious establishment, he confronted her amicably saying.

> it's because of problems of Kashrut of the meat slaughtered in our community.

Today it is not an issue in either family, they have found compromises which enable continued connection: Dov brings his own pots and pans to his mother's house when the family visits. Edna describes how when her extended family meet up for the Independence Day barbeque her father brings the wine and she brings the meat, together they celebrate their Aliyah to Israel.

When the Beta Israel community made Aliyah perhaps the most important component in their cultural baggage was their faith. In Ethiopia belief and practice were synchronized, there were no secular Jews, to be Jewish was to live according to Jewish customs and traditions passed between the generations for centuries. As Miki says:

> I can toy with what I want inside—Ethiopian culture or Israeli culture—but what envelops them, that's Judaism. To be Jewish, that is the essence of it all.

But even this very essence was challenged in the transition, as their very Jewishness was repeatedly debated and questioned. Requiring the immigrants to undergo symbolic conversion was a humiliating insult to their personal and collective history (Ben-Eliezer, 2008). The Rabbinical establishment has seriously undermined the traditional authority of the *Kesouch* as spiritual leaders, and for a long time refused to enable them to practice in Israel (Sharabi & Kaplan, 2014; Jaffe-Schagen, 2016). The Kosher slaughter of meat is totally controlled and supervised by the Rabbinical authority. But in the Ethiopian Jewish community are people whose traditional role has been to perform the slaughter of animals according to Jewish doctrine, to the elders of the community these people are more reliable than the Rabbinical establishment (Salamon, 2014).

Tareke also talks about the Kes as having unequivocal authority in the community, while in Israel there are many versions of Jewish law, interpreted by each Rabbi differently. Thus, being Jewish can take various forms, some more legitimate than others. Many immigrants of the older generation (G1) adhere to the words of the Kes, while the younger generation follow local Israeli Jewish law. Instead of Jewish tradition being a unifying force in the family, often it leads to bitter arguments between the generations. The struggle itself, between conservation and change, enhances the extremities—strict observance versus utter rejection of all religious practices. While the compromises which mark the middle road, such as the examples given by Edna and Dov (and those discussed in Shalom, 2018), enable families to celebrate Jewish festivals together (for further details on how these were celebrated in Ethiopia, see Ziv, 2017; Shalom, 2016).

As Shalom (2023) explains, trying to understand the Jewish community of Ethiopia through the lens of Jewish law as understood by the sages or through the prism of Orthodox *Halakha* has caused many misunderstandings. Shalom proposes using the instruments native to the Ethiopian community to understand their perception and practice of Judaism from their own perspective. To do so he has conducted extensive research which delves into the very foundations of the religious, practical and intellectual culture of the Ethiopian Jewish community, the only completely autonomous Jewish community outside Israel since the destruction of the second temple. His research reveals a perspective based on *Higigate Lemuse* (laws of Moses)—signifying all the Torah-based interpretations and rulings passed between the generations—rather than the established acceptable concepts of Oral law and rabbinic commandments. Shalom sees the Ethiopian Jewish community as unique, a living archive of Jewish history, whose perspectives and practices should be studied and learnt from rather than coerced into adhering to the doctrines created by the authority of an elite forming the religious establishment in Israel.

Shalom's bold vision brings us back full circle to the grandparents with whom this chapter began, as bearers of knowledge whose relationships with their grandchildren imbued them with cultural and religious traditions as well as self-efficacy and a clear sense of identity. In Israel their status and ability to instigate cultural transferal have been eroded beyond repair, even in the sphere of religion they have lost their authority. The Beta Israel of Ethiopia are becoming Ethiopian Israeli Jews by redefinition, negotiated by individuals, families and community between three binary contrasts: the old and the new, the particular and the universal, and the permanent and the temporary. The cultural and religious pathways open to the second generation contain convoluted combinations between these dichotomies, paved in the context of time and place by meaningful experiences and relationships.

References

Budowsky, D., Rosca, P., & Witztum, A. (2012). Alcohol and drugs among Ethiopian immigrants: Cultural sensitive aspects. In E. Witztum & N. Grisaru (Eds.), *Social and clinical aspects of Ethiopian immigrants in Israel* (pp. 153–184). The Jewish Agency for Israel and Ben Gurion University Press.

Foner, N. (Ed.). (2009). *Across generations immigrant families in America*. NYU.

Gezentsvey, M., & Ward, C. (2008). Unveiling agency: A motivational perspective on acculturation and adaptation. In R. Sorrentino & S. Yamaguchi (Eds.), *Handbook of motivation and cognition across cultures* (p. 2017). Academic Press Elsevier.

Jaffe-Schagen, J. (2016). Creating space. The construction of Ethiopian heritage and memory in Israel. *Annales d'Ethiopie, 31*, 81–105.

Keith, D., & Whitaker, C. (1988). The presence of the past: Continuity and change in the symbolic structures of families. In C. Falicov (Ed.), *Family transitions: Continuity and change over the life cycle* (pp. 431–448). Guildford Press.

Newman, R. (2007). Ethiopian Israeli grandmothers' stories. *Journal of Aging, Humanities and the Arts, 1*(3–4), 211–219.

Oyserman, D., & Lee, S. W. (2008). Does culture influence what and how we think? Effects of priming individualism and collectivism. *Psychological Bulletin, 134*(2), 311.

Salamon, H. (2014). Holy meat, black slaughter: Power, religion, Kosher meat, and the Ethiopian Israeli community. *Political Meals*, 273–285.

Shalom, S. (2016). *From Sinai to Ethiopia: The Halachic and conceptual world of Ethiopian Jewry*. Gefen.

Hebrew References

Ben-Eliezer, U. (2008). Cushi sambi bilibilibambo: How a Jew becomes black in the promised land. In Y. Shenhav & Y. Yona (Eds.), *Racism in Israel* (pp. 130–159). Van Leer Institute and the Kibbutz Hameuchad.

Shalom, S. (2018). *Conversations about love and fear: The dialogue between the Rabbi's daughter and the Kes's son*. Miskal – Yedioth Ahronoth and Chemed Books.

Shalom, S. (2023). *A living Genizah: Oral law in Ethiopian Jewish theology and religious practice*. The Open University of Israel press.

Sharabi, R., & Kaplan, A. (2014). *Like dolls in a window: Ethiopian leaders in Israel*. Tel Aviv.

Shmuel, N., & Rosen, C. (2007). From tele to Goldstar – The dangers of alcoholism amongst Ethiopian immigrants. *Quarterly of Amutat Efshar, 55*, 3–4.

Swidler, A. (1986). Culture in action: Symbolism and strategies. *Americal sociological review, 51*(2), 273–286.

Ziv, Y. (2017). *Festival and holiday in the Ethiopian Jewish tradition of Beta Israel*. Published by the Mofet Institute.

Chapter 13
Identity and Visibility

Mulu wants her daughter to 'be whoever she wants to be', expressing a desire to free her from the constraints of social or cultural expectations and provide her with the choice of creating her own identity based on abilities, desires, and aspirations. And yet identities are forged in context, guided by connections, fused with overt and covert social and cultural meanings. Today, it is recognized that cultures operate less from *within* the individual than *from the outside*, through the contexts in which we are embedded (Swidler, 1995). The narratives from my study reflect this, including the diversity of interpretations and perspectives defining self and other after immigration. Some of those interviewed initially answered my question on identity by stating personal traits, perhaps indicating that issues of community, ethnic or religious identity do not concern them, they are busy living their lives without analysing their place vis a vis socially classified categories. The 'boxes' so prevalent in Israeli society, distinguishing people according to ethnicity, religion, gender, location, seniority (referring to time spent in Israel) and other parameters are restrictive, each carrying a multitude of stereotypes (for example, Bokovoza, 2011). Everybody is aware of them; immigrants and their offspring are negotiating their self and other perceptions in the context of this convoluted mosaic of pre-definitions. As is evident in the narratives from my study, people find creative ways of coping with these 'boxes', by locating themselves inside, alongside, defining new boxes or refusing to play this game.

Before listening to these narratives, it seems pertinent to discuss briefly three important concepts related to identity: ethnicity, hybridity, and intersectionality.

© The Author(s), under exclusive license to Springer Nature Switzerland AG 2023
N. A. Shmuel, *Children's Wellbeing in Immigrant Families*, Children's Well-Being: Indicators and Research 26,
https://doi.org/10.1007/978-3-031-31917-4_13

13.1 Ethnicity

The term ethnicity is often used interchangeably for race or culture, providing a dangerous basis for generalizations about immigrants and overlooking the diversity which exists within immigrant groups. In most cases ethnicity refers to people who define themselves alike or are regarded so by others due to common origin or culture expressed through language and customs (Lam, 2013). In common language people in Israel are more likely to use the term ethnicity when talking about prominent minority groups (for example, dark-skinned immigrants) than when referring to white European immigrants. Thus, the subtleties of language contribute to create differential realities for people of different origins. If we look at Ethiopia, we can see a society comprised of a multitude of ethnic groups. Nigusie (2018) detailed Ethiopian history through the prism of Yang's integrated approach to ethnicity, showing that ethnic boundaries are simultaneously socially constructed and based on kinship, manipulated by state and politics, while subject to a degree of choice as people identify themselves with different ethnic groups.

When it comes to immigrants and their offspring, one might regard such identification as a strategy of action forged to facilitate a sense of belonging. After immigration ethnic identity is constructed by the host society in daily interactions which remould people's attitudes to themselves and others (Ari, 2012). 'Symbolic ethnicity' (Gans, 1994) as a means of identification with a group rather than intrinsic cultural connection may be simply part of the identity exploration of immigrants and their offspring, constantly negotiating their position in relation to local subcultures. For example, a study on Asian American adolescents found a difference between youth born in America or in Asia; the former showed more ethnic pride than the latter (Ying et al., 2008 from Ungar, 2011). The authors suggested that the immigrant youth were geared towards the promise of integration, while the Asian Americans were using their cultural heritage to protect against marginalization.

Immigration policies and attitudes in Israel have traditionally encouraged newcomers to relinquish their native culture and language in favour of becoming Israeli as soon as possible. And yet in recent years there is what might be called an ethnic revival of Ethiopian heritage as if this might be a 'miracle solution' to their integration problems (Jaffe-Schagen, 2016). I would argue that celebrating Ethiopian heritage and recognizing the heroism and sacrifices of the community to arrive in Israel will not combat racism and solve other problems but is important for the following reasons: firstly, to demonstrate empathy and appreciation for the rich cultural heritage and ardent Zionism of Ethiopian Jews. Secondly, to create social and spatial arenas of legitimate discussion of burning issues concerning this community. Thirdly, to give content to the ethnic identity of the younger generation, often detached from their family and community history, as demonstrated in previous chapters. Thus, although not resolving issues of racism, knowledge about and identification with Ethiopian heritage can buffer its effects.[1] Dana's narrative in this chapter supports this view.

13.2 Hybridity

Hybridity or biculturalism, as illustrated in Chap. 9, refers to cultural competency in two (or more) cultures (Bennet-Martinez et al., 2002, 2006). Hybridity is especially potent in countries like Israel, characterized by mass immigration, and creates a situation where it becomes increasingly irrelevant to speak about distinctly definable differentiated ethnic groups since there are many people with multiple identities, whose cultural toolkits contain elements from different cultural systems. The cultural pathways they are forging, as demonstrated by the narratives of the intermediate 1.5 generation, are full of combinations and compromises. Thus, although their lives may often be unsettled, they are already well equipped to deal with uncertainty and rapid change, they may even have learnt to thrive from it. As this study reflects, the path to hybridity can be forged or thwarted by interactions both within family and society.

13.3 Intersectionality

Intersectionality is a conceptual framework for understanding the ways in which aspects of human identity (such as gender, race and socioeconomic status, age, and sexual preferences) simultaneously interact and intersect to shape lived experiences and life chances through interlocking systems of bias and inequality that exist at the macro social-structural level, meaning sexism, racism, classism, ageism and homophobia (Crenshaw, 1989; McCall, 2005). An awareness of the effects of the intersection of identities highlights the multiple factors affecting people in their daily existence and reduces the individualistic tendency to analyse behaviour and outcomes based on individual attributes. It places the focus clearly on *interaction within context*—what happens between people and the societies they live in, revealing inherent structures of power that have an often seemingly invisible effect on people's lives. When discussing issues of identity these are crucial factors to bear in mind. As the narratives of Rachel, Habtam, and others will illustrate, power relations based on the intersection of identities are evident and potent in the lives of immigrants and their offspring.

[1] Further discussed in the next chapter.

13.4 Talking About Identity

Yaara looks at me indignantly when I ask her how she defines her identity, she waves her brown arm and raises her voice:

> How can I be Israeli? Look! I am Ethiopian! It is my colour, the way I talk, the way I behave.

But then she says:

> My children are both. When they are with Ethiopians, they are Ethiopian. With the Israelis they are Israeli. But not to forget they are Ethiopian. Who can forget?

She seems angry when she says this, she is insistent that only her children can be both, she herself can only be Ethiopian, signified by her colour. Many of the elder immigrants, although living in Israel for many years, have adopted what might be called a *diaspora identity* (Portes & Rumbaut, 2001) seemingly more connected to the country of origin than local culture (in spirit, not in any practical sense). But this term can be confusing, causing what Naujoks (2010) terms *identity fuzziness* or perhaps creating another identity box that confuses rather than aids our understanding. In the case of the Ethiopian immigrants in Israel, the difference between the way the various generations *talk* about identity seems the best way to clarify the complexity of their identity perceptions. Questions about identity led most of the G1 participants to tell me stories about their childhood, their ancestors, the village they grew up in. I came to understand that their very sense of self is embedded in community, the community was part of who they were, a part that has been lost after immigration together with communal living. Their desire to teach the younger generation genealogy comes from a wish to add them to the ancestral chain, to create continuance and meaning which are being lost to them. Moreover, as illustrated by my exchange with Yaara, they are acutely aware of their visibility in Israeli society. She was telling me that her colour *defines* her, prevents her from being anything other than Ethiopian, and yet her children can be both Ethiopian and Israeli. My impression is that this differentiation reiterates statements made by Mamu and Berihun, whose sense of personal irrelevance in the lives of their children and grandchildren excludes them from their world. In other words, the older generation perceive the younger generation as capable agents in Israeli society, while seeing themselves as competent and capable only within the remnants of their ethnic community.

Talking about identity with the younger generations, G1.5 and G2, was very different, for them introspection on their complex personal and collective identities was both legitimate and familiar. Edna attempts to thwart any effort to define her: 'I cannot fit into any of the categories' she says defiantly. The categories are socially created, she is avoiding making a choice that to her mind minimalizes who she is. Eventually, after much thought, she says:

> I am both [Israeli and Ethiopian] but today I feel no need to define or prove myself.

When I ask her what she means she says that she spent a long time:

studying myself, what am I, as part of my community, as a religious woman.

Time spent contemplating the issue of identity indicates its importance. Unlike in Ethiopia, where genealogy and community defined identity, in the new Israeli context people are more keenly searching for their identities, taking an active role in defining themselves in relation to the various sub-cultures around them. Edna experiences the intersection of several identities: as a woman, an immigrant (G1.5), and a religious person living in a peripheral area. She is highly competent in both Israeli and Ethiopian contexts, forging a gentle easy-going pathway for her children's hybridity. She is also acutely aware of the relative value society places on membership in different boxes—the social categories she refuses to be defined by. Identity has become both personal and pragmatic, defining not only a sense of self and belonging to a community but also a sense of visibility and social justice. Defining oneself according to set social categories is a statement of legitimacy and the right to belong, an affirmation by others provides reassurance of our very existence (Fanon, 1967). This is an on-going daily struggle of survival for the younger generation, Edna is keenly aware of all this and refuses to play the game.

13.5 Definitions and Self-perception

My question on identity did not include any categories, but was phrased 'how to you define yourself?' Most participants assumed I meant as Ethiopian or Israeli. Thirty-two participants gave full detailed answers, mostly G1.5 and G2. Three interviewees (Dana, Lee, and Orna) defined themselves as Ethiopian, seven (Avi, Teruneh, Shira, Matan, Noam, Yaniv, and Dov) defined themselves as Israeli, eleven participants (Ester, Genet, Addis, Shy, Shani, Liora, Noa, Aberash, Tsehai, Rachel, and Sarah) defined themselves as Ethiopian Israelis, eight (Habtam, Israel, Miki, Tigist, Lemlem, Mulu, Maayan, and Shimon) defined themselves as Israeli Ethiopian Jews. Aside from Edna, two other people refrained from using any of these categories; Yafit said she does not know, and her daughter Naama defined herself as 'universal'.

Habtam started her answer with a qualifier: 'another day I will define myself differently', and Naama said, 'it is something that is always changing'. This is an important and accurate observation: our self-perception and self-definition changes according to circumstances, connections, life experiences, and extent of self-awareness. Since identities are both dynamic and complex, the answers given in this (or any other) study can only reflect a momentary picture of chosen identities and current means of coping with the complexities of Israeli reality. The narratives can give insights into the *process* of negotiating self and other perceptions after immigration or as members of the second generation. This is an on-going process which can last a lifetime, with significant outcomes both within the family and in interaction with the outside world.

Addis introduced himself by saying he was a person who 'does not like to talk, does not advertise his emotions'. Later in the interview he defines himself as Israeli but qualified this by saying he does not have Israeli characteristics, such as 'impertinence'. In other words, in his understanding, to be Israeli one cannot be also emotionally reserved or excessively polite. Tsehai defined herself as 'responsible, very industrious, not afraid of hard work, with no social problems'. This list of characteristics indicates a high sense of self-efficacy and positive self-image. When asked specifically about her ethnic or community identity she said: 'I'm not bothered about that', then added that she has never felt discriminated against. It is an interesting question if her life experiences shaped her attitude or vice versa, meaning that her positive attitude blocked from her vision any evidence to the contrary. Either way, her ethnic identity does not concern her. One could argue that this is another way of 'not playing the game' or that her amicably diverse environment enables her to be comfortably hybrid, buffering the effects of intersectionality.

There are also cultural categories of identity from Ethiopia which intersect and create challenges, such as status based on age, gender, and the position in the family. For example, Shani is still struggling with 'being tenth in line' which taught her to minimize her presence, together with being a woman this has inculcated in her a certain reticence in the presence of others—quite opposite to Israeli assertiveness. In the individualistic world she lives in today she feels the need to 'develop oneself on a personal level', which includes rejecting the role of 'little woman' as she defines her family's traditional expectations of her. Like many of the younger generation Shani struggles to gain a sense of equality for herself and her children, her strategies of action bring her into conflict with the older generation. These latter interpret such behaviour, sparked by a reflective awareness of needs and desires, as an expression of audacity and selfishness totally unacceptable to them. What they are failing to see is that such behaviour is simply cultural adaptation.

Genet has been struggling with similar issues all her life, in training herself to be both a therapist and a role model to her children, she has invested in the sort of self-development Shani is referring to. In fact, she states explicitly; 'before I can be a therapist, I need to undergo therapy myself'. Her discussion of her own complex identity steers away from rigid social categories and opens a whole new perspective on the self, inclusive of personal choice and life changes. Thus, Genet describes herself as 'a baby' and 'a child' when she visits her mother:

> I invited myself to be a child here. I come here to be looked after.

With a bashful smile she admits that as a child she always dreamt of being 'a fairy'—a childhood fantasy that allowed her, at least in her imagination, to break away from the confines of rigid social categories and expectations placed upon her in Ethiopia. Today, her individualistic surroundings enable her to break free from social constraints in the real world, she explains that in Ethiopia 'dreaming of being a fairy was forbidden' and tells me how the childhood fantasy has come back to her repeatedly in guided imaginative therapy sessions. Now she can:

> tell him [her Ethiopian partner] that I never had this [the pampering at home] before and I want it now. All the neighbours know, they say *you are a grown woman, mother of three*, it's a joke to them.

Genet was a child-parent to her single immigrant mother, having to take responsibility prevented her from any option of being 'a child' or 'a baby' just as much as she was unable in Ethiopia to be 'a fairy'.[2] But as a grown woman with self-awareness today she can voice her need for pampering, and assertively tell her husband 'Don't say anything!' In the cultural transition restrictive cultural categories have been deconstructed, enabling a grown woman to choose as her identity, at least momentarily, to be a baby or a fairy.

Despite the differences and clashes between them, Dana describes herself often questioning her parents and trying to understand them. When talking about her own identity she says: 'I put the pieces together to form a personality', and thus appropriates an active role in forming her own independent identity.

The process of self-construction is embedded in the dominant cultural pathway and thus forged with the relevant social emphasis, on a sliding scale between individualism and collectivism. Thus, the primary focus is either on self-centeredness, individualistic desires, personal ego, self-expression, independence, and choice or on social harmony, humility, joint responsibility, interdependency, personal restraint, and the self as part of the collective, generally fitted into the appropriate social stratification (Greenfield et al., 2003; Kuhl & Keller, 2008). Of course, these are not dichotomies, most societies exist on a continuum between individualism and collectivism. But how people think about themselves is deeply related to these perspectives, for example if feeling good about oneself is the result of self-fulfilment or being part of a group, whether the focus is on oneself or others, if the predominant emotions are pride and anger (tending to be personal) or shame and blame (tending towards the social). Immigration rattles core self-perceptions and redefines the self in relation to others—familiar others within family and community as well as unfamiliar others in the new society. Balancing the ability to perceive and react according to two opposing cultural pathways—finding the equilibrium between individualism and collectivism—is a daunting task. Thus, the stress of immigration may enhance a sense of detachment or confusion, often reflected in the participants descriptions of their first years in Israel.

13.6 Complex Identities

Israeli society, like many Western societies, tends to encourage dichotomic categories based on analytical thinking, often creating the choice between two opposing alternatives. Thus, the needs of one are assumed to come at the expense of another, self-consideration is assumed to be instead of the consideration of others, and so on. However, in collectivistic societies considering others coexists internally with

[2] Similarly, Noa talks specifically about telling herself 'to stop being a child at this time' when shouldering responsibility for her brothers instead of her parents, discussed in the next chapter.

considering oneself—self-perception contains the perception of others—as Mamu and Berihun explained—the community was them and they were the community.

Sagiv's study on the offspring of bi-cultural marriages in Israeli (2014) found that often one identity was seen as cancelling the other, and the prevalent dichotomic social discourse left people feeling they had to choose one or the other. She notes that this applies not only to ethnicity, but also to religiosity—the expectation that Jewish people define themselves as religious, secular, or ultra-orthodox—leaving no room for a personal mix of religious affiliation and practice. Such a public dialogue of set pre-defined boxes precludes hybridity as an option, making it much harder for the offspring of bi-cultural marriages to appropriate and embrace a double-cultural heritage while regarding each of equal value. To return to the notion of cultural pathways, dichotomous thinking effectively blocks intertwining and merging different cultural pathways, rigidly set as opposing routes to different destinations. This reality within Israeli society has set the slippery slope leading to the current (January 2023) catastrophic situation. Within families it can be devastating—instead of members being able to set out comfortably supported along differing pathways (cultural, religious, or otherwise) they are often pitted against one another.

Holistic thinking enables a zooming-out view which makes visible the relationships between disparate elements of any given situation. The ability to switch from analytical to holistic thinking is dependent on the capacity to moderate emotions according to context (Williamson & Bray, 1988). If one's identity puzzle is composed both of permanent pieces and pieces that are adaptable to context, the balance between them is significant in dealing with stress and change. This is especially relevant when talking about immigrants, since the more independent people are from their traditional mainstream, the easier they will find it to adjust to the new society (Williamson and Bray). For example, people like Edna's father, Kabede, and Tareke, who were innovative in their behaviour in Ethiopia, adjust more easily to Israeli reality than people who have internalized the status quo that existed in Ethiopia as part of their own identity and now struggle with change. These latter, exemplified by Mamu and Berihun, are the epitome of interdependence—being part of their community *defines* them. After immigration, they are more vulnerable to the attitude of their surroundings towards them since their self-worth is dependent on being part of the collective.

13.7 The False Hope of Being Israeli

Most new immigrants long to be Israeli, so did Rachel, who arrived with her uncle when she was only 8 years old and was raised in various institutions. She speaks with bitter disappointment:

> I am angry with Israeli society. They demand that you give up everything you came with, disconnect yourself to be like them. But even if you do that, they don't accept you. You will always be considered different.

Rachel went on to talk about her long and perilous journey to Israel, the disconnection from her family and the loss of her childhood as the price she has paid for trying to be Israeli. Sadly, she adds: 'from all the effort to prove yourself, you forget where you came from!' Rachel feels detached from both cultures, and on this broken divide she is raising her five children.[3]

In another study on Ethiopian youth in Israel, Berhanu (2005) also found the younger generation often detached from both cultures, which he saw as a partial explanation for their underachievement in school. According to Berhanu, a clear identity is a psychological need essential as a base for learning. But despite their efforts to fit in through acquisition of language, change of clothes and behaviour, most of the youth in his study lacked a sense of belonging and like Rachel, felt they would always be treated as different.

In my study some of those interviewed spoke in past tense about wanting to be Israeli, explaining that the desire lapsed after repeated rejections or experiences of prejudice. For example, Shy:

> My wife and I arrived [separately] when we were young, she was fifteen and I was twenty. We thought we were completely Israeli, till we had to fight in all sorts of contexts... we saw that here each group keeps their own culture, so it's important that we keep our culture as well.

Shy is not bitter when he explains this, he is a realist who adapts to circumstances. Noa lives today in America, she says:

> I never suffered from prejudice; I was never discriminated against because I am Ethiopian. We were always welcomed, I had many Israeli friends, and I always tried to ignore my Ethiopian identity. Today I am returning to my roots. I listen to Amharic music, I show my son things from Ethiopia, I tell him you are Ethiopian and Israeli. He answers me: *I am American!*

Everybody wants to fit in, the easiest way to do so always seems to be by being like everybody else, Noa's young son has already figured this out. But in time it inevitably becomes clear that elements of our identity cannot be shed like old clothes. The fact that people try to do so is not always connected to harsh experiences, prejudice, or discrimination, sometimes it is just part of being an immigrant.

13.8 Partially Israeli

Four of the seven participants in my study who identified themselves as Israeli belong to the intermediate, 1.5 generation, the rest are second generation. Most of them qualify their Israeliness with a 'but', for example Avi:

> I am Israeli but not a full Israeli. An Israeli who knows part of him is Ethiopian, even though I was born here. I was born here, but my home is Ethiopian, a home that had only just arrived.

[3] Rachel's story is also discussed in chap. 12.

Avi is defining the context in which he grew up—an Ethiopian immigrant home—as an intrinsic part of his identity. In his narrative his own Israeliness precedes this, but he does not forget or deny that part of him will always be Ethiopian. That he describes himself as a child growing up in 'a home that had only just arrived' indicates the impermanence and inconsistencies of an unsettled reality, permeating his very sense of self.

Teruneh says proudly that he is 'Israeli by right', indicating his army service and reserve duty as proof of this. Serving in the IDF is for many young people an affirmation of their Israeli identity. Shy says explicitly that he can never be completely Israeli because he never served in the army.[4] Yaniv refers to himself as 'Israeli but' and explains that the 'but' refers to the way he is treated by Israeli society because of his colour (detailed later in this chapter).

When Avi describes his Israeli qualities, he says:

> When it is necessary to raise my voice I do so, most Ethiopians don't do that. When it is necessary to demand something, I demand it. I don't keep silent. Ethiopian Israelis have learnt to react, but not to talk…

Avi's assertiveness is presented by him as an acquired Israeli quality, it enables him to hold his own in the Israeli social arena. Yet, he uses this only when it is 'necessary', marked in striking contrast to Ethiopian polite silence. He makes an important differentiation between his ability to express himself and take control over the interaction, and the impulsive reaction of Ethiopian Israelis swamped by un-vent emotions.

Open assertiveness is the opposite of being polite, humble, and respectful, qualities highly valued by traditional Ethiopian culture. Many participants defining their Israeli qualities mentioned assertiveness. Noa said 'I will demand things, not remain silent', and Avi also talks about 'raising my voice'. These are new strategies of action mentioned as signifying an evolving Israeli identity. Avi, Noa, and others are replacing the polite passivity in their cultural toolkit for assertiveness, or alternatively maintaining both strategies, retrieved as appropriate according to context. This latter is an example of effective hybridity.

Matan says 'I feel like I belong here, over there [Ethiopia] is history'. Similarly, Noam states; 'I don't have knowledge of Ethiopia like I have knowledge of here'. Defining oneself as Israeli comes from a sense of belonging, enhanced by having local knowledge and being involved in Israeli society. Liora and Ester also talk about this and stress the importance of mixing with other cultural groups, to them living in a mosaic of different cultures is one of the unique qualities of Israel. Yaniv says that for him, going to the military boarding school, where he was the only youngster of Ethiopian origin:

> developed my way of thinking, something in me changed, I believe I became open to seeing things differently.

Yaniv is describing a formative experience stemming from inter-cultural mixing, one familiar to Dov from his Yeshiva boarding school:

[4] A comprehensive study on the significance of army service to a sense of belonging amongst Ethiopian immigrants was conducted by Shabtai (1999).

> I am very connected to this country, I am Jewish in every sense, Zionist-religious, I am not Ethiopian.

Thus, without once using the word 'Israeli', Dov defines himself as such through the specific sub-culture he belongs to. Dov has left no space in his life for Ethiopian culture, saying,

> What am I doing here, in Israel, if I feel Ethiopian?

He goes on to express the deep respect he has for his Ethiopian cultural heritage, which he sees as what led him to Israel. His daily decisions are forged in accordance with the Israeli religious community he lives in.

Even those who appropriate Israeli culture as their own find it difficult to explain what this is. Yisrael says he does not know what an Israeli identity is:

> Maybe there is no such thing! There are so many ethnic groups here. I don't have an answer on what it means to be Israeli.

When I ask Shira what her Israeli identity comprises, she talks of food, clothes, language, and behaviour. A similar answer comes from other second-generation participants when talking about an Ethiopian identity. Is this a symbolic identification with common cultural elements without the intricacies of cultural values and strategies of action? My feeling is that the answer is more complex. Firstly, it could just be the way people talk about identities, especially young people, who are more involved in *doing* than in analysing why they do what they do. Expressive elements of a culture are easy to latch onto, easy to describe, less committing than values and strategies of action, which are illusive and generally unspoken. The second point is illustrated by Lee, who talks of herself as able to wear or discard her Israeli identity, as if it was external to her, like a piece of clothing, while her core identity remains Ethiopian. Lee is bilingual, she lives and works with Ethiopian immigrants, native Israelis, and other immigrants. In many ways she has adopted a hybrid identity, and yet feels more comfortable in her Ethiopian identity, which is like a *home base*. Being hybrid can be akin to having two internal homes, two (or more) anchors of identity embedded in different cultures. The home base might change according to time and place, people can feel varying degrees of comfort, harmony, or tension about their various identities. It is this home base that many young people of the second generation seem to lack, perhaps because their primordial sense of self was forged on the invisible dividing-line between two cultures.

Mulu also says that Israel is 'not having one single culture, but a bunch of cultural contexts'. Sagiv (2014) reached the same conclusion, that Israel has not developed one collective unifying culture. In some ways this makes it easier for new immigrants to fit in, as Shy said; 'each group keeps their own culture, so it's important that we keep our culture as well'. But perhaps the opposite also applies; that the segmented nature of Israeli culture makes it even harder to feel attached, like many pieces of a puzzle that don't actually fit together to create a whole. Perhaps people like Dov who have integrated into a specific community sub-culture end up having more of a sense of belonging. And even then, these sub-cultures are also stratified and sub-divided by public perceptions of value (for example, according to ethnicity, gender, or other parameters) covertly prevalent in all social interactions. Moreover, the danger of 'cultural autonomy and communal tribalism' that President Rivlin spoke of when leaving office (July 2021) currently seems to be prevalent over national unity.

13.9 Ethiopian Identity

Lee arrived in Israel when she was 15:

> In the beginning I was Ethiopian from my roots. Because I grew up in Ethiopia, I always remained Ethiopian. I never really entered Israeli culture, well maybe a little bit.

As a teenager in a boarding school Lee struggled to reconcile the two different and opposing worlds she was living in. Out of respect and loyalty to her parents, she maintained many traditional customs even when out of their sight. Figuratively she never strayed from the cultural pathway they had assigned her to. Until today. Now she talks about her Ethiopian identity as expressed primarily in music and food, but she also says she chooses not to live where there are too many Ethiopians, so as not 'to remain always Ethiopian', and ends up by saying she would like to be 'a little of both'.

Lee's narrative illustrates that negotiating between two cultural systems is an on-going process even many years after immigration. Her strategies of action—choosing where to live, what to eat, what to wear, what music to listen to, and the larger decisions of life—are all guided by a conscious attempt to combine the two culture, to always remain 'a little of both'. Lee is aware that being embedded in a predominantly Ethiopian neighbourhoods enhances that side of her identity in every respect, thus to avoid remaining 'always Ethiopian' she chooses to intermingle with local sub-cultures.

Similarly, Genet describes herself as more of an Ethiopian woman at home—reserved, available for family requests, child-centred. Outside she is more loudly expressive and assertive. Shani also talked about this, distinguishing between herself in her parents' home—which:

> brought me back to the traditional, conservative, less ambitious, more authentic [Ethiopian woman].[5]

Shani in her parents' house was ruled by the intersection of two traditional categories of identity: 'the tenth-in-line' and 'the little woman'—in her terminology this is a move *backwards* in which she is unable to express or develop herself. Thus, for many women Ethiopian culture comes to represent the opposite of modernity (Salamon, 2003) but Israeli culture (whatever form it takes) also does not represent enlightenment. And so Naama is adamantly 'not Ethiopian', because she has 'shed too much' and 'disconnected from the source', but she also rejects Israeliness as

[5] These examples have been discussed in the chapter on gender.

minimizing and restrictive. Her conclusion is 'today more than ever I feel neither here nor there, I am universal'. Unable to place herself in any of the social boxes, she says:

> I have forged my own definitions, that are neither Ethiopian nor Israeli. They go beyond both.

Naama's sense of identity transcends constraining categories aligned with common stereotypes about ethnicity and gender to an all-encompassing sense of basic humanity. As she contemplates what she just said she adds quietly that she might even consider living somewhere else. This is a profound revelation from someone with her personal history, the fact that she lowers her voice when she says it even though we are alone attests to its potency. To consider living somewhere else is the ultimate break with tradition, an untethering from the moorings of her Jewish Zionist ethnic roots.

The young people who spoke of their Ethiopian identity as comprising the *Sigd, engera, buna* and music in Amharic (such as Ester and Maayan) experience these elements when visiting relatives, they do not *practice* these at home (most admit they do not know how to make *engera*). While Habtam states 'I can listen to Hebrew music and still be very connected to my ethnic group', it does suggest that these have become remnants of a culture they are no longer living, but literally sometimes tasting, hearing, and observing. Traditional ceremonies and tangible cultural expression have become symbolic reflections of Ethiopian culture, devout of their original value and moral contents (Kaplan & Rosen, 1998). They are no longer strategies of action for shaping their world. Although many young people mentioned eating *engera* as a cohesive element that binds the family together that they would like to adopt in the future, most of them would need to learn how to make it first.

In contrast the elders of the community talk about preserving their culture through core values and actions, not symbolism. Thus, Tareke sees as an essential part of Ethiopian Jewish identity a deep sense of morality which includes

> keeping the Sabbath, not stealing, not lying, being a good person.

Others mentioned group and family cohesion, mutual responsibility, and respectful behaviour. The terminology is of what one should or should not do, the elders are describing the cultural pathway they would like the younger generation to take. But this cultural pathway is no longer clearly visible or accessible to many of them. More recognizably present in their family homes are the symbols already mentioned and a strong sense of ethnic identification, at least partially inspired by common negative experiences in Israeli society. Ester and Avi spoke about this. Avi described an affinity to total strangers of Ethiopian origin 'as if we all came out of the same home'.

13.10 Public Representation and Generalizations

Visibility, being black in a white society, creates both the public and the self-image that is reappraised constantly according to experiences in the public arena, forging either a sense of belonging or more often a sense of detachment and 'otherness' (Abbink, 1984; Ben-Ezer, 2010; Salamon, 2001, 2003). Every Ethiopian immigrant and their offspring born in Israel are coping with this daily, their personal internal and communal dialogue on the subject incorporates own and other perspectives—this is the context in which they live, social categories and their implications can be negotiated or rejected but not ignored (Fanon, 1967).

The potency of cultural perspectives stems less from what people believe than from their knowledge on how others interpret their actions (Swidler, 1995). This is one of the reasons why living in a predominantly Ethiopian neighbourhood thwarts adaptation, as demonstrated, for example, by the men in my parent groups who wanted to help with domestic chores but did not want to be seen by their neighbours hanging out the washing. Thus, whatever is shared or institutionalized has great power over people in forming strategies for action suited to a sense of what is commonly regarded as appropriate or acceptable. This also applies to perceptions of identity—people want to belong, the easiest way to do so is to try and be like everybody else. But what if you don't *look* like everybody else?

> We came to a country where some accept us, and some do not. It depends where you landed. (Noam).

Noam has internalized a painful truth: in Israel, some sub-cultures accept the Ethiopian immigrants more easily than others. Identity is forged in context, in Ethiopia the Jews were differentiated by their Judaism, in Israel the Ethiopian immigrants are differentiated by their colour. This applies not only to the immigrants, but also to those born in Israel. The only participant in my study born in Israel who defined herself as Ethiopian was Dana. She reached this conclusion recently following her experiences and says sadly: 'they [Israelis] always manage to hurt us'.

As a child Dana wanted to be Israeli, a desire she has forsaken for a return to her Ethiopian roots. To her this means:

> First, I will work on my own identity, on the identity I see in the mirror, that I am black, so knowing where I came from.

In Ethiopia looking in the mirror did not arouse thoughts about colour, this awareness is a direct response to living in a predominantly white society (Antebe-Yemini, 2010). Jews in Ethiopian did not identify themselves as black but as red or brown, the category of black was limited to slaves (Salamon, 1995).

Dana recalls that as a child her mother told her:

> Do you think they are better than you? Look at these white people, they don't even know Arabic! Don't see them as an example, you can beat them in their own country.

At the time Dana was suffering from discrimination and exclusion at school, a fact she did not share with her parents. Her mother's words did not comfort her. More recently, after participating in demonstrations against racism, she began to make a connection between her personal experiences and the distress being voiced by the Ethiopian community in Israel.[6]

> Before the demonstration I felt differently. In the army I felt I needed to protect and serve. Now I think, what do I care? This is the truth: I don't care! Not like I used to. Suddenly I see those I was protecting turning on me and calling me *that Cushi what did she do for me?* So, it's just not worth it.

Dana used to care enough to serve her country, to see this as her duty. But realizing that she had experienced discrimination made her question this loyalty, the price she was paying for trying to fit in while often experiencing rejection or belittlement. This was a formative moment for Dana, in which she realized that it was up to her to fill the void within, to educate herself on her cultural heritage and give content to the Ethiopian identity which society was forcing upon her. She decided to embrace it as her own:

> Now I will fight for my own identity, defining myself as Ethiopian is *mine. Really mine.* Because I know Amharic, and you don't. I have something from my ancestors that is mine, not from here, because that is theirs—that is how the Israelis have defined it. I just could not see this before.

Dana's struggle to define her identity in positive terms that empower her is based on an awakening to the context in which she is living. To own the ethnicity which to other Israelis seems to define her, Dana is searching for her roots and learning about her cultural heritage.

Yaniv provides another example. Born in Israel, he says that he is always labelled as Ethiopian. He calls this his 'invisible ID card[7]' which prevents him from being completely Israeli:

> I cannot be Israeli. I can, I have fitted in very well. People who know me, they know exactly who I am. But people who walk past and look, or if I go to one of their parties, they see me as kind of exceptional.

The ambivalence Yaniv expresses resonates the paradox between *identity* and *identification* (Shalom, 2018). He probably has many exceptional qualities, but the one he is referring to here is the colour of his skin, which often prevents him from entering such parties with his friends, and if they were not paying attention at the entrance he remains outside. He tells humorous stories about this, but his expression bears witness to his pain. Repeated rejection scars him, shaking his confidence in his ability to belong here. Ziv (2012) coined this *persistent trauma*, common to most members of easily identifiable minority groups. The trauma is persistent because it has no time to heal, being reopened constantly by frequent encounters with bias and discrimination. In Israel Arabs and Ethiopians are most likely to suffer from this as

[6] Further detail on the demonstrations and their causes in the next chapter.

[7] Israelis above the age of 16 are obligated by law to carry identity cards.

they are more frequently stopped by police than other, white European, Israelis.[8] Many youngsters in Israel collect such experiences and live with this frustration, tending towards one of two options: continuously trying to prove themselves as Israeli or building themselves an Ethiopian identity (Mula, 2010; Ben-Eliezer, 2008). The middle road of hybridity is open primarily to people have had more positive experiences, whose surroundings are more amicably accepting of diversity and less concerned with fitting people into boxes.

Yaniv's expression that he is 'not a cry-baby' is a double entendre, invoking a stereotype based on the intersection of gender and ethnicity. The social norm is that men don't cry, and ethnic groups complaining of discrimination are often accused of unjustified whining thus undermining their claims of injustice (Shenhav & Yona, 2008). When Yaniv says he is 'not a cry-baby' he is simultaneously rejecting these stereotypes and asserting both manliness and ethnic pride. In defining himself as 'Israeli but' Yaniv is expressing both his desire to belong and his ambivalence about this possibility.

Even Dov, who adamantly defined himself as Israeli and 'gives very little space to my Ethiopian identity', says that his mother repeatedly tells him:

> Nothing can help you, you have the skin colour, you can't escape from it!

Abigail is using the category of colour to challenge her sons' efforts to fit into the Zionist-religious community, that which encourages him not to eat the food she cooks. He smiles bashfully as he recalls this, he feels embedded in this community and has never felt rejected by them because of his colour. Thus, social categories are flung like mud in family arguments, complicating the ability to accept personal choices by using ethnicity, culture, and above all colour, as symbols of group loyalty. But personal choices, however painful to other family members, are also legitimate coping methods in complex situations. Thus, personal allegiance to specific social categories tips the power balance between the boxes, reinforcing or undermining group affiliations by colour, gender, religious format, place of residence, or other parameters. Dov is persistently respectful and appreciative of his mother's point of view, she comments on this herself in her interview, it is his graceful manner which has enabled her to forgive and accept his choices. Abigail understands that Dov never rejected her, his ethnicity or his culture, his choices were not *against* anything, they were in favour of his need to belong, to embraced change and create the life he wanted for himself and his family. In other words, despite choosing a different pathway for himself than his mother would wish, Dov has maintained their connection by using suitable elements from his Ethiopian cultural toolkit, namely wax and gold communication, reverence, respect, and appreciation. Although sometimes strained almost to breaking point, relationships in this family are nurtured with care across the chasm of differing perspectives.

---

[8] A report by the State Comptroller of Israel (2021) shows the Ethiopian Israeli population disproportionately represented in 2019 in arrests (5.6% of all youth arrests, over three times their percentage in the population, 1.7%)

Shira adds the word 'normal' to her definition of herself as Israeli, three times in the same sentence she repeats this, but then when she turns to talking about herself at school suddenly in her own narrative she becomes 'Ethiopian'. The schoolchildren in Mula's study (2010) also referred to themselves as normal, attempting to be seen just like everybody else, as individuals without attached stigmatizing labels. The common expectation that they represent their immigrant community infuriates young people of the second generation:

> This is cumbersome, I don't want to represent anybody, I represent myself before I represent the community. (Yisrael).

Yisrael is a combat soldier, in his unit are young men from different places in Israel, he says:

> I had friends from remote moshavim [agricultural settlements] who had never met an Ethiopian before. They heard me say something and said, *listen, brother, you just shattered the stigma, I didn't know you were like this and like that…*

Many Ethiopian Israelis find themselves in the public sphere representing an entire community which they do not necessarily know or identify with. The vast diversity in this community is simply not reflected in the stereotypes about them. Addis, a recently discharged soldier, voiced a similar experience in a separate interview:

> Many friends said to me: *you represent the community with honour, they must be really proud of you for being in the navy commando unit.* But I didn't come here to represent anybody, I represent myself, my family, I don't represent other people.

Nevertheless, when finding himself the only Ethiopian Israeli in various groups, Addis was always expected to represent:

> Whenever I was with white people, including in the army, I was always *that Ethiopian*, even in high school. Once I was guarding with a friend in the army and I was shocked when he said to me: *first time I ever met an Ethiopian.* I asked him how come, and he said he grew up on a kibbutz and always negated us. When I asked him why he said that's what he learnt at home. I didn't know what to say to that, so I said OK.

Addis has taught himself not to react to prejudice, 'to let it glide past' him, as he put it. His attitude is one of self-preservation, when I ask him what about racism he shrugs:

> I came across it and kept going. Those who want to hurt us, really, they are hurting themselves.

These highly motivated young men, serving in combat units, forging their image as Israelis, do not let casually made remarks undermine their sense of belonging. Nevertheless, these moments have been scorched into their memory and surface during the interview.

Shira says of herself that she cannot stand generalizations of any kind and has to respond.

> I cannot remain silent. It's not just colour, I hate generalizations, about Arabs too, it drives me crazy. If one Arab did something they say all the Arabs are like that. I come across this a lot, directed at me and at others.

Like Addis and Yisrael, Shira would like to be seen as a person in her own right and not a representative of a group, neither does she accept generalizations about any group of people. Tigist is frustrated by the common generalizations made in the hospital where she works. She says that dark-skinned foreign workers or Eritrean asylum seekers are grouped together with Ethiopian immigrants in the perception of staff, who cannot differentiate between people of colour:

> They see someone the same colour as an Ethiopian, so [to them] he is Ethiopian, never mind if he is Eritrean or Sudanese. Just like people with slanted eyes are all Chinese.

Young parents of the intermediate (1.5) generation who understand the reality their children live in are trying to provide them with a viable identity that will defy prejudice and protect them against categorization by colour. Thus, Liora says that she wants her children 'to be proud of their colour'. In Ethiopia pride was based on ancestry, roots, courage, resourcefulness, and consideration of others. Liora and other parents are teaching their children to appreciate their cultural heritage, so that beyond difference, colour will represent all of these.

Generalizations are part of our attempt to simplify the world around us by categorization, putting people in pre-defined boxes gives us the illusion that we *know* something about others. Every society has their own stereotypes which obscure and negate the complexity of human identity and personal choice. Noam admits that 'we have racism in our community too', he is referring to discrimination against the Barya, dark-skinned people who in Ethiopia were commonly regarded as slaves (Salamon, 1995; Kaplan, 1999). Tsehai admits that Ethiopian immigrants also speak about the white Israelis in gross generalizations:

> There are many things in our community that I think are wrong and I don't agree with. Then people think I am racist towards my own community. But we also say the Israelis are like this, and like that, and it isn't true. [...] One should not generalize.

Some people in the Ethiopian community regard marrying white people as a sort of betrayal of the community and an attempt to improve social position (for example, Ungedaw-Wanda, 2019). Habtam, who married a white Israeli, says:

> I am very critical of seclusion in the community, when I first went out with a white person people said—*how do you dare?* I think it undermines them... then I became *the one who married a...* at my brother's wedding someone said *ahh you're the one with the white guy.*

The dichotomy of colour obliterates individuality and minimalizes people, enhanced when there is little or no intermingling, creating 'them' and 'us' narratives from a very young age. Some parents and several young people talked about this, for example Habtam said

> I see the way my nephews look at white people, like they'll say—*what is that white doing here?* Stuff like that. You don't want such a situation, to avoid it we need exposure.

But where whole neighbourhoods have become predominantly Ethiopian there is very little ethnic mixing. Ester referred to this as a factor in her parents' isolation from Israeli society and subsequent lack of integration. She also mentioned that her father was more exposed to Israeli society through his work, while her mother who stayed at home was not.

Generalizations about Ethiopian immigrants predominantly carry negative connotations, leaving them with a sense of being regarded as inferior. Rachel describes this:

> There is always this doubt about you, that maybe you don't know one hundred percent, you can see it, you're always on the margin, in parenthesis…

Rachel works in menial jobs, but even Habtam who is an academic employed by the Government expresses similar experiences:

> I often feel that I am proving to them that Ethiopians are much more talented than they imagine. I am not Israeli from their point of view. Often, I come to the office and participate in meetings and need to be much more eloquent and professional than other people, because I am being examined under a microscope. Especially when talking about something that has nothing to do with Ethiopians. You always need to know exactly what you are talking about.

Constantly needing to refute the common stereotypical assumption of 'not knowing' is frustrating and exhausting, Habtam goes on to say:

> You are Ethiopian, the image about you is minus ten, you need to work hard to get it to zero. They think all Ethiopian women are cleaners, you have to work hard to prove that Ethiopian women are not just cleaners.

The intersection of ethnicity and gender combine to stigmatize Ethiopian women as unknowledgeable and incompetent, expressed in the narratives as a growing frustration and sense of injustice. Habtam goes on to cite examples in which her boss introduced her as 'not just dealing with Ethiopian matters' and on another occasion asked her to explain the meaning of her name to the participants of a meeting. She talks about this with anger, her expectation is to be treated as a professional doing her job and asks why her origins need to be mentioned repeatedly in every meeting. It is these moments, when generalizations and prejudice surface unexpectedly, that challenge even calm and confident people like Habtam:

> My Israeliness is fractured when people remind me that I am Ethiopian, with all due respect to my feeling Israeli.

She goes on to say that the feeling is one of 'being pushed out', and it also occurs through tactless comments about her Hebrew such as:

> *Oh you are so fluent…* this is just such ignorance—if they opened their eyes and looked around them they might notice there are many people in different colours!

These experiences undermine the second generations birthright to feel that they belong. Any type of differential treatment emphasizing their origin is something that infuriates Maayan. She recalls how whilst working in a store she was always 'the Ethiopian worker', and how strangers would come up to her to say how much they loved Ethiopians:

I don't need you to come and tell me that you love me! I don't need it! I have my parents to tell me this, my brothers, my friends, my boyfriend... I don't need strangers in the street to tell me they love me!!

Maayan and Habtam reject the false affection of strangers expressing their admiration for the Ethiopian community in general, they want to be treated equally, as people in their own right, without being constantly reminded that they are Ethiopian. At work they wish to be judged by professional standards, according to their accomplishments, without unnecessary and irrelevant referral to their origins and ethnicity. Maayan says that in her current job in a boarding school for youth in danger she is very happy because:

I feel that I am just myself, they see me as one of the staff, in meetings I am asked for my opinion as Maayan.

It is the discussion of identity which brings to light these experiences, the effect of which is enhanced when they occur at home. Edna says that she finds any sort of discrimination sickening. As the intended bride of a white immigrant family, she soon came to realize how complicated things could be when her prospective mother-in-law requested to have her 'examined' before they even met. Looking up her in-law's history on the internet, she discovered that 'black people were slaves for his [her future husband's] grandfather'. As a young woman she was able to accept this disturbing reality with compassion, saying to her partner:

Your mother is right. What she knows about Ethiopians is that they have aids. That's what she knows! I told him I would invite her to see me give birth to show that I am healthy, I was not going to give her a health certificate!

But over the years her tolerance has subsided; 'I was easy-going then, today I have a problem', and she goes on to explain that her mother-in-law treats her children differently than the other grandchildren:

After the children were born, I have a problem with this [her mother-in-law's attitude]. I feel the discrimination. It seemed natural to me that they treated me differently because I am Ethiopian.

As a young new immigrant Edna accepted being treated differently by her in-laws, it did not bother her then. But today, seeing her children being treated differently than their cousins is something she cannot accept. Edna wants her children to feel equal, she goes to great efforts to include elements of the three cultures in their daily lives. But she will not let anybody, including her mother-in-law, rate between these cultures.

Ethnic rejection or undervaluation leaves a bitter sense of inferiority and affront, especially when it comes from an intersection of identities:

You're not Israeli enough, and you're not Ethiopian enough, and sometimes you're not Jewish enough! (Habtam).

A sense of 'not being enough' is undermining and demeaning. It takes strong inner resources to overcome such feelings and continue to function with confidence and efficacy. Habtam, Edna, and others manage to do so with great resilience, but not everybody does. These narratives illustrate the potency of social context in shaping both concepts about identity and strategies of action in face of stereotyping and discrimination. People create their identities in interaction with their surroundings, through a unique mix of cultures in a continuous on-going process that is always changing, leading to varying degrees of belonging or detachment (Maalouf, 2004).

References

Abbink, J. (1984). The Falasha in Ethiopia and Israel: The problem of ethnic, assimilation. *Social Antroplogische Cahiers, XV*. ICSA (Institute for Cultural and Social Anthropology).

Ari, L. (2012). North Americans, Israelis, or Jews? The ethnic identity of immigrants' offspring. *Contemporary Jewry, 32*(3), 285–308.

Bennet-Martinez, V., Leu, J., & Lee, F. (2002). Negotiating biculturalism. *Journal of Cross-Cultural Psychology, 33*(5), 492–516.

Bennet-Martinez, V., Leu, J., & Lee, F. (2006). Biculturalism & cognitive complexity: Expertise in cultural representations. *Journal of Cross-Cultural Psychology, 37*(4), 386–407.

Berhanu, G. (2005). Normality, deviance, identity, cultural tracking and school achievement: The case of Ethiopian Jews in Israel. *Scandinavian Journal of Educational Research, 49*(1), 51–82.

Crenshaw, K. (1989). *Demarginalizing the intersection of race and sex: A black feminist critique of antidiscrimination doctrine, feminist theory and antiracist politics* (pp. 139–167). University of Chicago Legal Forum.

Fanon, F. (1967). *Black skin white masks* (pp. 130–131). Grove.

Gans, H. J. (1994). Symbolic ethnicity and symbolic religiosity: Towards a comparison of ethnic and religious acculturation. *Ethnic and Racial Studies, 17*(4), 577–592.

Greenfield, P. M., Keller, H., Fuligni, A., & Maynard, A. (2003). Cultural pathways through universal development. *Annual Review of Psychology, 54*(1), 461–490.

Jaffe-Schagen, J. (2016). Creating space. The construction of Ethiopian heritage and memory in Israel. *Annales d'Ethiopie., 31*, 81–105.

Kaplan, S. (1999). Can the Ethiopian change his skin? The Beta Israel (Ethiopian Jews) and racial discourse. *African Affairs, 48*(393), 535–550.

Kaplan, S., & Rosen, H. (1998). Ethiopian immigrants in Israel: Between preservation of culture and invention of tradition. In E. Leshem & J. Shuval (Eds.), *Immigration to Israel, sociological perspectives*. Transaction Publishers.

Kuhl, J., & Keller, H. (2008). Affect-regulation, self-development and parenting: A functional-design approach to cross-cultural differences. In R. Sorrentino & S. Yamaguchi (Eds.), *Handbook of motivation and cognition across cultures* (pp. 19–48). Academic Press Elsevier.

Lam, V. (2013). Developing ethnic identities and ethnic attitudes in children: Theory and research in context. In C. Agymang, C. Airhihenbuwa, & D. Aikins (Eds.), *Ethnicity theories, international perspectives and challenges* (pp. 101–131). Nova Science Publishers.

Maalouf, A. (2004). *Les Identites meurtrieres*. France.

McCall, L. (2005). The complexity of intersectionality. *Signs, 30*, 1771–1800.

Naujoks, D. (2010). Diasporic identities–reflections on transnational belonging. *Naujoks, Daniel*, 1–21.

Nigusie, A. (2018). An integrated approach to the study of ethnicity and its relevance to Ethiopia. *International Journal of Social Science Studies, 6*(12), 38–46.

Portes, A., & Rumbaut, R. G. (2001). *Legacies: The story of the immigrant second generation*. Univ of California Press.

Salamon, H. (1995). Reflectors of Ethiopian cultural patterns on the Beta Israel absorption in Israel: The "Barya" case. In S. Kaplan, T. Parfitt, & E. T. Semi (Eds.), *Between Africa and Zion:*

Proceeding of the first international congress of the Society for the Study of Ethiopian Jewry (pp. 126–130). Ben-Zvi Institute. ISBN 9789652350589.
Salamon, H. (2001). In search of self and other: A few remarks on ethnicity, race and Ethiopian Jews. In L. Tessman & B. B. On (Eds.), *Jewish locations: Traversing racialized landscapes* (pp. 75–88). Rowman and Littlefield Publishers.
Salamon, H. (2003). Blackness in transition: Decoding racial constructs through stories of Ethiopian Jews. *Journal of Folklore Research, 40*(1), 3–32.
Swidler, A. (1995). Cultural power and social movements. In H. Johnston & B. Klandermans (Eds.), *Social movements and culture. Social movements, protest, and contention* (Vol. 4, pp. 25–40). University of Minnesota Press.
Ungar, M. (2011). The social ecology of resilience: Addressing contextual and cultural ambiguity of a nascent construct. *American Journal of Orthopsychiatry., 81*(1), 1–17.
Williamson, D., & Bray, J. (1988). Family development and change across the generations: An intergenerational perspective. In C. Falicov (Ed.), *Family transitions: Continuity and change over the life cycle* (pp. 357–384). Guildford Press.

Hebrew References

Antebe-Yemini, L. (2010). Marginal visibility: Ethiopian immigrants in Israel. In E. Lomsky-Feder & T. Rappaprt (Eds.), *Visibility in immigration, bòdy, outlook, representation* (pp. 43–67). Hakkibutz Hameuchad and the Van Leer Institute.
Ben-Eliezer, U. (2008). Cushi sambi bilibilibambo: How a Jew becomes black in the promised land. In Y. Shenhav & Y. Yona (Eds.), *Racism in Israel* (pp. 130–159). Van Leer Institute and the Kibbutz Hameuchad.
Ben-Ezer, G. (2010). A drop returning to the sea? Visibility in the absorption process of Ethiopian Jews. In A. Limsky-Feder & T. Rappaport (Eds.), *Visibility in immigration, body, outlook, representation* (pp. 305–328). Hakibbutz Hameuchad and Van Leer.
Bokovoza, G. (2011). Ethnic identity and stereotypes in Israel: Differences between Mizrachi and Ashkenazi and age groups. *Culture and Society, 4*, 607–633.
Mula, S. (2010). *The struggle to be normal: Ethiopian students meet racism in religious schools.* Thesis for main education, Hebrew University Jerusalem.
Sagiv, T. (2014). *On the fault line: Israelis of mixed ethnicity.* Hakibbutz Hameuchad.
Shabtai, M. (1999). *The identity journey of Ethiopian immigrant soldiers.* Cherikover.
Shalom, S. (2018). *Conversations about love and fear: The dialogue between the Rabbi's daughter and the Kes's son.* Miskal Yediot Ahronot.
Shenhav, Y., & Yona, Y. (2008). *Racism in Israel* (pp. 13–47). Van Leer Institute and the Kibbutz Hameuchad.
Ungedaw-Wanda, S. (2019). *Resilience in immigration* (pp. 81–83). Resling.
Ziv, E. (2012). Persistent trauma. *Mafteach, 5*, 55–74. Minerva Humanities Centre. Tel Aviv University.

Chapter 14
Resilience in Immigration

14.1 What Is Resilience?

Resilience refers to the capability of people and their immediate social and physical environments to cope in culturally meaningful ways (Ungar, 2011). This definition contains two crucial perceptions: firstly, that resilience is not a matter of personal strengths and capacities but is ecologically and socially produced and maintained. Secondly, that coping with life and achieving physical, mental, and social development are culture-specific constructs, in other words associated with different assumptions and meanings in different cultures. Resilience according to this definition is fostered by interaction between the individual and significant others, who include family, community and in a wider sense all social structures in which people's lives are embedded. Moreover, it depends on the availability and accessibility of culturally relevant resources to ensure wellbeing, and a negotiation of those resources sometimes under difficult and stressful circumstances (Ungar, 2015).

14.2 What Effect Does Immigration Have on Resilience?

If we look back at Chaps. 2 and 3 of this book, we can see that children's resilience in Ethiopia was built primarily on three crucial factors. Firstly, children were definitively anchored in family and community, through genealogical knowledge internalized at a very young age. In other words, children grew up with a clear sense of *identity* as part of their family and ancestral heritage. Secondly, children grew up with an intrinsic sense of *belonging* to family and community. In fact, the community as an entity was embedded in them to the same extent that they were embedded in the community. Thirdly, children grew into their social and familial roles as

© The Author(s), under exclusive license to Springer Nature Switzerland AG 2023

N. A. Shmuel, *Children's Wellbeing in Immigrant Families*, Children's Well-Being: Indicators and Research 26,
https://doi.org/10.1007/978-3-031-31917-4_14

significant *partners* who contributed to the wellbeing of the whole. This sense of all being in the same boat, so to speak, enhanced their self-efficacy and sense of worth.

Immigration changed all of this. In Israel children are surrounded by fewer family members who spend less time together. As demonstrated in Chaps. 7 and 8, there is less effective and affirmative communication in the family. The worlds of adults and children have been split as the adults disappear to work for many hours of the day and children attend day care, school, and after-school frameworks. In these institutions children spend most of their time with roughly same-age children, their play is predominantly object-oriented rather than people-oriented. In addition to all these changes children experience various forms of discrimination and racism as well as other difficulties, while traditional community and extended family support networks have effectively unravelled and diminished.

On the other hand, if we look at Chaps. 9 and 12 in this book, we can see examples of the strength and resilience of individuals, families, and children in this community. The ability to balance the demands of two (often opposing) cultural systems, to create viable pathways forward despite tensions and clashes involving cultures and contexts, reflects the intricate interactions between aspects of resilience (Ungar, 2008). Thus, we have seen examples of parents who diligently remain involved in their children's lives despite not always understanding what their children are experiencing. Families that use resourcefulness and creativity to maintain intergenerational relations when failing systems of language (spoken and unspoken) make communication difficult. We have seen examples of a caring, cohesive community struggling to help each other despite experiences of racism and prejudice (more on this in a moment). We have discussed the memory and narrative of the dangerous journey to Israel via Sudan as mentioned repeatedly by participants to indicate proof of personal and collective resilience. We have seen how faith and conviction can light the way ahead, and connection be maintained despite frequent and volatile clashes in the family. We have seen examples of the intermediate, 1.5 generation, sharing parental responsibility, taking affirmative action to encourage, empower, and inspire the younger generation (G2). All these and more attest to the strength and resilience within this community, who are involved in a constant ongoing process of negotiating cultural and contextual elements in their lives while maintaining family and community ties. The fact that this is not always successful, that connections may be unravelled to varying degrees and tragedies happen (depression, violence, suicide, etc.), does not negate the effort and successes that often go unnoticed when the focus is on the problems of immigrant communities.

Understanding resilience not as an individual quality but as forged by interaction and supported by nurturing environments (Ungar, 2013) changes the focus from the individual immigrant to the contextual surroundings after immigration. Aside from the family and the immigrant community itself, when talking about immigrant and second-generation children the most important factors seem to be neighbourhoods and schools (Ungar, 2011). This has also been the conclusion of other researchers, for example Motti-Stefanidi (2018) whose research on immigrant youth from collectivistic societies in Europe (including G2) encountering discrimination and prejudice indicates that resilience is dependent on a combination of cultural and personal resources as well as parental and community support.

Discussing the resilience of immigrants in Greek schools (Motti-Stefanidi, 2019) reveals a process across multiple levels of influence, which could be supported and enhanced by school policies. Specifically, by promoting inter-cultural competence in both immigrant and non-immigrant youth via carefully planned intergroup contact (Barrett, 2018 cited in Motti-Stefanidi, 2019), providing youth with invaluable skills of respectful and effective inter-cultural communication befitting our diverse and globalizing world.

Unfortunately, in Israel, as demonstrated in Chap. 10, methodologies for integrating immigrant children in schools are based more on personal initiatives of school staff, often lacking appropriate training, rather than on pre-directed professional policies based on cultural sensitivity and knowledge about pro-active diversity and anti-bias education. One prominent positive example of effectual resilience enhancement was provided by the Yemin Orde Youth Village in which Chaim Peri founded the idea of what has become known as 'the village way'—creating a supportive nurturing environment for immigrant youth to negotiate culturally meaningful pathways.

This emphasizes the significance of several paramount factors to enhance resilience in immigrant populations; an appreciation of the strengths and abilities of the immigrant community, an understanding of the issues facing this community in their new environment *from their own perspective*, and a synchronization between services or assistance offered and the community's needs. When the opposite applies, and the community is predefined as carrying a cultural deficit, as was often the case for Ethiopian immigrants in Israel, when the problems and solutions are defined by policymakers, whatever services or assistance offered are likely to be ineffectual. According to Engdau-Vanda (2019) this is exactly the case for the many projects which sprouted amongst the Ethiopian immigrant communities in Israel, based on what she terms 'the industry of risk' which resulted from official definition of Ethiopian immigrant children as 'at risk'. According to the narratives of her interviewees, many of whom worked in such projects, they were unsuccessful because they wasted too many resources on infrastructure, were not based on professional consideration of the issues and needs of the community by involving local people in defining their goals, and therefore also were not utilized effectively by the community.

Since resilience is contextually and culturally dependent, transition heightens the necessity for resourceful negotiation, providing many opportunities to assist immigrants in the transition. But resources offered are only useful if culturally valued (Ungar, 2011, 2013) and must be based on understanding, a relationship of trust, and community involvement. Otherwise, misunderstandings and a spiralling disharmony come to characterize relations between the immigrant community and the establishment trying to help them, in which the former experience despair and helplessness and the latter feel unappreciated. Thus, it is not a matter of how much money was spent on assisting an immigrant community, but what and how this was actually done.

14.3 Families and Resilience

Families are the primordial base of everything, through which children discover the world and forge their relationship with selves and others (DeFrain & Asay, 2014). Even child development is not intrinsic in the child but evolves through the interaction between child and context (Weisner, 1998). Inherent in families are two opposing processes that exist simultaneously: the flexibility to change and the stability to stay the same (Falicov, 1988). It is the balance between these that enhances endurance alongside adaptability. The primary elements that facilitate this are family cohesion and communication, rattled and undermined by immigration as lives become unsettled and uncertainties about everything become paramount. Contextually and territorially untethered, family members react differently to this new incoherence. The process of finding a new equilibrium, each individually and as a family, may bring them together or pull them apart, or both simultaneously to varying degrees (Joselevich, 1988). It is at this juncture that perceiving and utilizing personal and cultural resources becomes crucial, enhanced, or undermined by interaction with the host society. In a supportive, appreciative environment it is easier to feel capable and tap into personal, familial, and community resources. Whereas a critical environment that undervalues and diminishes people's cultural traditions and creates disproportionate dependency on state institutions undermines their confidence and effectively forestalls adaptability. This is why the strength-based approach when assisting families in crisis is so important and reflects the fact that resilience is a *process* forged between people and their immediate social and physical environments to cope in culturally meaningful ways.

The issues affecting families in Israel in general are added to the challenges that accompany transition itself for immigrant families. Using the strength-based perspective, Younes (2014) identifies the main challenges facing families in Israel as violence through terrorism and war on the backdrop of a diverse society fraught with ethnic tension, socioeconomic inequalities, and significant poverty. Nevertheless, Younes found that endurance seems part of the fabric of families in Israel; regardless of sub-culture or religions, all seem to share some intrinsic basic qualities that make them strong families: loyalty and commitment to family and traditions, religious beliefs, passionate communication styles, and plenty of energy to cope with never-ending challenges which keep everybody very engaged in familial, community, and national affairs. The differences between Arabs and Jews described in this study do not seem to take into consideration the various subcultures in each group which make it difficult to generalize in wider terms. But primary concerns of everybody seem to be both economic and security issues, each of these complicating life in different ways for all communities.

In this section, I will look at two aspects affecting family resilience in Ethiopian Israeli families that arose out of the interviews in my study. The first concerns a sense of belonging and feeling comfortable within the family, intrinsic to a sense of self-efficacy and self-worth fostering resilience. The second concerns filial responsibility and role reversal often paramount in immigrant families, considered here both from the various perspectives of the different generations (G1, G1.5, G2). A third aspect worthy of study which did not come up in my interviews (probably because most of the participants were veteran immigrants) is the relation between immigrant families and the institutions responsible for their integration (discussed in more detail by Engdau-Vanda, 2019; Herzog, 1998 and others).

14.4 Belonging to Family and Community

A sense of belonging to family and community is an asset for all children, especially since one of the most powerful forces affecting resilience is connection (Ungar, 2013). Family mythology—meaning the story people tell about themselves—is forged within the family and shapes relationships. New children are added into the family narrative in relation to formative events, enhancing their sense of belonging or sowing the seeds for their exclusion and marginality. Thus, in the Sehalu family, the story of the journey to Sudan was, for Habtam, a powerful indicator of her inherited strength. But to her younger sister Maayan, the fact that she was born in Sudan was a constant reminder of her inherent difference:

> I really don't look like any of them! My mother used to tease me saying *I don't know where **you** came from!* They always said, to insult me, *we found you in Sudan, you don't even have a birth certificate!*

Maayan laughs bitterly when she recalls this, the harshness of her mother's words is reflected in her expression. The family narrative jovially *excludes* her. A year after 13-year-old-Lee arrived in Israel her family arrived, visiting them from her boarding school she recalls

> feeling I was not their daughter. I wanted so much to be their daughter. But my brothers used to tease me *you're not our sister!* I wanted them to know that I was.

This sense of not fitting in at home made it difficult for these children to fit in anywhere. Whereas children who heard the family story as inclusive tend to feel connected and look to their parents as role models. Shira is one example, when I ask her 'who do you admire the most?' she says without hesitation; 'my parents [Shy and Liora] who made the effort to come here and fulfil their dream'. Shy recalls his son telling him:

> *I volunteered to a combat unit because of my grandparents, because of you, you all suffered so much in Sudan to come to this country, how can I not protect it?*

Shira and her brother are eager to take their part in continuing the story of heroism, the past is giving meaning to their life decisions today. Thus, past and present are processed by the next generation, the connection to tradition becomes both personal and collective (Noyes, 2012).

But what about Maayan and Lee who are not anchored securely in the family narrative in this way? And other children who have little or no knowledge about their parents' journey or their cultural heritage? Often these are the same children who suffer from *double rejection* discussed in Chap. 10. Disconnection thwarts resilience, and many of these children may experience multiple disconnection from their family, their ethnic community, their native Israeli peers, and wider society. Orna, Habtam, Genet, and Shy all talked about this, as members of the intermediate 1.5 generation they are keenly aware of this phenomenon. In fact, as demonstrated in previous chapters, it is often the intermediate, 1.5 generation who come to the rescue, taking responsibility for younger siblings and cousins, providing an attentive ear, emotional and practical support. But not everyone has someone who can step up for them in this manner.

14.5 Filial Responsibility and Role Reversal

I will first present examples from my study, followed by an analysis of the effect of filial responsibility and role reversal on the intermediate 1.5 generation and on the first G1 generation.

> In our community the siblings raised the children. Our parents' generation were not strong enough to raise their own children after they arrived.

This was said by Yaniv, who frequently seeks advice from his elder sister Mulu, who 'to this day is the most important person in my life'.

Filial responsibility is a common denominator affecting many immigrant families (Bergelson et al., 2015). Mulu explains:

> I was what professionals today call a child-parent to immigrant parents. Yes, I was a child-parent to my brothers. Because of the language, the cultural change. It wasn't easy, but it is in the past. I was the bridge between two different worlds.

Being a 'bridge between two different worlds' to four younger brothers with whom she shared a mother struggling with transition was often a full-time job for Mulu, who was just 12 years old when her family arrived in Israel. During her sibling's adolescent years, she was often instrumental in providing guidance and mediating between them and their parents. Yaniv explained how:

> when I was in eighth grade, I wanted to go to a youth village, a military boarding school. My mother just said no.

It was Mulu and another brother (later killed in a car accident) who took him to the open day and persuaded the parents that this was a good choice for him. Noam also found Mulu as supportive during his turbulent youth, especially when he was dropping out of school and getting in trouble with the police:

> I got in trouble when I was sixteen, Mulu used to call and take me to stay with her. I used to think, *what will I do there?* But she persuaded me with the computer. So I waited for her till she came home from work, and the next day she took me to the safari. She actually took time off to be with me. She was attentive to all my problems… if I talked to my parents in Hebrew, they never understood me, and anyway they couldn't help me or explain things, because they lacked the knowledge, but my sister could, she could help me.

Mulu effectively stepped up and kept her brother off the streets. He is grateful for her support to this day. Many of the intermediate, 1.5 generation are hybrid, fluent in both languages, and sensitive to the distress of the second generation as well as the world view of the first generation. As Mulu said, and Avi reiterates, they effectively act as *bridges* between the generations:

> If there is a gap between oneself and the grandmother or the mother, they [G1.5] are an excellent bridge, because they understand, they arrived young and they understand both sides, me and those who raised me.

It was common for brothers and sisters to take responsibility for their siblings in Ethiopia, but there was a difference in scope and extent, as available adults could still give guidance and in complex situations take the burden of responsibility. Whereas in Israel the full weight of responsibility is often shouldered by siblings alone, when they themselves are still very young. Noa provides an example:

> Sometimes it was a burden. When I had to go with my parents to the offices… I used to go to my brothers boarding school. Sometimes I didn't even tell my parents that they had called, I just went by myself. […] every time I went I used to think that I have to stop being a child at this time.

Noa was only 3–4 years older than her next sibling, nevertheless, she travelled alone to their boarding schools, sometimes without her parents' knowledge. She explains that she wanted to save them the worry and frustration, and to do so told herself 'to stop being a child'. She was parenting not only her younger brothers but herself as well, a daunting double responsibility, as Genet's narrative illustrates. Genet (at the time in her late teens to early twenties) tried to be an authoritative aunt to her sister's children:

> They used to be very attentive. There were times when I overdid it, taking too much responsibility, at my own expense, to raise my siblings and help my sister raise her children…. At some point I understood what a burden I was carrying, to maintain such a presence in their lives.

In time Genet began to feel it was all too much:

> It scared me, how it was affecting me. I talked to each one of them to see how it affected them, [and asked myself] from what perspective I was taking such responsibility—with no knowledge, no skills, no experience.

Genet had been trying to actively enforce her authority over the younger members of the family as an older sister and aunt, in tune with Ethiopian tradition. Her intentions of helping them were good, but her methods, based on a hierarchy no longer relevant, lead to power struggles that escalated their negative behaviour. At some point Genet realized her intervention might be causing more damage than good, including to herself. With great courage and determination, she initiated conversations about this with each one of them:

> It was not an easy thing to open this up for discussion with my sisters and my nephews. What exactly happened there, how there was over interference on my part…

Genet was only 12 when she arrived in Israel, her adolescent years were fraught with challenges which she dealt with on her own. There was no one to listen to her, she says of herself 'I had to drown'. Because of these experiences she wished to help her younger siblings and nephews, figuratively to save them from drowning. But her authoritative attitude, based on the cultural hierarchy she knew, did not leave room for attentive consultation. She has learnt a valuable lesson from these experiences, now implemented on her own children, with whom she has shifted her base of authority from status to connection. In her nephew's interview, Addis mentions both Genet and her brother as people he can always rely upon to be attentive and helpful, indicating that despite her misgivings that was what she was.

Tigist, the eldest daughter in the family, is very involved with her younger brothers' upbringing, when she talks about them, she inadvertently refers to them as '*my children*'. She states that her motivation is twofold; to save her parents frustration and to advance her brothers education.

> I know my parents would be disappointed. Often, it's silly things they get in trouble for, like their behaviour. How hard can it be to behave?! Really! Often, they hide the notes the teacher sends.

The situation has become such that these notes are now hidden from the sister as well, because 'sometimes they say I am even harsher than our parents!' But she is careful to keep an open channel of communication with them:

> I always ask them, *did something happen?* They say, *no nothing*. They know our parents can't read the notes, they just hide them.

One of her brothers, a teenager, was at her home when I arrived for the interview. She said they practically live with her; it is a second home to them.

When Habtam's older siblings moved to boarding school, she became the eldest child at home:

> If they need something in the family, they always call me. It's not just the emotional connection, it's the responsibility, I am the centre of the home.

Habtam no longer lives at home, but over the years her academic success and job promotions have enhanced her role as 'the centre' in their perception. Habtam says:

> They see it like this—*she already finished her degree, she can help.*

Often families will choose one child as the responsible one, and all requests will be channelled his or her way. For Habtam, despite now living further away from her family than all her other siblings, this is still the case:

> My younger brother needs help because of his medical condition. I actually raised him, I used to change his diapers. Now I want him to make the right choices. Sometimes the big sister has to say tough things, then he doesn't talk to me for two weeks, but overall, our connection is strong. The other two sisters, who were there all our childhood, are attached to my veins.

Newly married and trying to make her own life, her parents' attempts to keep her involved in what is going on at home, via frequent telephone updates carrying implicit expectations of her, she finds irksome:

> When they tell me, say, *this sister did that, and the other one did this, and your brother doesn't feel well,* and I'm here, it's exacerbating, because why are you telling me this? I have my own problems…

Her sister Maayan says in her interview:

> The people most attentive to me are Orna and Habtam. I can talk and share with them.

Sometimes this might be a burden, but Habtam is happy to help her siblings, for example:

> My elder sister is completing her undergraduate degree at the age of forty. She needed a lot of encouragement, there were many crises of *why do I need this?!* So I am always there for her.

Many studies have found that although filial responsibility may sometimes be a burden, it also enhances self-worth, providing a sense of purpose and self-fulfilment (for example Kashi, 2010; Bergelson et al., 2015). This is a good example of resilience being contextual and dependent on connection, since in these studies it was the intermediate 1.5 generation, whose parents appreciated and encouraged them, who felt a sense of purpose and fulfilment, which does not in itself negate the burden. In other words, protective processes associated with resilience are not either good or bad, it is the context which will shape the outcome (Ungar, 2011). And part of the complexity associated with resilience is that the same process may simultaneously be enhancing and cumbersome.

Tareke (G1) states explicitly that when he arrived in Israel he transferred the responsibility for the younger children to his older children. Liora, his daughter, remembers this, being told to go to her siblings' parent evenings instead of her parents. She sighs and pulls a face indicating this was hard, but also makes a dismissive gesture with her hand. Perhaps one has to remember that in Ethiopia teenage children were expected to participate in many chores, they often took care of their siblings, and some were already becoming parents themselves. With this in mind, filial responsibility in Israel seems proportionately a piece of cake.

Ester is the second child in her family, but the first girl. When I asked her who influences her most, she thought for a while and then answered; 'I think I do. I influence the others at home'. Even her older brother asks for her advice, and when he had issues with the army she says:

> I talked to my father and told him what needed to be done. My father said *you are right*. Also, when something bad happens at home I tell my father he needs to do this and that and he says *yes you are right.*

Coping with the authorities, whether it is school or the army, inevitably brings the older siblings to the aid of their parents. Choosing a suitable school, preparing preschoolers for the transition, parent evenings, buying the necessary books and notebooks, keeping tabs on their progress, all these and more often become the responsibility of older siblings. As Naama explains:

> It's very hard, I think it's too much to leave my mother to cope with all that on her own.

Naama shares the burden with her mother, because she does not want to 'leave her alone with it all' as she says repeatedly. Even though her father is at home, Naama is adamant that he would never take a role in relation to these things.

Shy has an extensive extended family of siblings, nephews and nieces, he says unequivocally:

> Amongst the Ethiopians, you don't just raise your biological children, you raise the whole family.

Members of Shy's extended family often turn to him for help:

> God-be-blessed there have been children who got into trouble. I can't say I got them out of it, but I did *help* them get out of it. When they quarrelled with their parents. Or got in trouble in nightclubs, or ran away from the army, or secluded themselves at home... God forbid there are a lot of children who choose suicide.

Aware of the many risks facing youth effectively detached from their families, Shy has been attentive and actively helpful to youth of the second generation for years. Liora has always supported him in this, to the extent that they fostered two orphaned brothers for a long period of time, one of them even came with them to visit Ethiopia.

Few participants in my study mentioned their responsibilities as primarily that of translation, in other words filial responsibility is not just a matter of language. In fact, those who spoke about translating in parent evenings described this as *cultural translation*. As Ester explains:

> What translation? It's not that they spoke in Amharic and I translated for them, because my parents knew Hebrew. It wasn't that my mother could not speak Hebrew, she could. I just understood better, so I explained things to them, in such a way that they would understand. In Hebrew, not in Amharic.

This situation, of a teacher conversing with a child in the parents evening, and having the child explain to the parent in simple Hebrew, is absurdly common. Tigist talked about it with indignation:

> Every time one of my brothers got a letter from school, my mother asked me to go with her, because she did not understand what it was about. I entered the classroom with her, and the teacher would talk to me not to her, telling me *tell your mother* ...I said to her: ***you** tell her! And if she doesn't understand I'll explain some more.*

14.6 Dana and Her Brothers

Most siblings did not express any special hardship in their filial responsibilities, beyond what was mentioned above. Dana was the exception. Repeatedly during her interview Dana described the pain inflicted upon her by taking care of her sick brothers:

> I am raising children who are not mine and paying for my mother's mistakes.

Dana's three older brothers are mentally ill and have spent many years in and out of mental institutions. Her mother has been struggling with this alone since her father effectively 'left her alone with this' as Dana says. In the beginning of the interview, in describing her family, Dana spoke of her brothers as 'not very successful', it was only towards the end of the interview that she found the words to describe the very difficult situation in her family. With no one else there to help her mother cope, Dana has been taking sporadic responsibility for a long time and paying a heavy price, as her narrative shows:

> Sometimes I feel I am falling together with them. [....] They try to save themselves through me.

Three years ago, Dana moved away from home to study for her degree, but her mother still often calls her back to help (a 2-h bus ride). On one such occasion Dana became ill, 'with both physical and mental pain', she adds 'I killed myself', explaining that the effort of trying to help was what damaged her.

There is also a younger brother, Dana's face lights up as she talks about him:

> He always compliments me, he calls me *the normal one*, he is sweet, he is wonderful. I was the first one he called when he passed his driving test. He said *because of you, I did it for you, you were the one I thought of.*

After saying this she fell silent for a while, and when I reflected that she was available and supportive for her younger brother in a way that nobody had been for her, she smiled and said:

> I never thought of that, you know... I never thought that he talks to me, shares things, and it helps him. I was taught that if you tell, you need to do something. Now that you say that it really empowers me to think that just talking about things can help. He would never talk to our mother, only to me. I have a different attitude.

Dana is struggling on the fine divide between her desire to help her older brothers, and her own need for independence and time to study, support herself and build a relationship with her partner. But she is also struggling with the fear of 'what is their effect on me?' which has become an anxiety about 'losing myself'. Her understanding, following our conversation, that she is a tremendous help to her healthy, younger brother, seems to fill her with optimism and self-efficacy. I think what a tremendous burden this young woman carries, and how courageous of her to move away and begin her own life, challenging herself with work and studies. When I compliment her on her academic achievements she smiles again.

Dana is extracting herself from an impossibly difficult family situation with great efforts while not turning her back on either her mother or her siblings. The context in which she grew up was unsupportive both at home and at school, repeatedly she refers to herself as 'an unprotected child' when describing her childhood. Dana experienced *double rejection*,[1] she also fits Mulu the social worker's description of vulnerable siblings born into a family of 'people who are broken'. Her resilience under such circumstances is remarkable, and a testament to the complexity of family dynamics, able to be simultaneously both stressful and supportive. Although there is obvious tension between Dana and her mother, of whom she is very critical,

[1] Described in Chap. 10.

the relationship also seems symbiotic. Even the father, whom Dana says is 'not functional as a father', has been significant in strengthening her ethnic roots by teaching her Amharic, she talked about them reading together as their 'warm connection'. It is these roots she leans upon to buffer the effects of experienced racism and develop her ethnic identity.[2] Although her supportive role in the family from a young age is cumbersome to Dana, sometimes to breaking point, she also derives self-esteem from her ability to help. Her most positive and empowering relationship seems to be with her younger brother, she positively glows when talking about him. He seems to be a great source of joy to Dana, providing her with encouragement, optimism, and a sense of self-worth. Thus, although challenged by her family situation, paradoxically this has also forged her resilience along culturally meaningful pathways that enable her to overcome and even develop as a role model for her younger brother.

14.7 The Effects of Role Reversal on the Intermediate 1.5 Generation

For families to be inclusive and attentive to the needs of all their members, they must each create what Bergman and Cohen (2004) have coined *the golden pathway*, ensuring equilibrium between family members' differing needs. This *golden pathway* is constantly re-evaluated and re-defined according to personal development and changing circumstances. After transition, at the meeting point of cultures with opposing cultural pathways, when life becomes unsettled, this *golden pathway* may be impossible to find. It is dependent upon a unique balance, specific to each family, on the continuum between differentiation and fusion. The difference is the degree of autonomy; differentiation enables family members to function without feeling responsible for or hindered by other family members. While fusion limits autonomy, stressing mutual responsibility and influence (Williamson & Bray, 1988). The balance between differentiation and fusion is also culturally determined, therefore the transition from a collectivistic to an individualistic society upsets any pre-established equilibrium. As the balance of knowledge and coping abilities between the generations shifts with immigration, roles are reversed, and filial responsibility coupled with cultural changes displace parental authority. The interviews in my study reflect several effects of this on Ethiopian immigrant families in Israel:

- Traditional family cohesion enhances the sense of responsibility felt by G1.5 to help their parents and siblings. But since they were raised to see themselves as part of a community, this is generally not perceived by them as making a great personal sacrifice.

[2] Described in Chap. 10.

- The traditional family hierarchy and inter-generational respectful distance effectively annihilated by role reversal and filial responsibility after immigration enhance the sense of inferiority and helplessness in the older generation.
- Culturally flexible families provide a more supportive atmosphere that enables role reversal and filial responsibility to coexist alongside a mutually supportive relationship between the generations. This is inclusive of supporting networks crisscrossing the family structure vertically and horizontally (in other words, support can come from cousins, siblings, aunts, uncles, etc.).
- It is striking the extent to which G1.5 take responsibility for family cohesion and actively perceive themselves as inter-generational and inter-cultural bridges.

These findings are reiterated by other studies, showing many factors effecting the benefits or detriments of role reversal. For example, Kashi (2010) in his study of Ethiopian immigrants of the intermediate, 1.5 generation, asked about their experiences in the family before and after immigration, especially regarding changes in family roles. Their answers reflected that new roles adopted after immigration (such as translation, giving advice, mediation, financial help, and educational supervision of younger siblings) was anchored in the culture, and therefore had no negative effects. In fact, quite the opposite, most of his interviewees felt that these roles gave them independence, responsibility, and self-worth and that their parents were proud of them.

Similarly in a study on Russian immigrants in Israel, Kosner et al. (2014) found that what helped young people cope with role reversal was family and community support, a sense of self-fulfilment and personal strength. Another study by Oznobishin and Kurman (2009) on Russian immigrants in Israel found that role reversal created psychological stress and difficulty in adjustment, but that this was mediated by supportive parenting. Bergelson et al. (2015) identified three parameters affecting G1.5 in coping with role reversal; clarity (understanding their surroundings and being able to give meaning to events), optimism, and support networks. The former two were found most significant, and the emotional reaction to role reversal most important for long-term psychological adjustment. An important finding was that role reversal can arouse both positive and negative feelings, as young people felt personal importance and capability in helping their families, but at the same time often struggled with too much responsibility.

14.8 The Effects of Role Reversal on the First Generation

'Our era is over, this is the time of the children', says Mamu, and Genet explains her uncle's statement:

> This is the role reversal, there [Ethiopia] he was the leader, here he is led [by the younger generation].

While her grandfather Berihun talks of 'not having a voice' and lacking local knowledge. These men have lost their traditional authority in the community, as their wisdom is often undervalued as irrelevant, and the younger generation educated in Israel have taken the lead in decision making. Berihun says:

> We have become the ones who don't know, our minds and our hearts are closed.

In Ethiopia the elders of the community could even make decisions about the grandchildren against their parents' wishes, for example to keep the grandchildren with them when the parents left for Israel (as in the case of Dov and Naama). But in Israel the younger generation, knowledgeable and competent in their new surroundings, are now making decisions for their elders. Thus, Abynesh's teenage daughters found themselves boarding schools against her will, and later found her a job, and Naama tells Yafit how to do things 'the right way'. The younger generation have also taken over symbolical functions at home, for example in most families they are the ones to initiate and implement the traditional *kiddush*[3] normally performed by the head of the household. As described by Yaniv, Matan and Dov, in many homes it is one of the sons who initiates the ceremony, while the final act of blessing the bread is reverted to the father or grandfather as an act of reverence. This is a significant compromise in tradition which breaks the hierarchy, its acceptance enables the elders to save face, maintaining the semblance of their status while conceding to their new position and effectively accepting the role reversal. But the acceptance is provisional, becoming dependent on their children for translation and guidance makes the older generation feel that 'we left our dignity in Ethiopia', as Eneye put it. Even Yafit (G1.5) who respects and admires her parents does not see them as her primary source of guidance, saying:

> I have nothing to learn from them except how to love my family.

The younger, second generation, do not even necessarily admire or respect their elders. Yaniv describes his father as 'innocent' and like 'a small child', their relationship is summarized by his statement that 'I hardly feel his presence'. Addis describes his father as 'introverted' and 'living in his own bubble'. These are sad examples of first-generation immigrants who have relinquished their role in the family, shutting themselves off in defiant silence against the changes over which they have no control. They are trying to maintain their dignity by making themselves unavailable, effectively at the price of severed or tenuous connections. Yet, there are families in which the older generation struggle to adapt and remain involved in the lives of their children and grandchildren. For example, Tareke says:

> We arrived in a country populated not only by people but by God. We need to be present and mingle with the population. I want to be with all of them, not to differentiate myself as Ethiopian. I am part of the Jewish people.

Tareke is an optimistic man, he sees Israeli reality as providing endless opportunities for young people and encourages them to study and get ahead and not bother

[3] Ceremonial reception of the Sabbath before the Friday evening meal

themselves with differentiation, a sense of inferiority and prejudice. Tareke is not concerned with his lost status or maintaining the traditional hierarchy, he wants the younger generation to fit in and demand equality through hard work and ambition:

> You can be anything, even prime minister, just study, mingle, get involved.

Similarly, Dany has relinquished his status for connection; 'I am like the child, they are like the parents', he says smiling as he talks about his children. He describes his relationship with them as 'not like a father, like a friend'. Dany has embraced change to his advantage to remain an influence in his growing children's lives. He does so amicably, no longer expecting his children to follow his lead. For example, he has come to terms with the fact that none of them are religious, saying:

> I don't want to burden them. If you burden them [with demands] it comes in the way of love.

This father is focused on maintaining connection with his children, not controlling them. He goes on to explain how parents who try to limit their children and make decisions for them reach the point where:

> The children don't tell their parents anything, they have no connection with their parents.

Historical and technological developments inevitably lead to changes in power relations and the balance of knowledge between the generations, regardless of immigration. But the latter adds instability and cultural collision *within* the family, the resultant stress often coexists with loving, caring relationships. For example, Naama frequently advises her mother, even 'sometimes I preach morality, which is really inappropriate'. The boundaries of legitimate role reversal are tricky. She says Yafit 'gets annoyed', when her daughter crosses it, but they manage to stay on good terms. Yafit has given up on maintaining a respectful distance between the generations, their communication is open and direct. And yet her daughter says that because 'of her ego' her mother refuses to ask for help, although she does share her feelings with her daughter, who listens without reciprocating. A similar pattern exists between Orna and her mother Eneye, it appears that there is a role reversal in this respect as well: parents are leaning on their children but not vice versa—it is a one-sided support system. The younger generation are practical and realistic, acting upon current events and circumstances, while the older generation often act according to fixed cultural norms and expectations. Thus, Naama says explicitly:

> I don't really listen to them because I'm not sure from what perspective they are passing judgement.

Naama is aware that her father's advice is based on 'wanting to be like everybody else'. Orna says that her husband tries to educate his children according to what other people will say, and not according to a persistent educational doctrine he has chosen. In Ethiopia the cultural norm determined behaviour, as in many societies, people were very concerned with 'what others will say'. Thus, culture shapes behaviour less through personal conviction on values and ethics and more through concern about how other people in the same culture perceive this behaviour (Swidler, 1986).

Yaniv says about his mother that she:

> cares a great deal what other people think about her, what they might say… my father is much more closed up. That's their generation.

Yaniv's description gives a concise summary of the first generation: women attuned to Ethiopian traditional norms and men who have fallen silent. Edna is furious about this pattern of behaviour; '*what others will say*. If I judge my community, it is for this!' As has been described in previous chapters, her father, Kabede, persistently ignored 'what others will say' even in Ethiopia, and instead raised his children according to his own conscience and opinions. Thus, families navigate cultural pathways in constant dialogue with tradition, convoluted by immigration which adds personal and collective negotiation of more than one cultural system. 'What others will say' becomes a dubious basis for determining strategies of action, as the various 'others' will all say different things.

It might be postulated that for the older generation, living in ethnic enclaves might be more supportive and conducive to wellbeing than pressuring for their increased integration. This was the conclusion of a qualitative study on Egyptian immigrants who came to America above the age of 60 (Girgis, 2020). All participants spoke Arabic as their primary language and identified nationally as Egyptian, living in ethnic enclaves provided them with space to comfortably practice their culture and religion as well as resilience to cope with their unsettled lives post-immigration. The immigrant community acted as a protective factor that buffered prejudices and discrimination experienced outside it and enabled the immigrants to maintain traditional lifestyles.

Many of the elders in my study reminisced about their lives in Ethiopia, Girgis (2020) notes that reminiscence can serve as a way for enjoyment and remembering good and happy times, as well as serving as a life review process enhancing a sense of reconciliation. If resilience is context based, it seems that the context of immigrant enclaves has the upside of enhancing resilience by providing a safe place of belonging, especially for the older generation whose adaptation to new and often somewhat hostile environments is that much harder.

14.9 Resilience in Face of Bias, Stereotyping, and Discrimination

One of the biggest challenges to immigrants is coping with prejudice and discrimination, or as Lamont et al. (2013) put it 'being over scrutinized, overlooked, underappreciated, misunderstood, and disrespected'. Obviously, this is also a challenge for other, indigenous minority communities. Handling this is both an individual and a communal task, involving a renegotiation of personal and group identity as well as a constant struggle for social inclusion and equal access to local and national resources. Historical and political contexts create shared narratives that buffer the effects of exclusion and stigmatization and forge common group processes for dealing with all this. For Jewish ethnic groups in Israel such as immigrants from African and Arab countries, these narratives are rooted in Zionism, emphasizing their inherent legitimacy of arrival and citizenship. Whereas for Arabs in Israel these narratives are rooted in common humanity and universal human dignity (Mizrachi & Herzog, 2012).

In a recent newspaper article (Steinberg, 2023) Shmuel Yilma, who founded the Yerusalem Forum in 2016, is quoted:

> Ethiopians don't get equal treatment in Israel. There was a problem of low expectations, a lack of opportunities, racism, I understood that in order to fix all that, it had to come from the community itself.

Yilma quotes a survey[4] conducted in Israel in 2019 showing that 33% of Jews responded as not wanting their children to marry Ethiopian Israelis, 22% still doubting the Judaism of Beta Israel, 16% not wanting to live near Ethiopian Israelis, 15% considering the Ethiopian immigration a mistake, 10% who refuse to work with an Ethiopian superior, and 9% who object to their children even learning about the Ethiopian community. Since then in the space of 4 years Israel has had five elections, fierce political rivalry playing on common fears and ethnic loyalty consistently add fuel to an already volatile situation, affecting especially minorities and marginalized groups.

According to Engdau-Vanda (2019) general social and economic inequalities coupled with the prevalent public discourse on ethnicity and open expressions of racism are the main challenges facing the Ethiopian community in Israel. In addition, the dissolution of traditional community and family support networks after immigration, the dependency fostered by state policies, and sending teenagers to boarding schools, have weakened family and community support networks. Many members of the community experience social exclusion causing marginalization and feelings of alienation. The participants in her study, who arrived as children via Sudan 30 or so years ago, speak of various coping methods, like the narratives in my study and roughly corresponding to Lamont et al.'s (2013) coping strategies: enhancing individual autonomy and self-definitions, enhancing group identification, adopting a universalistic narrative, or some combination of all of these. This is still an on-going process that has far from been resolved.

The first major protest by Ethiopian Jews in Israel took place in 1985 over recognition of their Jewish identity, in which elders of the community undertook a hunger strike in a massive demonstration opposite the Chief Rabbinate Council in Jerusalem.

Since then, various overt expressions of racism have sparked collective protests and demonstrations:

- In 1996 after it became public knowledge that blood donations by Ethiopian immigrants and their offspring were discarded without their knowledge, 10,000 members of the community demonstrated opposite the prime minister's offices,

[4] By Midgam Research & Consulting.

41 policemen and 20 demonstrators were injured, parked cars in the vicinity were vandalized.

- In 2006 when it was publicized that blood donations by Ethiopian immigrants and their offspring were still not being used, the protests instigated a change in this policy brought into effect in 2007, but only with respect to the offspring of Ethiopian immigrants born in Israel.
- In 2013 a team collecting blood donations from Members of Knesset refused to accept a donation from an Ethiopian minister, sparking further demonstrations attended this time by many veteran Israelis and other immigrants. The rules regarding the blood donations were effectively changed only in 2017.
- In 2012 a television documentary reported a secret agreement between homeowners in Kiriyal Malachi not to sell houses to Ethiopian immigrants so that their properties would not be devalued. This sparked a local protest and a big demonstration in Jerusalem in 2013.
- In 2015 an Ethiopian Israeli soldier was beaten up by policemen for no apparent reason, an incident inadvertently caught on camera that led to a series of massive demonstrations all over the country. Prominent in these demonstrations were also pictures of a teenager who had mysteriously been found dead after controversy with the police. Frequent altercations between Ethiopian Israeli youth and police brutality familiar to the immigrant community nationwide were the triggers that fuelled the anger, frustration, and even violence in some of these demonstrations. Following these protests, the police instigated a plan to improve relations with the Ethiopian Israeli community including enlisting more Ethiopians, opening community policing centres and training for cultural competence. Another result of the demonstrations was the establishment of an interministry team to consider ways of reducing racism, which in turn led to the formation of a government unit for coordinating efforts against racism based in the Ministry of Justice in 2016, headed by a talented young Ethiopian Israeli lawyer.
- In 2019 two tragic incidents sparked further nationwide demonstrations, some of them violent: the death of a disturbed young man shot by police who were summoned by his family after he left home with a knife, and the death of an 18-year-old shot by an off-duty policeman. The Ethiopian community count various other cases of young people who mysteriously found their death after altercations with the police.

In a study conducted before the 2015 demonstrations, Abu et al. (2017) examined perceptions of Ethiopian Israelis regarding the police. They attempted to explain the apparent paradox between these negative perceptions based on felt discrimination and their relatively high levels of trust in the police. It seemed then that despite the frustrations of the community in feeling stigmatized, their strong desire to integrate and gain membership of Israeli society on an equal basis inspired coping strategies that enhanced confidence in the establishment and even specifically the police. But the events since then seem to have changed this situation. A more recent report by the State Comptroller of Israel (2021) shows the Ethiopian Israeli population disproportionately represented in 2019 in arrests (5.6% of all youth arrests, over three times their percentage in the population, 1.7%), in the opening of police files (almost twice as many police files opened for adults 3.2%) and indictments (32.6% compared to 26.8% in the general population, while files referred to a non-criminal resolution for youth 34% compared with 43% from the general population). Perhaps, it is therefore not surprising that this study found only 13% of the Ethiopian community answered positively to having confidence in the police, in contrast to 56% of the general population. It is also worth noting that now (2023) there are significant numbers of Ethiopian Israeli policemen, who make an important contribution to instigating change in the relations between the community and the police.

My interviews were conducted between 2014 and 2017, the issue of relations with the police and resultant demonstrations entered the narratives,[5] but were not the focus of conversation, which concentrated more on how people cope with discrimination on a personal and familial basis. What follows is a discussion on this, followed by a discussion on common themes in community leadership attempting to thwart the effects of discrimination and enhance the wellbeing of the Ethiopian Israeli community.

14.10 Personal and Familial Strategies for Coping with Discrimination

Many second-generation participants in my study spoke of ignoring and overlooking prejudicial remarks as their preferred coping method. Thus, Addis talks about 'moving on' and focusing on his own goals and aspirations rather than getting bogged down in feeling discriminated against. It is something he tries to teach his mother (G1) when she gets upset about incidents of discrimination, which happens often:

> My mother adjusted quickly [to Israeli society], but anything they say to her she takes it personally and gets offended, if they mention her skin colour she takes it really hard. My father, in contrast, he doesn't care. He says *so such and such happened, forget it, just keep going, let them explode not you!* My father is very introverted, apathetic, he just doesn't react. I think this attitude saves our community.

Apathy is generally not regarded as positive behaviour, but it can be a protective mechanism in face of discrimination. As Ungar (2008) noted, all reactions to discrimination can be seen as a manifestation of resilience, even if they result in maladaptive behaviours. By using apathy Addis's father is distancing himself from insult and hurt, he is figuratively putting on a suit of armour made of indifference. In contrast his mother gets upset repeatedly in face of felt discrimination, while her son Addis tries to persuade her just to 'let it go', his own methodology to remain

[5] See especially Dana's comments in the last chapter.

focused and not succumb to despair and self-pity or anger and aggression—two alternatives he regards as self-damaging. Addis adds astutely that one cannot educate others, so it is better to take care of oneself and avoid confrontation.

Matan takes the same attitude, it serves him well both in his personal life and at work:

> To let things slide, to look at things differently… at work, when they round corners, I can ignore it. I don't have to fight it or say something. This is how we were educated in Ethiopia.

Emotional restraint proves to be a powerful element in the cultural toolbox, it is something Tareke (G1) strongly recommends young people to embrace, enabling them to concentrate on their studies, army service, and jobs to counteract discrimination. He sees this as much more effective and self-enhancing than participating in demonstrations, which he fears arouse antagonism against the community.

Noam has the same sentiments following his experiences on the kibbutz, which tends to be a very closed community:

> It's like in the kibbutz, not everybody likes Ethiopians. Some people are racist. But I say, well, in our [Ethiopian] community we also have racists. So why should I argue with people? I just ignore them. Head down and that's it.

Noam is struggling for economic and social survival, he prefers to concentrate on his family's wellbeing, which is much improved on the kibbutz, rather than getting upset about bias and discrimination. His 'head down' is a choice not to see this and not an expression of despondency. Once, as a teenager, he behaved differently[6] and even got into fights, but today he says he doesn't 'get worked up about everything'. He adds that if his daughter comes home and says she was called *cushi* he tells her not to worry about it. Today Noam is practical and optimistic, not wanting to deal with the flaws of Israeli society, pointing out that the Ethiopian community has flaws too.

Addis feels that 'looking for racism everywhere, making a fuss about it', averts people from their life course and weakens them. He advises others not to go down this path:

> I have friends in combat units, and they're always frustrated, telling me that they are discriminated against. I always say to them: this is not a good attitude, you need to show them what you're worth, show them your best side, don't think like that all the time.

I heard such stories from my own children, about Ethiopian Israeli soldiers in their units who felt discriminated against. My sons voiced the opinion that this attitude made their service harder, that the service was hard for everyone, that feeling resentment just made it worse, which reiterates the adage that if one cannot change reality better to change one's attitude towards it, which is precisely what Addis admires about Genet and her brother:

> They are people who moved out of the box—*I am Ethiopian and it is hard for me*—and now they are like, *I'll show the world what I can do…*

---

[6] Discussed in Chap. 10.

There is no doubt that the narrative of the underdog is a self-fulfilling prophecy which makes it much harder to get ahead, Addis feels that the answer is excelling and not giving up on one's dreams, thus proving that the stereotypes are not true. Orna (G1.5) reiterates this and criticizes the second generation for giving up too easily and blaming their failings on discrimination.

Teruneh (G1.5), a highly competent computer engineer, was sent to mend computers in a classified security office and almost thrown out because they did not believe he was the expert sent to assist them. He tells this story with a smile, choosing not to be bitter, and says that the change will come when there are more experts of Ethiopian origin in different fields. He sees himself as a role model, saying 'I am a pioneer in my field, I hope to pave the way for others'.

Some participants, such as Tsehai and Yisrael, said they never experienced discrimination. Yisrael was often the only person of Ethiopian origin in various situations:

> Sometimes I think it would be nice if there was another Ethiopian, but even if I am the only one, I've learnt to have a sense of humour about it. I was the only one in my grade for three years, it didn't kill me. I can survive without [other Ethiopians]. Most of the time I don't worry about it, I never experienced or was never aware of any discrimination.

Either these are the lucky ones, or their attitude sheltered them from unpleasant experiences. Edna sighs as she says:

> I thank God that one day I got the revelation to stop worrying about our community… If I do meet racism, it rattles me to the core, but then I remember one [white] child at school was in great distress because his parents didn't understand him, and that rattled me too.

Human suffering, whether induced by racism or other circumstances, irrespective of categories of identities, is upsetting to Edna. Unfortunately, there are always examples of this, in Israel and elsewhere, children who are not properly cared for, victims of tragic family or political situations, refugees, immigrants, homeless and unprotected. Resilience is built on interaction, whether it be a sound home-base and attentive relatives, or other people who come to the rescue in lieu of these, such as an attentive teacher like Edna.

14.11 Leadership and Activism in Face of Discrimination

Several participants in my study mentioned the journey from Ethiopia to Sudan repeatedly as a testament to personal, familial, and community resilience. Sometimes the story of the journey was what they chose to tell me when I asked them to describe their families, inevitably containing painful memories of losses and separations. Habtam specifically distinguished the narrative of heroism and personal initiative she heard at home from the narrative of Israelis rescuing a weak stranded community which she heard at school. It was this dissonance in the narratives that caused Shmuel Yilma to found the Yerusalem Forum in 2016, which has since produced various educational materials, conferences, and annual activities emphasizing the bravery and heroism of the leaders in the community who initiated and implemented the journey at great risk to themselves.[7]

Engdau-Vanda (2019) interviewed 20 people in their late 20s or early 30s who emigrated to Israel by walking from Ethiopia to Sudan when they were 4–10 years old. This qualitative study examines their coping mechanisms for the journey and after arrival through their own narratives. The emphasis falls on collective identification and action while appropriating the story of the journey as symbolic of collective resilience. The journey to Israel which included walking from Ethiopia to Sudan and overcoming all odds to arrive is a source of ethnic pride. The children who made this journey and are adults today would like this story to be better known as part of the Zionist narrative imprinted in collective Israeli history, giving them legitimacy to belong and reflecting the bravery and resilience of the community. At the same time there seems to be a dissonance between their personal integration, regarded by the participants as positive, and their view of the community as failing to integrate. Engdau-Vanda explains this as a result of the many challenges facing the community, these being primarily poverty, racism, and the struggle with bureaucracy and the Israeli establishment which often does not understand them or treats them in paternalistic ways.

Yilma and many other leaders and activists from the Ethiopian Israeli community regard the story of the journey as effective in elevating self-esteem in the second generation and combating persistent discrimination and racism, together with other initiatives such as adding the history of Beta Yisrael to the school curriculum, leadership programs for youth and trips to Ethiopia. Jaffe-Schagen (2016) suggests that re-creating Ethiopian heritage 30 years after their arrival will not undo all the mistakes made by the establishment in their absorption or counteract discrimination. Which of course is true, but what it can do is give the second-generation valuable cultural knowledge they are not necessarily getting at home, a sense of belonging to a thriving resilient community with a rich cultural heritage, as well as creating a cultural bridge between the two worlds they are living in and often finding difficult to negotiate between.

I have discussed transition as involving a process of negotiation with change that occurs in the gaps between cultures, between social structures, and between the possibilities of change and continuance. When this process involves the merging of religious and cultural beliefs, customs, and practices it is called syncretism, and the result is the creation of new tradition (Sharaby, 2021). I have also described the intermediate generation (G1.5) as often acting as a bridge between the older and the younger generations, being culturally competent in both the home and the host culture, able to mediate between the two and provide valuable support to the second generation. Sharaby analysed the process whereby four prominent leaders in the Ethiopian immigrant community, all from the intermediate 1.5 generation, instigated this change. Their strategies of action involved creating partnerships, gaining recognition, and funding from national institutions as they combined protesting

[7] https://www.forumyerusalem.org/english

discrimination with transforming the Sigd[8] into a national Israeli holiday recognized by the Israeli establishment since 2008. Effectively, they elevated this specifically Ethiopian festival into Israeli mainstream culture in a way that enhanced ethnic self-esteem as well as the public image of the entire community. As Sharaby has noted, this radical change is very significant for several reasons: firstly, it reshapes and preserves ethnic identity while emphasizing Jewish ancestry and customs, strengthening the position of this immigrant community whose very legitimacy as Jews has often been doubted. Secondly, the celebration itself has been reformed as a bridge between the generations in this community, enabling new joint negotiation of traditions within families. As we have seen in previous chapters, the breakdown in communication between the generations is a major crisis in many families. We have also seen that traditionally emotional expression is based on actions rather than words (Chap. 7). Joint celebrations of the Sigd festival combining traditional and new customs provide new channels of connection within the family based on *doing* rather than *talking*. An additional dialogue between the young G1.5 leaders and the Kessoch enabled an adaptation of the celebrations to formats suiting both the older and the younger generations. Thirdly, achieving the official status of the Sigd as a new national holiday in Israel creates positive interaction between the immigrant community and the host society while enabling continuity of traditions. Today the Sigd is celebrated all over Israel in schools and community centres, tens of thousands of people (not only of Ethiopian origin) arrive every year to the main event in Jerusalem. In Tel Aviv the 'Sigdiyada' event gives prominence to Ethiopian artists, performers, and film makers, attended by thousands of people every year. Smaller events are held all over the country, on many occasions celebrating the Sigd has become a symbol of both appreciation and acceptance of the Ethiopian community alongside a much-needed atmosphere of general inter-cultural tolerance.

The importance of the trips to Ethiopia undertaken by the second generation, most of whom either were never there or were so young when they arrived that they have no tangible memories of Ethiopia, can be illustrated by Maayan. Her parents were very opposed to her journey:

> They tried to persuade me not to go. They said *what have you got to do over there? We have no family there!* After they realized I was really going they started giving me tips… when I came back and showed them photos, they got emotional and also understood how important it was for me to go, what it meant to me…they kept saying, *now you understand, now you know…'*

Maayan was born in Sudan and arrived in Israel as a baby, I have discussed in previous chapters her sense of *double rejection*, feeling often that she did not belong either at home or with her peers. The journey was a healing process in which she re-connected both to her roots, and on her return, to her parents:

> I re-evaluated my life here, things came into proportion […] Suddenly I understood my parents better. Why they are so hard, so unavailable… I understood the great transition they have made and the difficulties they had…

[8] An explanation on this festival and discussion of Sigd celebrations in schools appears in Chap. 10.

Maayan's journey included a deep identification with her family's story and seeing herself as part of that story strengthened her self-image. The fact that she had initiated and executed the journey by herself also built her self-confidence.

> Only at university I began to understand how important it is to be connected to one's home, one's parents… until you go there [to Ethiopia] you cannot understand. Not via picture or videos. To be there was to understand that if I had grown up there, I would have been like them, those children.

Maayan's descriptions of her childhood were full of difficulties forged on the cultural divide included many misunderstandings with her parents. Understanding them, getting a glimpse of the world through their eyes by visiting the place they came from, enabled Maayan to sense that any rejection she felt as a child was *cultural* and not *personal*. Coming to terms with her own complex identity through her journey to Ethiopia has been a milestone in her personal development. Mok and Morris (2009) explain how environmental stimulation, such as odours, taste, or vision, arouse subconscious associations of cultural knowledge which trigger appropriate thought processes. Oyserman and Lee (2008) call this cultural priming. Being in Ethiopia had this effect on many young people who made the journey, awakening dormant memories and arousing a deep connection with their parents and their past.[9] This effect is also described by Kalnisky et al. (2015) who accompanied groups of students training to be teachers on this journey, which unfolds as a process enabling internal acceptance of their complex mixed identities. This last study followed both personal and professional development and considers the effect of the journey to Ethiopia as crucial in both, clearing away ambivalent feelings and inconsistencies and helping the students live harmoniously with a healthy hybrid identity. Not being accepted, feeling rejected because of discrimination or prejudice, has powerful personal and collective effects (Montalvo & Gutierrez, 1988). It was precisely this, recognizing the personal and professional significance of self-acceptance and developing resilience out of a viable hybrid identity, that inspired the staff at Ahva academic teaching college to initiate the journeys as part of the study program to become teachers.

In this chapter, I have attempted to delve into the intricacies of resilience in immigrant families coping simultaneously with many changes, especially role reversal and filial responsibility on the backdrop of bias, stereotyping, and discrimination. The narratives of participants in my study as well as examples from other

[9] Only three people from my study travelled to Ethiopia for a visit (Maayan, Shy, and Tigist). Since this seemed an important issue, I posted a request on Facebook to contact young people who were born in Israel (or arrived as infants) and had travelled to Ethiopia as young adults. Twelve people (ten women and two men, eight G2 and 4 G1.5) answered me and agreed to share their experiences about this. Nine of them were in their twenties when they made the journey, the others were in their thirties. All but one described the journey as a formative experience which changed both their relationship with their parents and their own self-image. Many of them spoke of the overwhelming sense of homecoming even though they had either never been there before or only as infants. This subject is worthy of further detailed study. Another interesting source on this matter is Anteby-Yemini (2005).

studies have been used to illustrate how individuals, families, and communities negotiate such complex, often very stressful, situations using culturally specific tools such as reciprocity, joint responsibility, and emotional distancing as well as sheer determination and innovative methodologies such as creativity in maintaining connections, syncretism, shared protest, and visits to the country of origin. All these examples reflect the social basis of resilience and the interplay of interaction with context to create culturally meaningful pathways towards wellbeing.

References

Abu, O., Yuval, F., & Ben-Porat, G. (2017). Race, racism, and policing: Responses of Ethiopian Jews in Israel to stigmatization by the police. *Ethnicities, 17*(5), 688–706.

Anteby-Yemini, L. (2005). From Ethiopian villager to global villager: Ethiopian Jews in Israel. In A. Weingrod & A. Levy (Eds.), *Homelands and diasporas: Holy lands and other places* (pp. 220–244). Stanford University Press.

Bergelson, Y. P., Kurman, J., & Roer-Strier, D. (2015). Immigrant's emotional reactions to filial responsibilities and related psychological outcomes. *International Journal of Intercultural Relations, 45*, 104–115.

DeFrain, J., & Asay, S. (2014). An introduction to the families strength perspective. In J. DeFrain & S. Asay (Eds.), *Strong families around the world: Strengths-based research and perspectives* (pp. 1–10). Routledge.

Falicov, C. (1988). Family sociology and family therapy contributions to the family development framework: A comparative analysis and thoughts on future trends. In C. Falicov (Ed.), *Family transitions: Continuity & change over the life cycle* (pp. 3–54). Guildford Press.

Girgis, I. (2020). Protective factors and processes fostering resilience and buffering psychosocial distress among later-life Egyptian immigrants. *Journal of Gerontological Social Work, 63*(1–2), 41–77.

Jaffe-Schagen, J. (2016). Creating space. The construction of Ethiopian heritage and memory in Israel. *Annales d'Éthiopie, 31*(1), 81–105.

Joselevich, E. (1988). Family transitions, cumulative stress and crisis. In C. Falicov (Ed.), *Family transitions: Continuity and change over the life cycle* (pp. 273–292). Guildford Press.

Kashi, A. (2010). *Ethiopian immigrants: Perception on role reversal in the family following immigration*. PhD thesis, Hebrew University Jerusalem.

Kosner, A., Roer-Strier, D., & Kurman, J. (2014). Changing familial roles for immigrant adolescents from the former Soviet Union to Israel. *Journal of Adolescent Research, 29*(3), 356–379.

Lamont, M., Welburn, J., & Fleming, C. (2013). Responses to discrimination and social resilience under neoliberalism the United States compared. In P. A. Hall & M. Lamont (Eds.), *Social resilience in the neoliberal era* (pp. 129–157). Cambridge University Press.

Mizrachi, N., & Herzog, H. (2012). Participatory destigmatization strategies among Palestinian citizens of Israel, Ethiopian Jews and Mizrahi Jews. *Ethnic and Racial Studies, 35*(3), 418–435.

Mok, A., & Morris, M. (2009). Cultural chameleons and iconclasts: Assimilation and reactance to cultural cues. Bicultural expressed personalities as a function of identity conflict. *Journal of Experimental Social Psychology, 45*, 884–889.

Montalvo, B., & Gutierrez, M. (1988). The emphasis on cultural identity. In C. Falicov (Ed.), *Family transitions: Continuity and change over the life cycle* (pp. 181–210). Guildford Press.

Motti-Stefanidi, F. (2018). Resilience among immigrant youth: The role of culture, development and acculturation. *Developmental Review, 50*, 99–109.

Motti-Stefanidi, F. (2019). Resilience among immigrant youths: Who adapts well, and why? *Current Directions in Psychological Science, 28*(5), 510–517.

Noyes, D. (2012). The social base of folklore. In R. Bendix & G. Hasan-Rokem (Eds.), *A companion to folklore* (pp. 15–39). Blackwell Publishing.

Oyserman, D., & Lee, S. W. (2008). Does culture influence what and how we think? Effects of priming individualism and collectivism. *Psychological Bulletin, 134*(2), 311–342.

Oznobishin, O., & Kurman, J. (2009). Parent-child role reversal and psychological adjustment among immigrant youth in Israel. *Journal of Family Psychology, 23*(3), 405–415.

Sharaby, R. (2021). Between cultures and generations: Ethnic activism of 1.5 generation immigrant leaders. *Journal of Ethnic and Cultural Studies, 8*(1), 270–290.

Steinberg, J. (2023). Shedding image as bystanders to history, Ethiopian Jews reclaim their exodus saga. *Times of Israel.* https://www.timesofisrael.com/shedding-image-as-bystanders-to-history-ethiopian-jews-reclaim-their-exodus-saga/

Swidler, A. (1986). Culture in action: Symbolism and strategies. *Americal Sociological Review, 51*(2), 273–286.

Ungar, M. (2008). Resilience across cultures. *British Journal of Social Work, 2008*(38), 218–235.

Ungar, M. (2011). The social ecology of resilience: Addressing contextual and cultural ambiguity of a nascent construct. *American Journal of Orthopsychiatry., 81*(1), 1–17.

Ungar, M. (2013). Resilience, trauma, context, and culture. *Trauma, Violence and Abuse., 14*(3), 255–266.

Ungar, M. (2015). Practitioner review: Diagnosing childhood resilience – A systemic approach to the diagnosis of adaptation in adverse social and physical ecologies. *Journal of Child Psychology and Psychiatry, 56*(1), 4–17.

Weisner, T. (1998). Human development, child well-being and the cultural project of development. *New Directions for Child Development., 81*, 69–86.

Williamson, D., & Bray, J. (1988). Family development and change across the generations: An intergenerational perspective. In C. Falicov (Ed.), *Family transitions: Continuity and change over the life cycle* (pp. 357–384). Guildford Press.

Younes, M. (2014). The resilience of families in Israel: Understanding their struggles and appreciating their strengths. In J. DeFrain & S. Asay (Eds.), *Strong families around the world: Strengths-based research and perspectives* (pp. 101–118). Routledge.

Hebrew References

Bergman, Z., & Cohen, E. (2004). *The family in search of equilibrium.* Tel Aviv.

Engdau-Vanda, S. (2019). *Resilience in immigration. The story of Ethiopian Jews in Israel from a perspective of 30 years.* Resling.

Herzog, E. (1998). *Bureaucracy and Ethiopian immigrants: Dependency in absorption centres.* Cherikover.

Kalnisky, A., Millet, S., & Cohen, N. (2015). *Travels of hope: Ethiopian Jews in the paths of education, academic studies and success.* Published by the Mofet Institute.

Chapter 15
Children's Wellbeing in Immigrant Families

I started this book with a personal introduction, because I feel there is a deep connection between life stories and academic research trajectories. Certainly, my own personal and family history has shaped the subjects I have chosen to prioritize in my life. Research on other families as well as introspection on my own has enabled me to see these patterns more clearly as they relate to myself, my siblings, my children. The subtle often invisible ways in which historical, social, and economic processes have deep formative influences on our lives. Even our most intimate relationships, in our families of origin and in the families we create, are embedded in social systems, shaped by cultural pathways forged between the generations over time and space. And those relationships are also not immune to the interplay of identity boxes, the stereotypes and stigmas of the societies in which they were formed, the unspoken demons lurking behind the scenes in every family. To understand family dynamics, they need to be taken into consideration, especially when discussing families in transition, building new cultural pathways forged between two or more cultural paradigms. The very nature of family relationships, the covert distribution of power and discrete stratification between family members, gender roles and expectations, concepts of childhood and adulthood, family cohesiveness, joint responsibilities and individual freedoms are all forged in wider contexts of family history and on-going interaction with places the family has lived and called home. Recognizing this is part of the process of extracting ourselves from the narrow confines of social categories which damagingly try to define us as one thing or another, mistakenly assumed to be part of who we are in some intrinsic way. To understand that what were perceived as clashes between individual family members may often have been forged not by personalities or individual traits but by social processes, assumptions, and misconceptions based on the collision of cultural pathways. That even rejection, lack of communication, painful family crisis are linked to larger scenarios of historical and social change, the making and breaking of tradition through everyday acts of construction and dissolution.

© The Author(s), under exclusive license to Springer Nature Switzerland AG 2023

N. A. Shmuel, *Children's Wellbeing in Immigrant Families*, Children's Well-Being: Indicators and Research 26,
https://doi.org/10.1007/978-3-031-31917-4_15

People are often negotiating their lives in the spaces between opposing forces pulling in opposite directions; being settled and unsettled, the paradigms of collectivism and individualism, belonging and feeling excluded, embeddedness and disconnection in family and society. These negotiations also take place in the spaces between cultures, generations, places people call home. Children of the second generation are growing up on these narrow divides, which form their habitus, it is the world they know—intricately complex and full of ambiguous, often conflicting meanings or harmoniously integrated into a variously bumpy pathway towards hybridity. It is on these narrow divides these children learn their place in family and society, their sense of self-worth, methods, and styles of communication, acquire an inherited and constantly evolving cultural toolkit. The children are not passive receptors but active agents on the family stage, introducing the host culture into immigrant families, challenging traditional assumptions by their very being, an embodiment of the changes after immigration. Natural processes that instigated gentle inter-generational transferal alongside change in settled lives have been replaced by massive multiple and sudden drastic changes which rock the family boat after immigration, often lasting throughout the childhood of the new generation. The ensuing family turmoil coupled with the challenges of the host society, segmented and confusing, including varying degrees of discrimination, form the context for growth and development.

The narratives from my study presented in this book reflect all of this, alongside the resourcefulness of families and individuals, building resilience through connection under difficult and challenging circumstances. The very building blocks for communication, verbal and non-verbal, lost or intrinsically altered in the transition, create a new fog around meanings, covert and overt messages now convoluted and misunderstood. The very process of family living, forming and maintaining the delicate balance of relationships, becomes challenging, sometimes painful. In the intimacy of the family home, where understanding and empathy are expected to be paramount, misunderstandings and conflict may thrive and take over. Differences between family members now conceived of in terms of birthplace or cultural affiliation forge deep chasms in the very fabric of family living, variations in perceptions and strategies of action create rifts between the sexes and between the generations. As the narratives from my study demonstrate, negotiating reconciliation and compromise becomes increasingly difficult, nevertheless the cultural toolkit provides various solutions, such as evasiveness, restraint, patience, reciprocity, and shared responsibility. Cultural flexibility becomes a powerful factor in family and community dynamics, buffering the culture clash, creating new options.

The fear of losing connection inspires innovative ways of maintaining family cohesion. As roles shift, the intermediate, 1.5 generation, often step up as viable cultural and inter-generational bridges, connecting family ties before they unravel, providing valuable support to both the younger and the older generations. Where they are absent a dangerous path to *double rejection* may be forged for youngsters experiencing repeatedly an impossible dissonance between themselves and their surroundings, both at home and at school. A deep vulnerability becomes an intrinsic part of their makeup, the fragility of people unanchored in ancestral heritage and social networks. And even then, sometimes people manage to overcome, to compensate by being significant in some invaluable role or by excelling in some way.

The changing balance of power within the family, defined by age and gender, creates powerful undercurrents of dissention in daily living. Often articulated in the narratives from my study using the terminology of war, the overt and covert expression of this effects patterns of communication, mutual expectations, and relative status. As *wax and gold* communication is replaced by direct unfiltered expression and the *respectful distance* is erased, each family negotiates a new equilibrium or wallows in frequent conflicts. All this takes place in the context of adjustment to a new society, alongside the challenges and pressures of social and economic survival. The narratives demonstrate that disputes and clashes between family members can exist alongside cooperation and caring, but also that this applies more where the intermediate, 1.5 generation are involved as go-betweens. Tensions between the first generation and the second tend to be more acute, interwoven into the very fabric of their childhood. In adjusting to the new society strategies of action through neccesity often change faster than core values, sometimes leading to fierce parental disputes on how to raise the children (and other matters). The narratives suggest that children of the second generation find it easier to communicate with their mothers, while at best the fathers are characterized by a range of behaviours from absenteeism and apparent indifference to active involvement and a facade of traditional status. In some families creative innovative ways are found to maintain cohesion, for example by evasive behaviour (fathers who pretend not to see their children taking unconventional pathways) or by initiatives encouraging the grandparents to make things with their grandchildren (usually initiated by the intermediate, 1.5 generation).

The axes of contention between two cultural systems are thus expressed through collisions within the family, voiced as personal struggles between liberalism and conservatism, between concern for the self-image of a child and the demand for reverence, between protection and restriction, between obedience and consultation, between faithfulness to tradition or personal ambitions. Even the very basis for making the perilous journey to Israel, the Jewish faith, frequently becomes a source of dispute, as different versions of Judaism enter the family home, challenging traditional doctrines and practices, pitting the generations against one another in adherence to Ethiopian Jewish heritage or local versions of Jewish practice.

Social definitions stressing ethnicity and colour, slotted into the common existing stratification of Israeli society, are challenged by segmented assimilation and self-perceptions stubbornly defying categorization. Perhaps the greatest challenge for all immigrants from Ethiopia and their Israeli born offspring is dealing with discrimination, prejudice, and the expectation to represent their ethnic group. And yet there were participants in my study who attested never to have felt discrimination, who refused to play the game in which identity and identification are one, who insist on being seen for who they are and not judged by the colour of their skin.

We have seen that resilience is born out of a combination involving both connection and context, challenged by the many changes that accompany immigration. In many ways the resilience of this immigrant community was demonstrated by overcoming the challenges of the journey, often their strengths and abilities were underestimated after their arrival. Listening to their narratives enables an in-depth understanding of their experiences and concerns from their own perspective. Since resilience is contextually and culturally dependent, transition heightens the necessity for resourceful negotiation, theoretically providing many opportunities to assist immigrants, if culturally meaningful pathways to do so can be found. This book has demonstrated the importance of understanding the full complexity of diverse immigrant experiences, the intricacies of family dynamics as they change after immigration, and the value of appreciation for inherent strengths and capabilities prevalent in immigrant communities.

The research presented in this book, based on the narratives of Jewish Ethiopian Israelis, attempted to provide a unique perspective on immigration and the meeting of cultures within families. Any attempt to summarize or categorize immigrant experiences is likely to create an oversimplistic representation of these, while the reality is both complex and dynamic. As other researchers have explained (for example, Lam, 2005; Perreira et al., 2006) qualitative analysis using interviews provides invaluable insights into peoples' perceptions of reality. The narratives of the participants in my studies, belonging to G1, G1.5, and G2 generations, reflect multiple factors affecting families in transition, their varied coping mechanisms, and significant aspects and circumstances influencing children's wellbeing.

The differences between the families represent a range of experiences; from families who manage to support each other through the process of change, incorporating into their repertoire local customs, language, and behaviour, to families in which the disintegration of traditional structures and support networks create a crisis preventing mutual support, hindering effective communication, and blocking avenues for cultural transferal between generations. This latter scenario may be temporary, applying just after arrival or to families undergoing particularly stressful events, or may be a long-term situation.

The friction between the subtle, often invisible, forces of change and conservation provides the backdrop for daily living, infiltrating every area of life and shaping family relationships. Focusing alternately on the individual, the family, and the community enables observation of the effects of the meeting of cultures and how these are negotiated. In transition the interplay between personal choice and social expectations and limitations is clarified, as the balance between cultures is constantly challenged and redefined. If the receiving society is open to diversity, the resultant mix may be both personally and communally enriching, if not it may be both challenging and stressful.

The journey made by Ethiopian Jews to Israel has been fraught with difficulties, initiated and implemented by heroic members of this community, aided by brave Israelis. My personal experience with the community as well as this study and others (for example Engdau-Vanda, 2019; Shatu, 2011) attests to the great personal and collective resilience of the Ethiopian Jews, an enduring faith, personal and collective resourcefulness, and mutual responsibility. The immigrants who came to Israel brought with them a rich cultural heritage based on community cohesiveness and philanthropic attitudes. Other researchers such as Landau (2007) have stressed the importance of perceiving immigrant families and communities in their inherent strength, recognizing resilience and intrinsic capabilities as the basis for their adjustment to the new society. Similarly, it is important to understand the cultural and contextual nature of resilience fostered in family and community, as formed and maintained through consistent supportive connection and enhanced by a clear sense of identity (Ungar, 2008). These factors are essential in fostering the confidence of new immigrants to engage and cope through personal and collective endeavours, rather than promoting dependency, apathy and increasing marginality as a minority group.

Maholmes (2014) has stressed the importance of hope as a cognitive process fostered by supportive, encouraging relationships with family and friends. Hope enables an optimistic perspective, which together with resilience—the capacity to adapt in face of adversity—provide the way to move forward, create motivation and agency to set personal goals and work to achieve them. Meaningful connections empower self-esteem, self-awareness, and self-confidence, whereas conflict, criticism, and disconnection are discouraging and hindering. When comparing the experiences of the Ethiopian Jews in Israel with other immigrant communities throughout the globe, another important factor is the recognition of diversity *within* immigrant communities (including diverse coping mechanisms). Many researchers before me have emphasized the heterogeneity of the Ethiopian Jewish community in Israel (for example: Ben-Ezer, 2011; Berhanu, 2005; Bodovski, 1989; Kaplan & Salamon, 1998; Rosen, 1985; Salamon, 1999; Weil, 2012), warning of the dangers of generalizations. This point is also reflected in my study, where there was no *typical* Ethiopian immigrant family, but many different families each negotiating their own way through the changes which come with immigration. Moreover, this research also emphasizes the necessity for caution when using common terms such as family, community, childhood, responsibility, authority, etc. We are all subjects of the cultures we grew up in and make automatic assumptions about the meaning and significance of such terms, which need re-examining in the context of inter-cultural qualitative research. In fact, my own perspective and understanding has been deeply influenced by other scholars whose research reflects the diversity of the human experience, enabling stepping out of the narrow confines of a Western perspective (such as Lancy et al., 2012; Hrdy, 2011; Meehan & Hawks, 2014; Otto & Keller, 2014; Weisner, 2014; Weisner & Gallimore, 2008).

The voices from my study are not representative, they provide a momentary glimpse into the lives of immigrant families at a specific time and place. Coping strategies are varied, as demonstrated by their narratives, which present a range of examples; adults living as Ethiopians in Israel or incorporating elements of Israeli culture into their repertoire, young people marginalized by exclusion or alternately determined to forge a place for themselves via army service, academic studies, or affiliation to religious communities. Individual choices create new social alliances within the family or alternatively new rifts to be negotiated or lead to disconnection. As evidenced in other studies (see Chap. 4) immigrants and their children are active agents in the process of adjustment. Parents are sometimes able to integrate new practices into their parenting toolbox, showing understanding towards the challenges facing children in the new environment and demonstrating a degree of cultural flexibility (for example Gorman, 1998). This study and others (for example Perreira et al., 2006; Newman, 2007; Usita & Blieszner, 2002) show the creative means used by families to preserve and enhance inter-generational connection despite problems of language.

The experiences and wellbeing of the children of the new generation to immigrant families are affected by many factors, perhaps foremost the delicate fragile balance between the various cultures as expressed in their daily lives and family relationships. Their experiences are shaped by the multiple contexts of their lives:

- The specifics of their family history and life experiences, including the nature of the journey and the availability of responsive, capable caring adults.
- The presence or absence of the family story in their childhood, including their immigration story, as giving meaning and context to their life experiences.
- Knowledge of language (verbal and non-verbal) as opening or blocking inter-generational communication.
- The absorption policy of the receiving country as it influences family management, language use, and child education (including the policy of sending teenagers to boarding schools).
- The changing balance of power in the family after immigration—especially in relation to gender and age—and how the adults in the family negotiate this.
- The cultural flexibility of family members, and their willingness or ability to relate to the child and the moment as opposed to adhering to cultural models of normative expected behaviour.
- Experiences in the public and educational spheres which effect the self-image of children and their parents, especially overt and covert discrimination.

Every family contains an invisible axis of cultural transferal linking the generations to their cultural heritage and ancestral past. Often immigration results in changing communication patterns as well as changing or adding new languages, all of which may sabotage this natural cultural transferal and create a new complexity in communication between the generations. As has been presented through these narratives, some families manage to overcome this, creating a new viable equilibrium between the generations which enables the simultaneous coexistence of continuity and change. In other families (or during difficult times), a rigid inflexible adherence to tradition or a sense of losing control further impairs family communication and may lead to withdrawal and disconnection. In such cases immigration itself is one context of many jeopardizing children's wellbeing.

The case of the Ethiopian Jews in Israel may be unique in many respects, but there are also many similarities with the cultural transition of other communities around the globe, most specifically families from collectivistic societies from African or Asian countries transferring to Western, educated, industrialized, rich, and democratic countries (WEIRD—an acronym coined by Weisner, 2020). As detailed throughout this book and in various examples in Chap. 4 (such as Gorman, 1998; Lam, 2005; Vu et al., 2019; Usita & Blieszner, 2002) many families find creative ways to maintain the connection between the generations. This is not to negate the many difficulties and challenges families face after immigration, but to stress that their experiences and coping mechanisms are varied. When cultural flexibility is evident, families manage to contain and negotiate the subtle and long-term cultural changes in the fabric of their daily lives while minimizing conflict, paving the way to hybridity for the younger generation.

On a personal note, it has taken me almost a lifetime to come to terms with my own hybrid identity and see this as a positive thing. I often thought that my life would have been easier if I had grown up in once place, that my experiences of transition added a complexity to my sense of identity and belonging at times painful and difficult to negotiate. Today I am more aware of the advantages, this study and others reflect the benefits of hybridity on both a personal and a family level. Unrestricted by rigid cultural dictates, accepting oneself as containing varied and constantly changing identities provides a certain sense of freedom—an internal uninhibited legitimacy to be ourselves.

Embracing hybridity invites the natural dissolution of all assumptions, a readiness to watch and listen before responding, as cultural knowledge is triggered by context. This breeds in hybrid parents the unique ability to accept the slow discovery of each child, rather than the rigid determination to mould children in a certain way. Children who grow up steeped in more than one culture often develop an inbuilt acceptance of complexity and the legitimacy of being more than one thing. Where diversity—between and within people—is acceptable and valued—children can develop multiple identities and yet feel whole. They may gain not only a better relationship with their parents but also learn to be more accepting of the diversity within themselves and others.

The pathway to hybridity may be fraught with difficulties, dependent on context and an inherent openness to the new and unexplored in ourselves and others. The receiving context, in which immigrants make their first steps in the new society, is full of overt and covert messages on the value and legitimacy of their culture of origin. Discrimination and xenophobia are powerful hurdles to overcome, even simple narrow mindedness and stereotyping can have very devastating effects. Positive attitudes to pluralism and diversity, especially in educational frameworks, ease the way for children (G1.5 or G2) towards an acceptance and appreciation of their evolving culturally mixed identities. In my opinion schools should be encouraging hybridity and appreciation of diversity as national policies backed by the appropriate training of educational staff. Especially here in Israel, much needs to be done to move away from the common assumption that children's problems at school are intrinsic to their origins or home cultures, towards a perspective which sees immigrants and their offspring simply as people in transition (Shmuel, 2015). Both home and school can provide viable pathways to hybridity, devout of judgement or comparison of cultures, familial and social acceptance enabling self-acceptance as a key to wellbeing.

I am completing this book in troubled times; the worst political and social crisis Israel has ever known. And yet this crisis also proves how deeply the people of Israel feel about our country, as tens of thousands take to the streets to safeguard our democracy. They come from all the various sub-cultures, have different identities and political affiliations. It is a grass-roots protest of ordinary people who want to live in a sane, equitable, just society. To live and let live. One can but hope the future will enable this simple vision to be our reality.

References

Ben-Ezer, G. (2011). Cross cultural misunderstandings: The case of Ethiopian immigrants in Israeli society. *International Journal of Adolescent Medicine and Health, 11*(1–2), 21–38.

Berhanu, G. (2005). Normality, deviance, identity, cultural tracking and school achievement: The case of Ethiopian Jews in Israel. *Scandinavian Journal of Educational Research, 49*(1), 51–82.

Gorman, J. (1998). Parenting attitudes and practices of immigrant Chinese mothers of adolescents. *Family Relations, 47*(1), 73–80.

Hrdy, S. B. (2011). *Mothers and others* (pp. 77–85). Harvard University Press.

Kaplan, S., & Salamon, H. (1998). *Ethiopian immigrants in Israel: Experience and prospects* (Vol. 10). Institute for Jewish Policy Research.

Lam, C. (2005). Chinese construction of adolescent development outcome: Themes discerned in a qualitative study. *Child and Adolescent Social Work Journal, 22*(2), 111–131.

Lancy, D., Bock, J., & Gaskins, S. (Eds.). (2012). *The anthropology of learning in childhood* (pp. 146–162). Alta Mira Press.

Landau, J. (2007). Enhancing resilience: Families and communities as agents for change. *Family Process, 46*(3), 351–365.

Maholmes, V. (2014). *Fostering resilience and wellbeing in children and families in poverty: Why hope still matters*. Oxford University Press.

Meehan, C., & Hawks, S. (2014). Maternal and Allo-maternal responsiveness: The significance of cooperative caregiving in attachment theory. In H. Otto & H. Keller (Eds.), *Different faces of attachment: Cultural variations on a universal human need* (pp. 113–141). Cambridge University Press.

Newman, R. (2007). Ethiopian Israeli grandmothers' stories. *Journal of Aging, Humanities and the Arts, 1*(3–4), 211–219.

Otto, H., & Keller, H. (2014). *Different faces of attachment: Cultural variations on a universal human need*. Cambridge University Press.

Perreira, K. M., Chapman, M. V., & Stein, G. L. (2006). Becoming an American parent: Overcoming challenges and finding strength in a new immigrant Latino community. *Journal of Family Issues, 27*(10), 1383–1414.

Rosen, C. (1985). Core symbols of Ethiopian identity and their role in understanding the beta Israel today. *Israel Social Science Research, 3*(12), 55–62.

Salamon, H. (1999). *The hyena people: Ethiopian Jews in Christian Ethiopia* (pp. 66–74). University of California Press.

Ungar, M. (2008). Resilience across cultures. *The British Journal of Social Work, 38*(2), 218–235.

Usita, P., & Blieszner, R. (2002). Immigrant family strengths: Meeting communication challenges. *Journal of Family Issues, 23*, 266–286.

Weisner, T. (2014). The socialization of trust: Plural caregiving and diverse pathways in human development across cultures. In H. Otto & H. Keller (Eds.), *Different faces of attachment: Cultural variation on a universal human need* (pp. 263–277). Cambridge University Press.

Weisner, T. S. (2020). Still the most important influence on human development: Culture, context, and methods pluralism. *Human Development, 64*(4–6), 238–244.

Weisner, T., & Gallimore, R. (2008). Child and sibling caregiving. In R. LeVine & R. New (Eds.), *Anthropology and child development: A cross-cultural reader* (pp. 264–269). Blackwell Publishing.

Hebrew References

Bodovski, D. (1989). *Customs and culture: Consequences for professional connection.* Asi Community Resources.

Engdau-Vanda, S. (2019). *Resilience in immigration. The story of Ethiopian jews in Israel from a perspective of 30 years*. Tel Aviv. Resling.

Shatu, S. (2011). *The different narratives of the journey made by Ethiopian Jews.* Master's dissertation, Hebrew University of Jerusalem.

Shmuel, N. (2015). Transitions and not gaps: Integrating Ethiopian immigrant children in the education system. *Gilui Daat*, 137–146. Seminar Hakibbutzim.

Vu, K., Castro, K., Cheah, C., & Yu, J. (2019). Mediating and moderating processes in the associations between Chinese immigrant mothers' acculturation and parenting styles in the United States. *Asian American Journal of Psychology, 10*(4), 307.

Weil, S. (2012). Ethiopian Jews: A heterogeneous community. In E. Witztum & N. Grisaru (Eds.), *Social and clinical aspects of Ethiopian immigrants in Israel* (pp. 17–36). The Jewish Agency and Ben Gurion University of the Negev.

Appendix: Family Genograms Table of Participants

People interviewed in the second study (Shmuel, 2018)							
Family name	First name	Age	Gender	Time in Israel in years	Generation	Education	Relationship to first person interviewed
Demse	Dana (H)	28	F	Born	G2	Undergraduate student (teacher)	
	Yael (H)	52	F	29	G1	None	Mother
	Dany (H)	56	M	30	G1	Partial high school	Uncle (mother's brother)
Abebe	Ester (H)	26	F	Born	G2	Undergraduate student (teacher)	
	Modesh (E)	51	F	30	G1	None	Mother
	Leah (H)	22	F	Born	G2	High school completion	Sister

© The Author(s), under exclusive license to Springer Nature Switzerland AG 2023

N. A. Shmuel, *Children's Wellbeing in Immigrant Families*, Children's Well-Being: Indicators and Research 26,
https://doi.org/10.1007/978-3-031-31917-4

People interviewed in the second study (Shmuel, 2018)

Family name	First name	Age	Gender	Time in Israel in years	Generation	Education	Relationship to first person interviewed
Desta	Genet (E)	35	F	23	G1.5	Undergraduate degree (social worker)	
	Almaz (E)	64	F	23	G1	None	Mother
	Berihun (E)	90	M	23	G1	None	Grandfather
	Mamu (E)	87	M	23	G1	None	Uncle (grandfather's brother)
	Avi (H)	23	M	Born	G2	High school completion. Recently discharged soldier	Sister's son
	Addis (E)	21	M	16	G2	High school completion. Soldier	Cousin
Fekre	Naama (H)	35	F	30	G2	Graduate degree	
	Yafit (H)	52	F	31	G1	Courses (child minder)	Mother
	Mahari (E)	58	M	14	G1	None	Father
	Yisrael (H)	20	M	Born	G2	High school completion. Soldier	Brother
	Shani (H)	37	F	29	G2	Undergraduate degree	Cousin
	Teruneh (E)	38	M	25	G1.5	Undergraduate degree	Cousin's husband
	Abraham (H)	56	M	31	G1.5	Partial high school	Uncle
	Gebre (E)	90	M	30	G1	None	Grandfather
	Fasika (E)	80	F	30	G1	None	Grandmother
Shmuel	Shy (H)	53	M	30	G1	One year of university	
	Liora (H)	47	F	30	G1.5	Course in community work	Wife
	Tareke (E)	85	M	30	G1	Partial high school	Father-in-law
	Emebet (E)	75	F	30	G1	None	Mother-in-law
	Shira (H)	13	F	Born	G2	High school student	Daughter

People interviewed in the second study (Shmuel, 2018)

Family name	First name	Age	Gender	Time in Israel in years	Generation	Education	Relationship to first person interviewed
Gebray	Noa (H)	39	F	30	G1.5	One year of university	
	Worknesh (E)	76	F	30	G1	None	Mother
	Lee (H)	45	F	31	G1.5	One year of college	Sister
	Matan (H)	43	M	30	G1.5	High school completion	Brother
	Miki (H)	39	M	34	G2	Undergraduate degree	Husband
Solomon	Lemlem (E)	38	F	23	G1.5	Graduate degree	
Aharon	Mulu (E)	42	F	30	G1.5	Undergraduate degree (social worker)	
	Noam (H)	32	M	31	G2	Partial high school	Brother
	Yaniv (H)	24	M	Born	G2	High school completion	Brother
Metiku	Aberash (E)	33	F	23	G1.5	Courses (professional)	
	Rachel (H)	39	F	31	G1.5	Courses (professional)	Sister
	Tsehai (E)	35	F	23	G1.5	Academic courses	Sister
Sahalu	Habtam (E)	32	F	30	G2	Graduate degree	
	Eneye (E)	60	F	30	G1	None	Mother
	Fentahun (E)	67	M	30	G1	None	Father
	Orna (H)	40	F	30	G1.5	Undergraduate degree	Sister
	Maayan (H)	31	F	28.10	G2	One year of university	Sister
	Sarah (H)	29	F	Born	G2	Undergraduate student	Sister
	Shimon (H)	19	M	Born	G2	Awaiting national service	Brother
Anbesa	Dov (H)	30	M	22	G1.5	Undergraduate degree (teacher)	
	Abigail (H)	61	F	28	G1	Courses (professional)	Mother
Matan	Edna (H)	35	F	23	G1.5	Undergraduate degree (teacher)	

People interviewed in the second study (Shmuel, 2018)

Family name	First name	Age	Gender	Time in Israel in years	Generation	Education	Relationship to first person interviewed
Tafere	Tigist (E)	32	F	24	G1.5	Undergraduate degree (nurse)	
	Abynesh (E)	55	F	24	G1.5	None	Mother

Abbreviations: *G1* The first generation refers to people who emigrated as adults over the age of 21, *G2* The second generation refers to participants who were either born in Israel or Sudan (emigrating as babies) or emigrated up until the age of seven, *G1.5* The one and a half generation are people who emigrated between the ages of eight and 20 and were thus educated both in Ethiopia and in Israel, *H* Hebrew, *A* Amharic, *F* Female, *M* Male

People interviewed in the first study (Shmuel, 2010)

Musherit (H)	55	F	27	G1	None	Mother to Ziv
Ziv (H)	40	M	25	G1.5	Police academy & practical engineering	Husband to Bossana
Bossana (E)	36	F	23	G1.5	Undergraduate degree	Wife of Ziv
Takele (E)	42	M	25	G1.5	Undergraduate degree	Husband of Nava
Nava (H)	34	F	23	G1.5	Undergraduate degree	Wife of Takele
Rinat (H)	45	F	25	G1	None	
Neta (H)	38	F	25	G1.5	Undergraduate student	

Glossary

Amharic words	
antu	Plural of 'you' to a man as a sign of respect
balebet	The woman of the house
berekete	Special bread made for the Sabbath
Beta Yisrael	Ethiopian jews
beta-saab	People who live under the same roof, which can also mean people who are not blood relations.
bedilu yadigal	Fate dictates how a child will grow (proverb)
ballena-mist	A married couple
be-ikul gabbicha	Of equal status in marriage
buna	Coffee
dabbo	Traditional bread used for the blessing to receive the Sabbath
engera	Traditional Ethiopian flatbread with a spongy texture, generally made from Teff
Ferunge	Non-Ethiopian, white people
gebeta	A traditional game, mancala
irswo	Plural 'you' to a woman as a sign of respect

Amharic words	
Kes	Rabbi and spiritual leader
Kessouch	Rabbi and spiritual leader—plural
kita	Unleavened bread ate at Passover
lidge	Child
maret	Soil
mergem godjo	Menstruation/impurity hut
natele	Scarf
quontats	Pinches
sam enna warq	Wax and gold
seyt	Woman
setaset	A boy who behaves like a girl—girlish
shmagele	Adult intermediary concerned with keeping the peace
teff	A fine-grained cereal which grows in Ethiopia
tele	Homemade beer from cereal, water, and yeast
terut terut	Stories
unjera-lidge	Adopted child
unkulba	Baby-carrier
unkoklish	Riddles
wond	Man
wondawend	A girl who behaves like a boy—boyish
zamad	Relatives in a wider sense

Hebrew words	
dugri	Direct speech
Haggadah	Jewish text that tells the story of Passover
Halle	Traditional bread used for the Kiddush
ish	Man
isha	Woman
Kiddush	Traditional Jewish blessing preceding the Friday evening meal to receive the Sabbath
cushi	Negro, black person, although *kcush* is a term used in the bible, the word today is commonly regarded as derogatory, the equivalent of Nigger, and not to be used
kiddush	Ceremonial reception of the Sabbath
lo ba li	I don't want to
Matzah	Unleavened bread ate at Passover
mohel	The person who performs the Jewish custom of circumcision for boys (traditionally eight days after the birth)
Pesach	Passover
shivah	Seven days of mourning
ulpan	Hebrew classes

DEMSE FAMILY

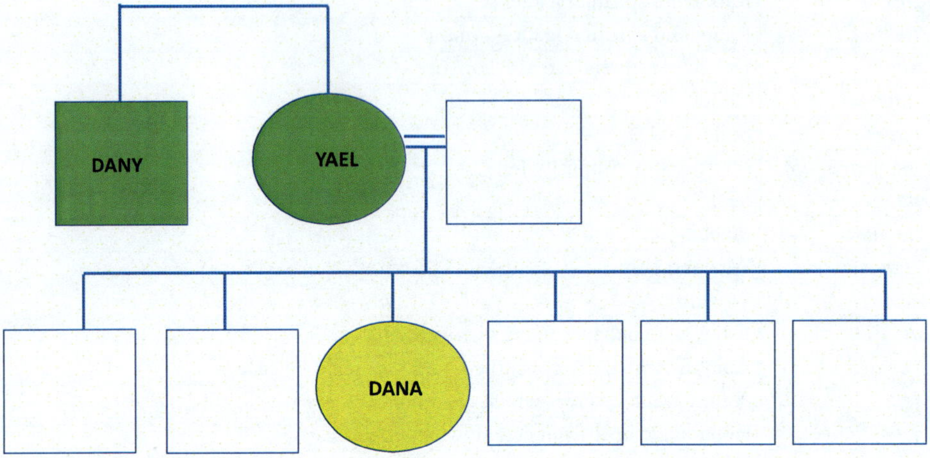

ABEBE FAMILY

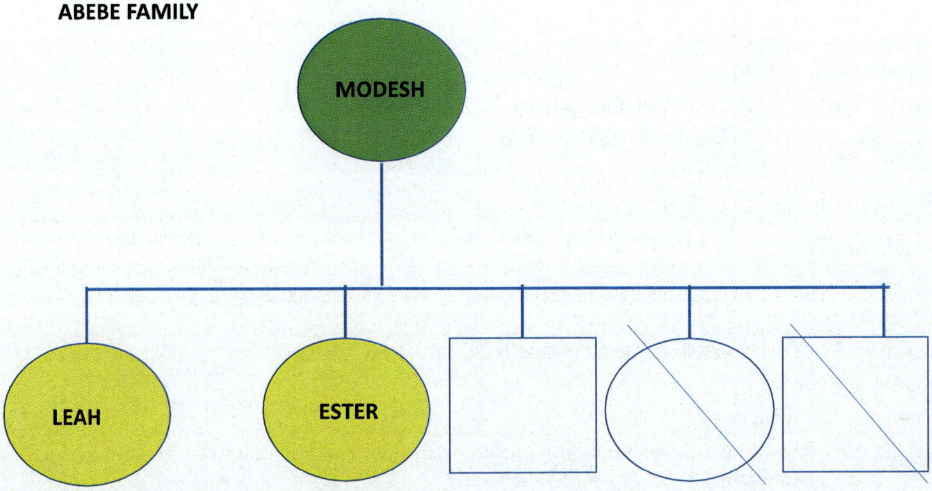

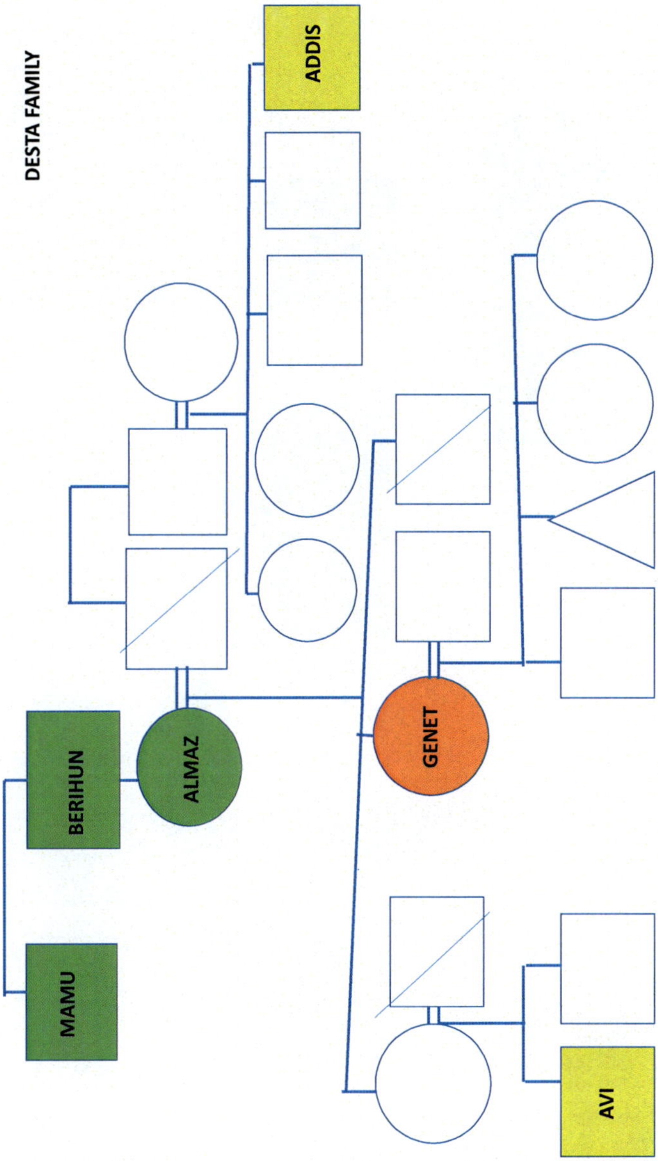
DESTA FAMILY
ADDIS
BERIHUN
ALMAZ
GENET
MAMU
AVI

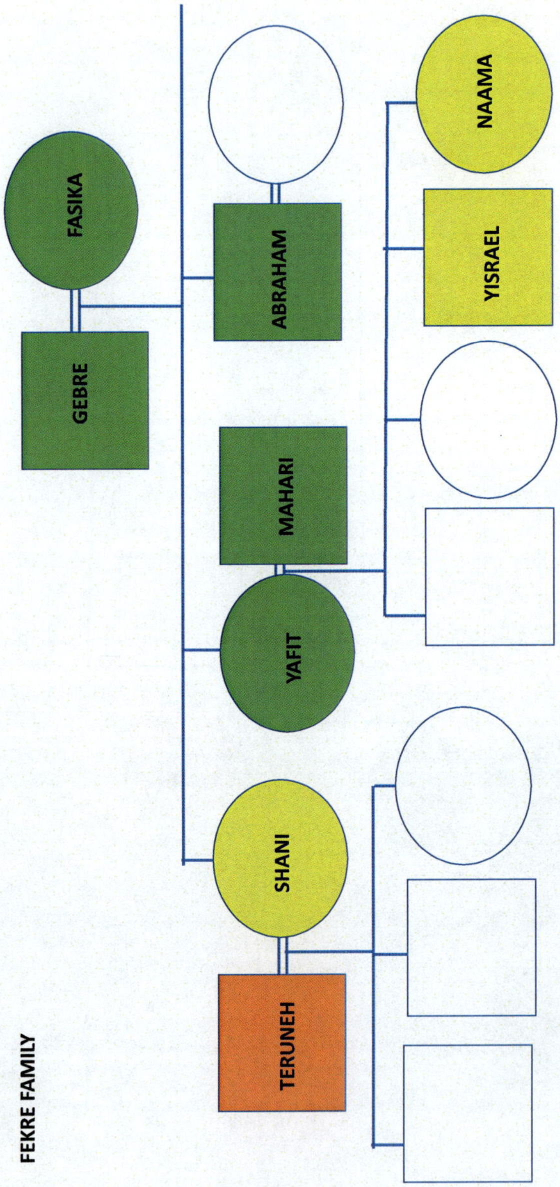
FEKRE FAMILY
GEBRE
FASIKA
ABRAHAM
MAHARI
YAFIT
SHANI
TERUNEH
NAAMA
YISRAEL

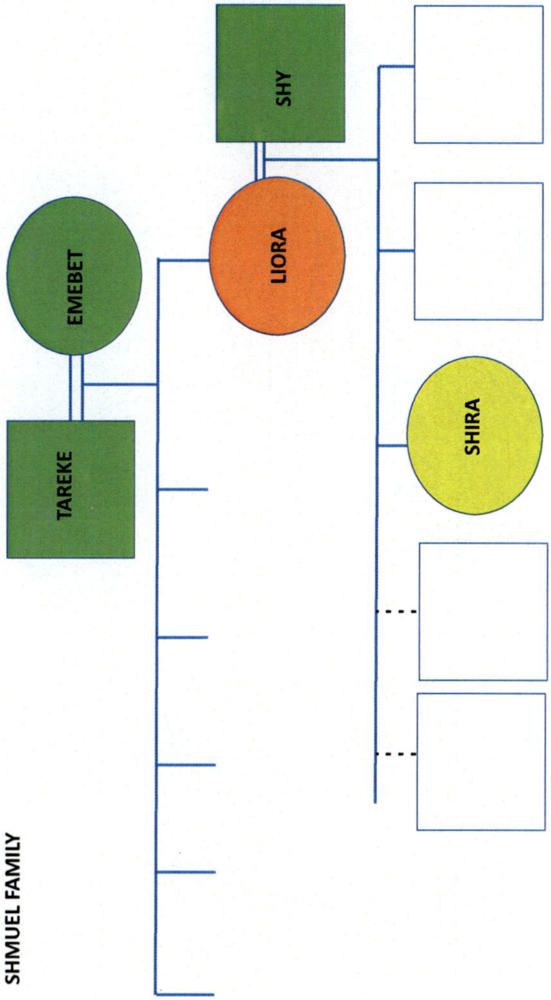
SHMUEL FAMILY
TAREKE
EMEBET
LIORA
SHY
SHIRA

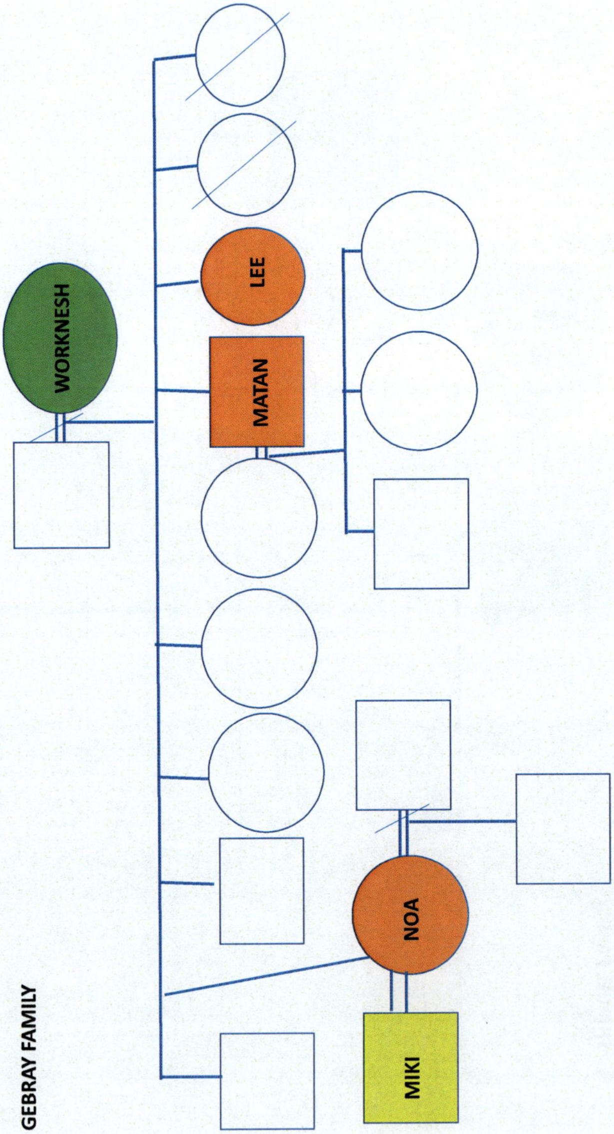
GEBRAY FAMILY
WORKNESH
LEE
MATAN
NOA
MIKI

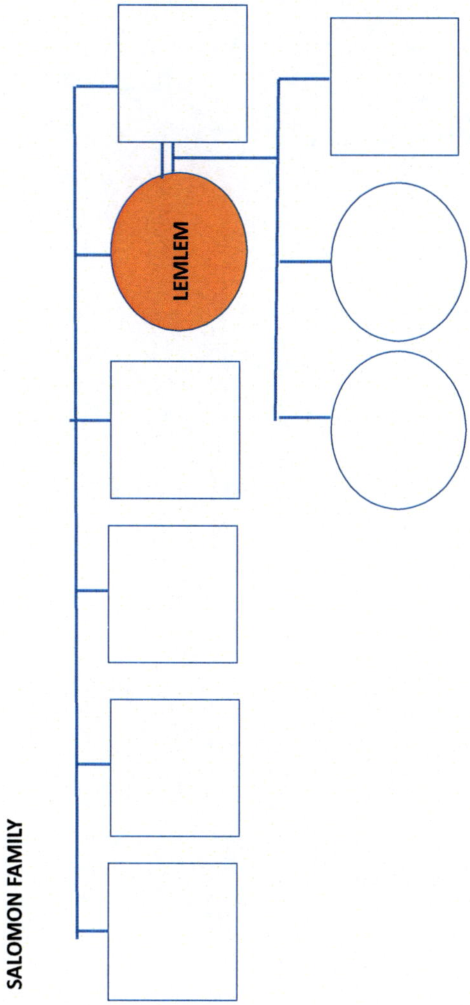
SALOMON FAMILY
LEMLEM

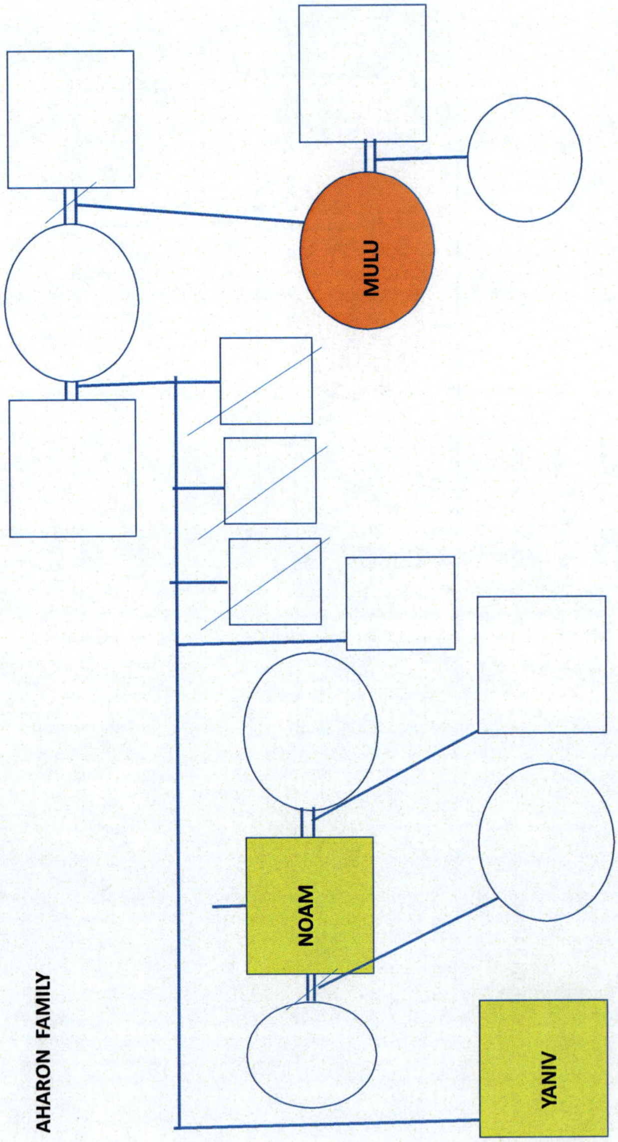
AHARON FAMILY
MULU
NOAM
YANIV

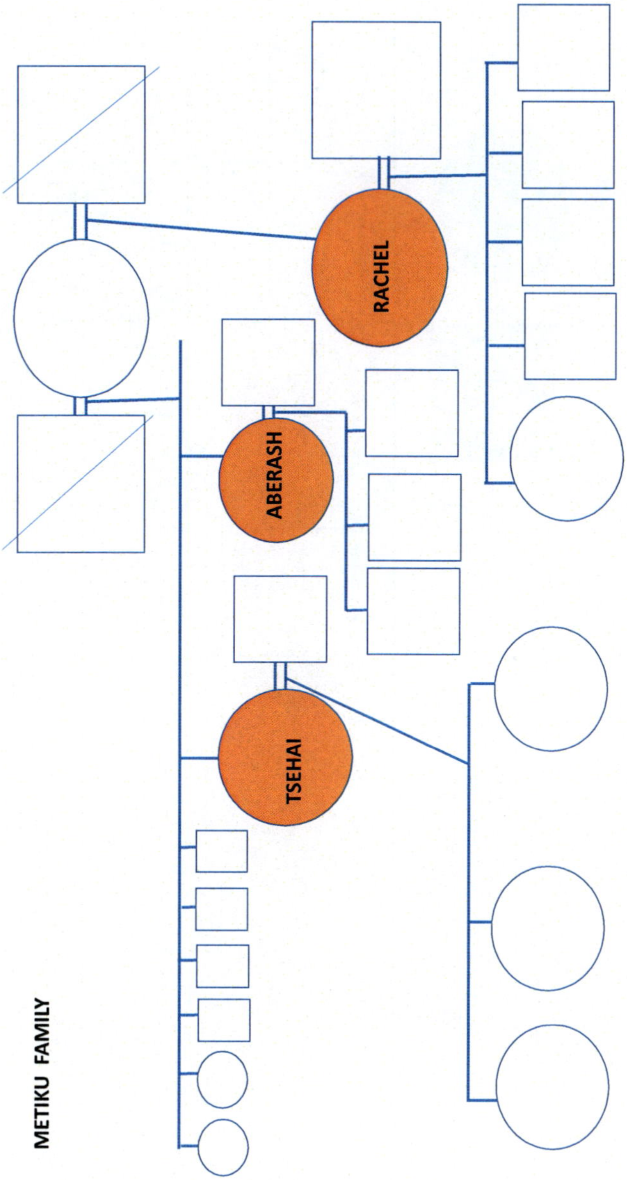
METIKU FAMILY
RACHEL
ABERASH
TSEHAI

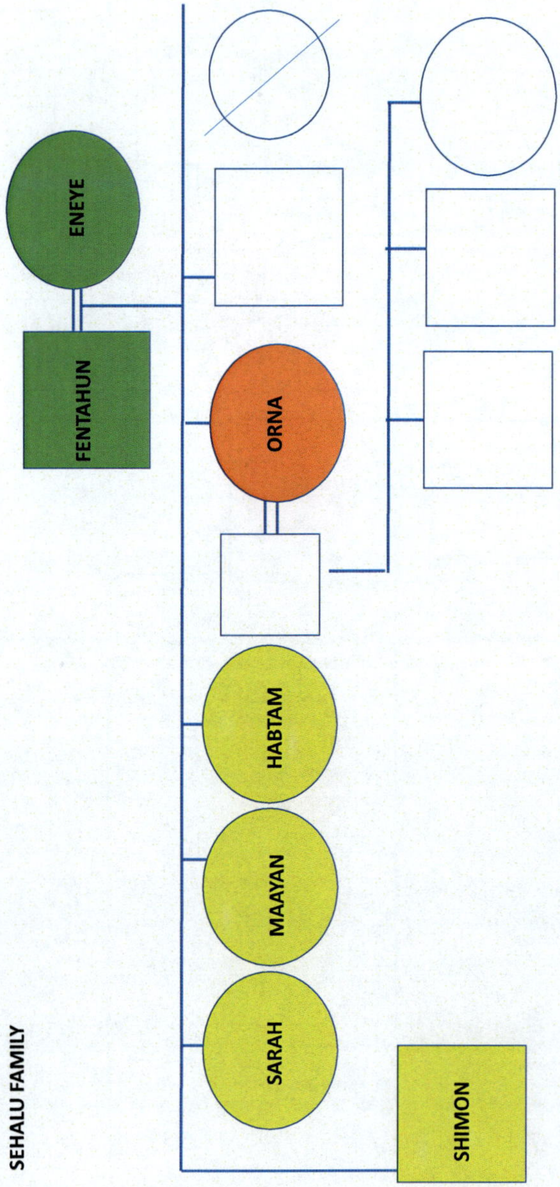
SEHALU FAMILY
ENEYE
FENTAHUN
ORNA
HABTAM
MAAYAN
SARAH
SHIMON

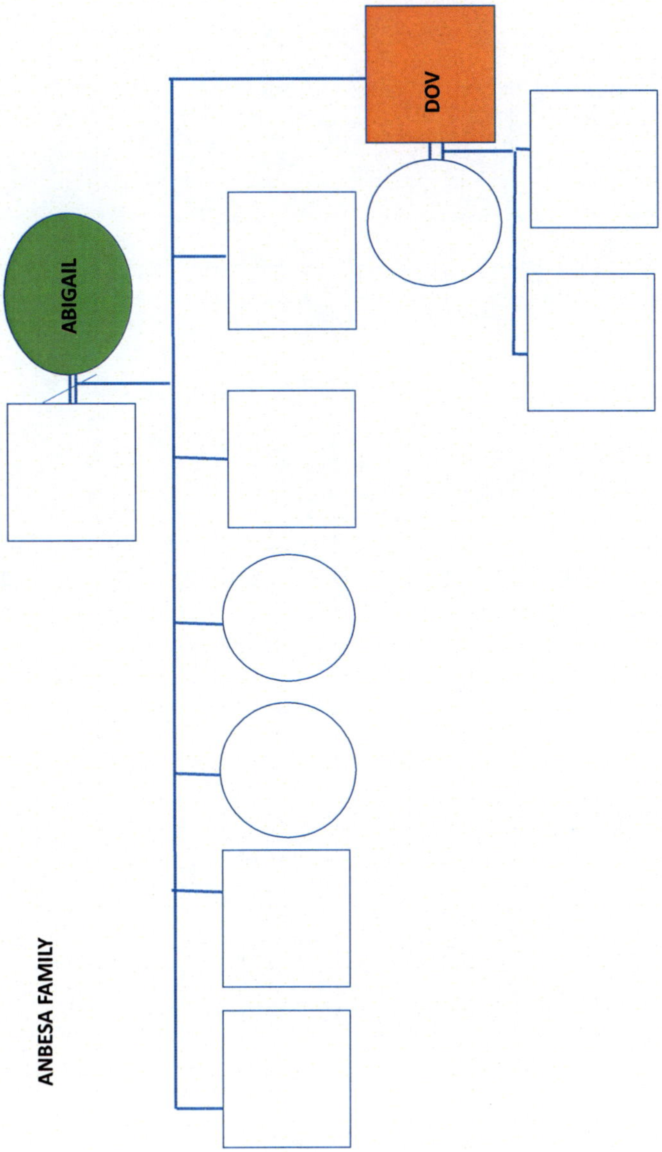
DOV
ABIGAIL
ANBESA FAMILY

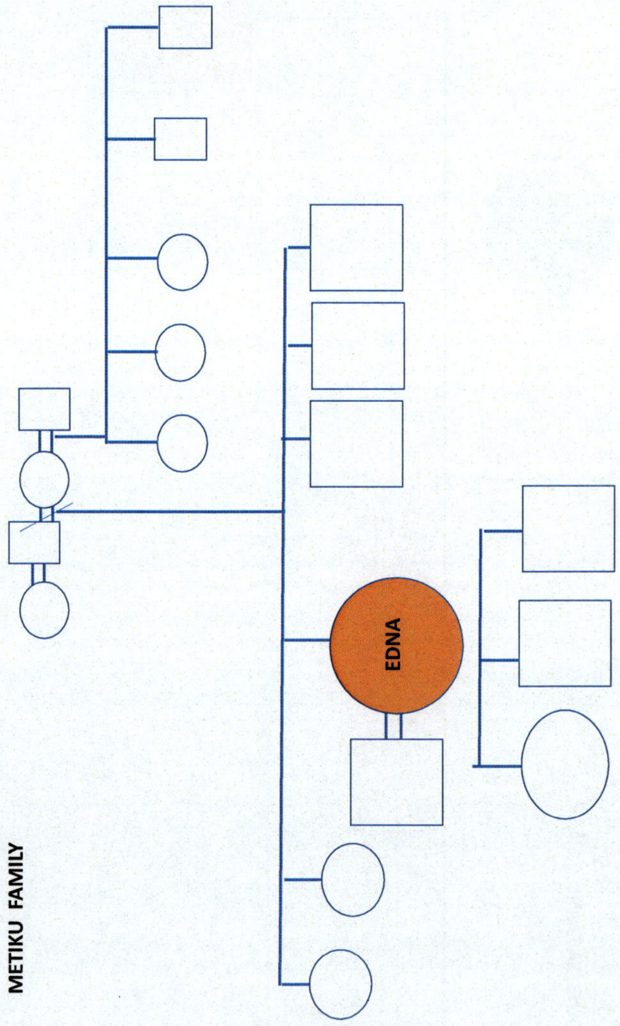
METIKU FAMILY
EDNA

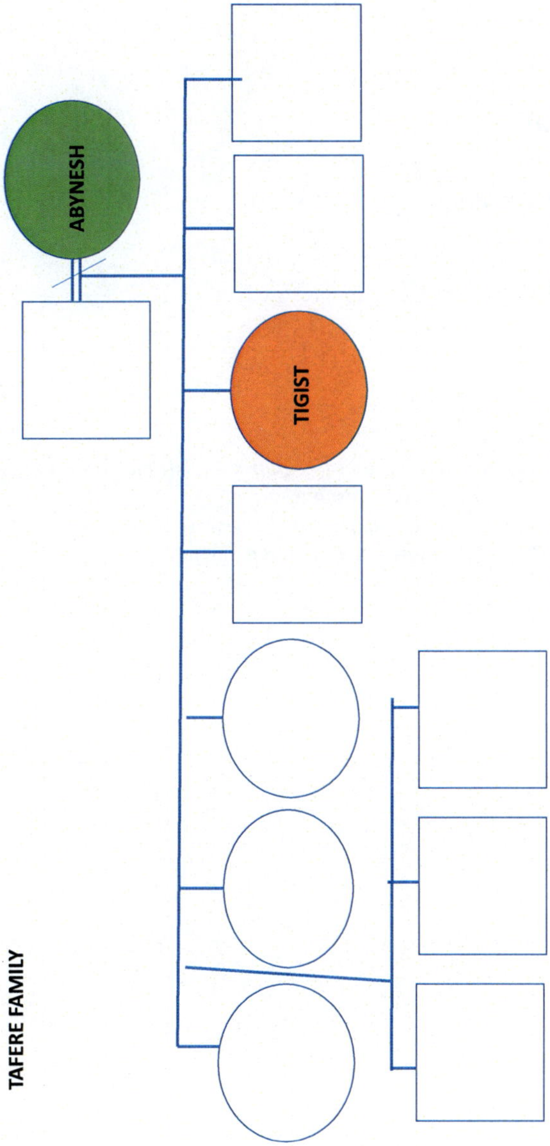
TAFERE FAMILY
ABYNESH
TIGIST

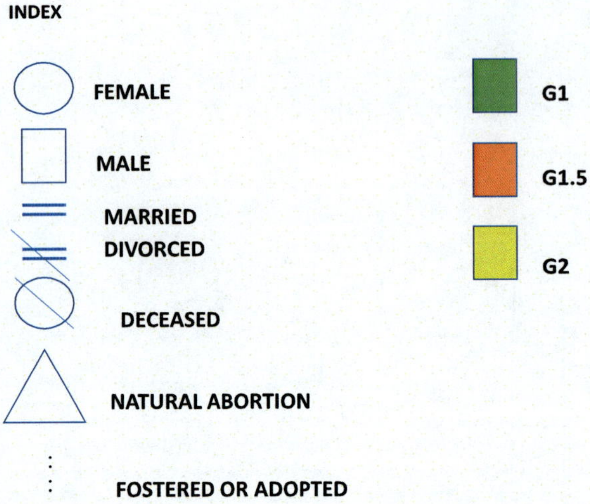

References

Shmuel, N. (2018). *Family and tradition in cultural transition: From Ethiopia to Israel*. Doctoral dissertation. Hebrew University Jerusalem.

Shmuel, N. (2010). *Educational traditions of Ethiopian Jewry: The dynamics of continuity and change*. Masters thesis. Hebrew University Jerusalem.